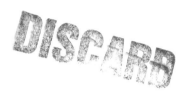

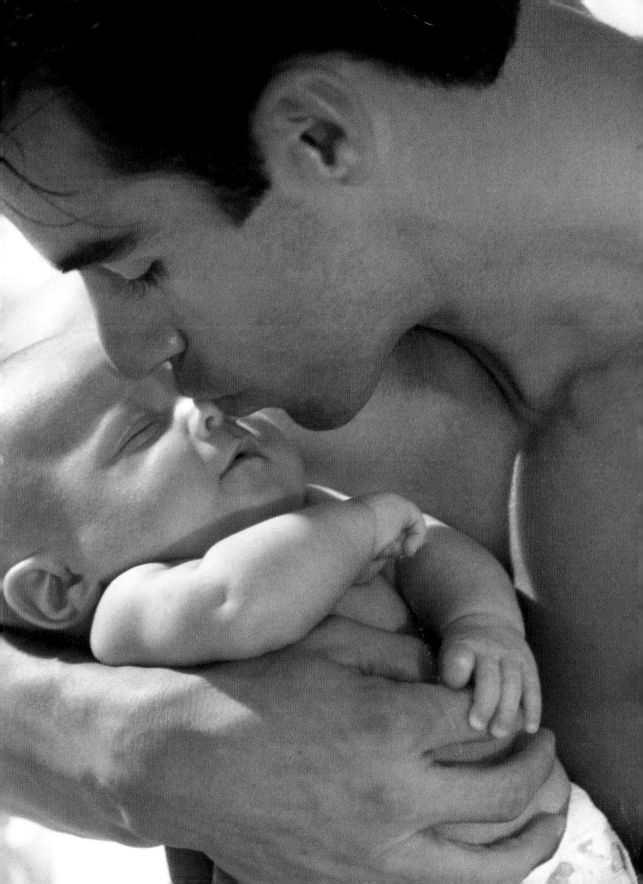

conception, pregnancy & birth

Dr. Miriam Stoppard

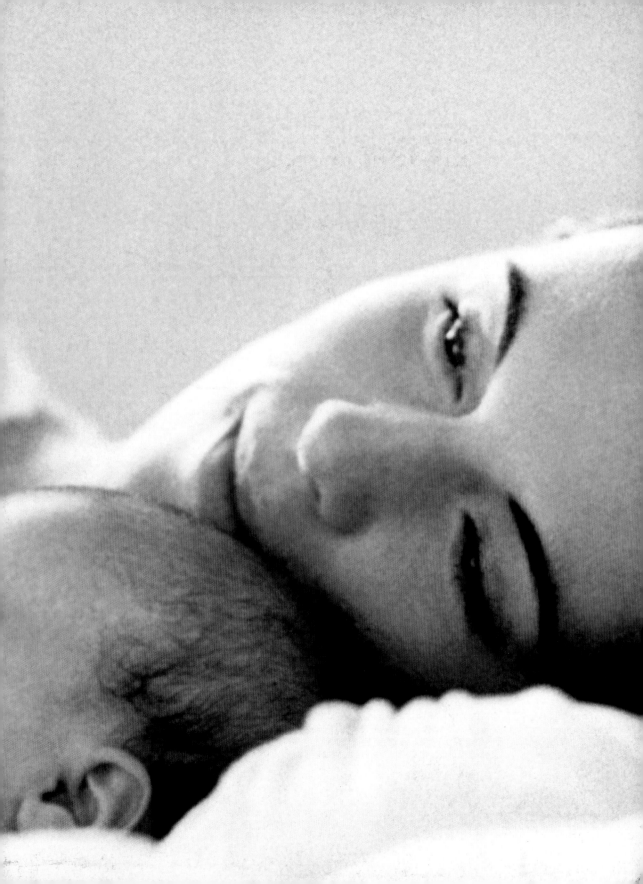

For Linzi & Will

London, New York, Munich Melbourne, Delhi

Revised edition

Brand Manager for Dr. Miriam Stoppard Lynne Brown
Publishing Director Corinne Roberts
Senior Managing Editor Jemima Dunne
Senior Art Editor Helen Spencer
Editor Jinny Johnson
US Editors Jennifer Williams, Christine Heilman
US Medical Consultant Dr. Courtney D. Stephenson
Designer Edward Kinsey
Picture Researcher Franziska Marking, Anna Bedewell
DTP Designer Traci Salter
Production Shwe Zin Win

First published by DK Publishing, Inc. in 1993

This revised edition published in 2005

Published in the United States by
DK Publishing, Inc., 375 Hudson Street,
New York, New York 10014

05 06 07 08 09   10 9 8 7 6 5 4 3 2 1

618.2

DK books are available at special discounts for bulk purchases for sales promotions,
premiums, fund-raising, or educational use. For details, contact: DK Publishing
Special Markets, 375 Hudson Street, New York, NY 10014 or SpecialSales@dk.com

Cataloging-in-Publication data is available from the Library of Congress.

ISBN 0-7566-0956-9

Reproduced by Colourscan, Singapore
Printed and bound in Singapore by Tien Wah Press

Discover more at

www.dk.com

Preface

Conception, pregnancy, and birth are the most amazing events in any couple's life. There's so much information to absorb, so many choices to make, and all the time your body's changing in a million marvelous ways. From your first positive pregnancy test to your very last push, I've written what I hope is a practical and accessible guide for you to dip into throughout your pregnancy, helping you and your partner to navigate your way smoothly into parenthood.

With this revised edition of *Conception, Pregnancy & Birth*, I've taken the opportunity to give the whole book a refreshingly lighter and more modern feel, with new full-color pictures wherever possible. Page by page, I've worked with top medical consultants to bring every word up to date, including all the latest medical research, hospital practices, and new treatments. I've also paid special attention to the real-life case studies, with brand-new material on induced births and on becoming a new dad—a little reassurance for all anxious fathers-to-be!

Although the majority of pregnancies are straightforward, it's true that some can be less so. This book contains lots of information, written with the aim of reassuring you, on fertility treatments, complications of pregnancy, special deliveries, and all the special medical interventions available in such cases. I always think that forewarned is forearmed—it's better to know about what might happen, and to plan accordingly, than to be taken by surprise.

Notwithstanding all the updating, my overall goal in this book remains the same: that you should have the birth you both want, in the circumstances you both want, helped by caregivers who put your needs and the needs of your new baby first.

With very best wishes for your pregnancy, and beyond!

Contents

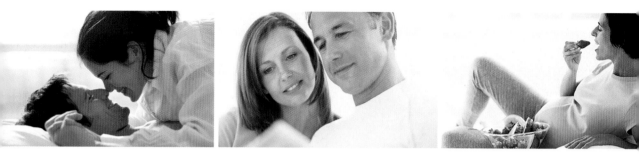

Introduction 8

CHAPTER 1
Preparing for pregnancy 14
· Fit for parenthood 16 · Case study: The importance of folic acid 20 · What is a gene? 22 · Genetic counseling 26 · Conceiving a baby 28 · The man's role 30 · Fertilization 32 · Problems in conceiving 34 · Seeking advice 36 · Male infertility 38 · Male tests 40 · Female infertility 42 · Female tests 44 · Treatments for female infertility 46 · ART (assisted reproduction technology) 48 · The typical pattern of an IVF treatment 50 · Advanced ART 52 · Using donors 54 · Case study: Infertility 56

CHAPTER 2
You and your developing baby 58
· Pregnant! 60 · Your rights 64 · First trimester 66 · Second trimester 68 · Third trimester 70 · First 6 weeks 72 · Up to 10 weeks 74 · Up to 14 weeks 76 · Up to 18 weeks 78 · Up to 22 weeks 80 · Up to 26 weeks 82 · Up to 30 weeks 84 · Up to 34 weeks 86 · Up to 40 weeks 88

CHAPTER 3
Preparing for fatherhood 90
· Becoming a dad 92 · The expectant father 94 · Fathers at the birth 96 · Learning about your new baby 100

CHAPTER 4
The birth of your choice 104
· The choices in childbirth 106 · Childbirth philosophers 112 · Birthing centers 114 · Hospital birth 116 · The care available 118 · Professional attendants 120 · Birth plan 122 · Childbirth classes 124

CHAPTER 5
Food and eating in pregnancy 126
· Food in pregnancy 128 · Essential nutrition 132 · Nutritional values 134 · Case study: The vegetarian mother 136 · Nutritional and food-related problems 138 · Case study: The diabetic mother 140

CHAPTER 6
A healthy pregnancy 142
· Exercise for a healthy pregnancy 144 · Stretching 146 · Body exercises 148 · Shaping up for labor 150 · Massage for relaxation 152 · Emotional changes 154 · Body care 158 · Avoiding problems 160 · What to wear 162 · A working pregnancy 164 · Case study: Choosing single parenthood 166 · Avoiding hazards 168

CHAPTER 7
Your prenatal care 172
· Prenatal care 174 · Routine checks 176 · Ultrasound scan 180 · Case study: Twins 182 · Special tests 184 · Case study: Testing for abnormalities 188

CHAPTER 8
Caring for your unborn baby 190
· In touch with your baby 192 · Your baby's movements 194 · Fetal problems 196 · Fetal surgery 200 · Case study: The Rh-negative mother 202

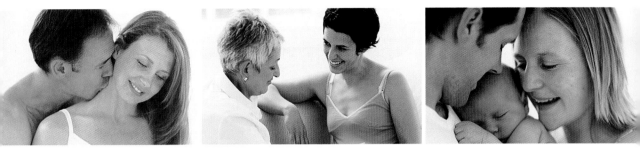

CHAPTER 9

Common complaints 204

· Common complaints 206 · Case study: The mother who has MS 214

CHAPTER 10

Medical emergencies 216

· Medical emergencies 218 · Case study: The mother who has miscarried 220 · Case study: The mother with preeclampsia 226

CHAPTER 11

A sensual pregnancy 228

· A sensual pregnancy 230 · Sensual massage 232 · Making love 234 · Sexual problems 236

CHAPTER 12

Getting ready for your baby 238

· Preparing for your baby 240 · Choosing equipment 242 · Baby clothes 244 · Breast or bottle? 246 · Choosing a name 248 · Preparing siblings for a new baby 252 · Arranging childcare 254 · Case study: The working mother 256 · The late stages of pregnancy 258 · Are you overdue? 260

CHAPTER 13

Managing your labor 262

· Getting ready for the birthing center 264
· Going to the hospital 266
· Comfort aids for labor 268 · Prelabor and labor 270
· The first stage 272 · Hospital procedures 274 · Partner's role in labor 276 · First stage positions 278 · Pain relief 280
· The second stage: delivery 284 · Giving birth 286
· Partner's role at birth 288 · The third stage 290
· Baby's first hours 292

CHAPTER 14

Special deliveries 294

· Special labors 296 · Induction of labor 300 · Case study: An induced birth 302 · Sudden birth 304
· Complications at delivery 306 · Cesarean section 308
· Case study: An emergency cesarean 310 · If a baby dies 312

CHAPTER 15

Getting to know your newborn baby 314

· Your new baby 316 · What your new baby can do 320
· Your stay in the hospital 322 · Holding and handling 324
· Beginning to breastfeed 326 · Breastfeeding your baby 328
· Bottlefeeding 332 · Giving the bottle 334 · Choosing diapers 336 · Changing a diaper 338 · Bathing baby 340
· Newborn health 342 · Special care baby 344
· Neonatal Intensive Care Unit (NICU) 346
· Case study: Premature baby 348

CHAPTER 16

Adjusting to parenthood 350

· The first weeks 352 · Postnatal health 354
· Postnatal exercises 358 · Your changing emotions 360
· Case study: The depressed mother 362
· Making love again 364 · Changes to your lifestyle 366
· Case study: The new father 368

Useful addresses 370

Index 371

Introduction

PREPARING FOR PREGNANCY

Now that we're discovering more and more about what can damage eggs and sperm, it's all the more important to prepare for pregnancy with some lifestyle changes. Stopping smoking at least three months before trying to have a baby is essential for everyone, and giving up alcohol is a good idea, too. A healthy and fit body is the best possible place to conceive and carry a baby to term. Not everything is always straightforward, of course: genes and chromosomes may be imperfect and fertilization may be difficult, but doctors now know about many of these problems, and some of them can be successfully treated.

One in six couples has difficulty conceiving, but that doesn't necessarily mean you'll never have a baby. Most couples who think they're infertile are only subfertile, and with help, can manage to conceive. At least half of all problems with conception are due to male fertility problems, something some men have difficulty coming to terms with, but that simple fact means that infertility can only be investigated as a couple. And the first test to be done is semen analysis.

Couples starting on fertility treatment deserve and should get counseling support right from the start—their own doctor can refer them to a counselor who specializes in dealing with the stress of infertility. There's a bewildering number of treatments available for all kinds of infertility, which is why I've gone into detail on fertility testing and treatment from simple drug therapies to the latest complex assisted reproductive technologies (ART).

YOUR DEVELOPING BABY

For convenience, the stages of your baby's development can be roughly divided into three phases: the first, second, and third trimesters. They're divided this way because of the particular changes happening to mother and baby in each of the three stages. In the first trimester your baby's organs form, in the second these organs become complex, and in the third they grow in size.

For you, the first trimester is when your body becomes primed for pregnancy: your breasts grow, your internal organs adapt, and your muscles and ligaments start to slacken in preparation for labor. High levels of pregnancy hormones bring on morning sickness, the desire to go to the bathroom more often, and tenderness of the breasts. During the second trimester, the body goes into a phase of consolidation. The third trimester sees your body preparing for delivery and making sure that your baby is growing healthily.

PREPARING FOR FATHERHOOD

Nowadays even the most hardworking dad wants to share childcare and be there for his kids. On the other hand, there are still some men who worry that taking a greater part in child-rearing would somehow be feminizing, and that sits uneasily with them.The result is that some men become disillusioned and anxious. Men feel they're on the horns of a dilemma; society, especially mothers, seem to know what sort of guy they want New Dad to be, but often men feel driven into a corner by being pressured into a hitherto unfamiliar role.

Long ago it was established that children can do perfectly well with only one parent of either gender. So even though some children are fine without a father, perhaps we need to encourage New Dads by offering fathers a proper New Deal. For this reason, I've included all aspects of fatherhood and fathering in the hope that, after reading it, more men will feel free to liberate their fathering instincts.

THE BIRTH OF YOUR CHOICE

Labor and birth can be managed any way you choose. There are many decisions for you to make, and it's important to be aware of all your options. In theory, it's possible to have exactly the kind of birth you want, but this involves lots of reading, soul-searching, and talking with your partner. You'll also have to talk things over with your nursing and medical attendants so that any difficulties that might come up later on can be dealt with.

A more relaxed and cooperative approach to childbirth has made birthing centers a popular alternative to hospitals for many couples. But for those who feel more comfortable with— or whose pregnancies require— more medical attention, hospitals provide all the facilities, the staff, and even many of the comforts of birthing centers, to meet your needs. It's important to make a birth plan outlining the kind of birth you'd prefer, and by talking this through with your attendants, you should be able to have the birth you want. It's up to women and their partners to take a more assertive role in the way the delivery and birth of their baby will be handled.

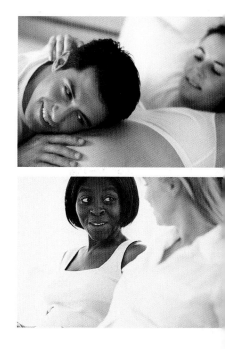

FOOD IN PREGNANCY

Eating healthily in pregnancy is mainly a question of choosing a wide variety of foods that contain plenty of essential nutrients. Make sure you eat lots of fresh fruit and vegetables, whole grains, and raw food and that you have a healthy intake of protein by eating fish, poultry, and low-fat dairy products, with red meat and eggs now and then. Fish is a good source of vitamin B12 and vitamin A, which is also found in green and yellow vegetables.

Your baby uses iron up fast and needs fresh supplies every day, so it's vital for you to eat plenty of iron-rich foods, such as red meat, apricots, raisins, prunes, and fish. Ideally, a woman should start taking daily folic acid supplements three months ahead of getting pregnant and then all the way through pregnancy to avoid neural tube defects like spina bifida. So it makes sense to add folic acid-rich foods to your diet at all times—green leafy vegetables, nuts, and cereals.

HEALTHY PREGNANCY

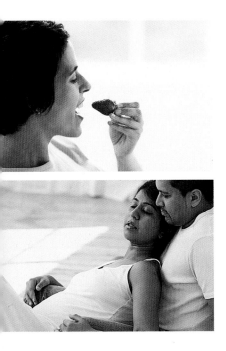

Regular exercise keeps you mentally and physically in good shape—when you exercise, the body releases tranquilizing chemicals, helping you to relax, and soothing away tension. The fast circulation of the blood during exercise means that your body and your baby are well oxygenated. Your labor will probably be easier and more comfortable if your muscles are in tone, and many of the exercises taught in prenatal classes, combined with relaxation and breathing techniques, will help you to be more in touch with what's happening to you during labor and delivery. Learn to save your energy, sleep as much as you can, and catnap whenever possible.

YOUR PRENATAL CARE

Good prenatal care is usually rewarded with healthy mothers and babies. At the prenatal clinic, routine tests are done to spot potential problems, avoid them where possible, and get treatment promptly if needed.

Tests such as ultrasound scanning and amniocentesis are carried out for mothers and babies with special needs. The social and personal aspects of prenatal care are as important as the medical ones. You'll probably find that talking to other mothers, doctors, and midwives reassures you about any worries you have and helps you feel confident about labor and birth. The clinic gives you the chance to ask questions, explore the different circumstances in which you can have your baby, and plan ahead for the kind of birth that you and your partner want.

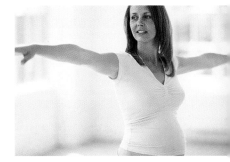

CARING FOR YOUR UNBORN BABY

You can be in touch with your unborn baby all through your pregnancy. The first time that you really feel you're in touch is when you feel your baby move. Keep talking to your unborn child. Babies have very sensitive hearing and at birth recognize both their mother's and father's voice from simply having heard them as they were growing and developing in the womb. Most parents really enjoy talking and singing to their unborn child, and gently massaging him through the abdominal wall.

Not all babies develop normally, but modern techniques are so advanced that we can even care for a developing baby in the womb. Advanced surgery can be carried out while your baby is still inside you so that he has every chance of being born normal and healthy. Not all babies enjoy the perfect conditions for development, but even so, diabetic mothers and mothers with Rhesus incompatibility, for example, can, with careful monitoring and treatment, have healthy pregnancies.

COMMON COMPLAINTS

Very few women go through pregnancy without some minor health problems. Most of these are uncomfortable rather than serious. There's a group of complaints particular to pregnancy. Being prepared and knowing about the treatments you can have is half the battle in coping with them. Most are easily dealt with and have no long-term effects.

MEDICAL EMERGENCIES

The risk of medical emergencies tends to be concentrated in the first and third trimesters of pregnancy. Nearly all of the classic emergencies are accompanied by classic symptoms, so if you experience any of them, call your doctor immediately. These symptoms include severe abdominal pain, vaginal bleeding, a fever of more than 100°F (37.8°C), severe nausea or vomiting, unremitting headache, blurred vision, swelling of the ankles, fingers, and face, no movement of your baby for more than 24 hours, and rupture of your membranes. In the first trimester, most emergencies are linked with loss of the baby due to hemorrhage or miscarriage, or to the pregnancy implanting in the wrong place, as in an ectopic pregnancy. Later on, an emergency might be brought on by very high blood pressure

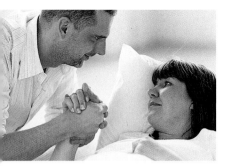

leading to preeclamptic toxemia, by recurrent late abortion, by Rhesus incompatibility, and by abnormalities of the placenta, such as placenta previa. Nonetheless, the vast majority of babies are delivered safely.

A SENSUAL PREGNANCY

Most women find that certain parts of the body, such as breasts, nipples, and the genital area, become more sensitive in pregnancy and their sexual organs are more easily aroused. This increased sensuality is due to high levels of pregnancy hormones and means that a woman may find she enjoys all aspects of sex, including sexual intercourse, even more than usual. Making love can be better than ever, with more heightened sensations, earlier arousal, and intense orgasms. Some women may orgasm for the first time, while others may find they are now able to have multiple orgasms. As your abdomen swells, you may find some positions uncomfortable.

GETTING READY FOR YOUR BABY

From the thirty-sixth week, nesting begins in earnest. There's lots to do—getting your baby's room ready, choosing clothes and equipment, deciding on your baby's names, working out how long you're going to take off work, and what kind of care you'd like for your child and for your other children.

Whether you're planning to have your baby in a hospital or a birthing center, you'll want to make a checklist of what to bring, including your medical insurance card, ID, and birth plan. Also, if you familiarize yourself with admission procedures at your hospital or birthing center, you'll feel less anxious and more in control when you actually arrive to have your baby.

MANAGING YOUR LABOR

Labor is the culmination of your pregnancy, and it can be divided into well-defined stages. Prelabor is a time before labor when you might have a dull backache or pass a "show." Your membranes may also rupture painlessly before your true labor begins.

The first stage of labor is entirely taken up with dilatation of your cervix to a size that lets your baby make her way from your uterine cavity into the birth canal. This stage is usually straight-forward, particularly if you're able to keep moving around and, by staying in an upright position, use the force of gravity to help your cervix to dilate.

Very few labors are pain-free, but there are many methods and types of pain relief from which to choose. And some labors aren't straightforward, so I've devoted a whole chapter to "Special deliveries," with information on inductions, breech babies, and sudden births.

GETTING TO KNOW YOUR NEWBORN BABY

Building a relationship with your baby begins the second she's born, and you and your partner will want to be left alone with her. Parents who bond closely with their children are more constructive, more sympathetic parents. The importance of fathers bonding cannot be overemphasized, and it's important for your partner to have the chance to hold his baby right after her birth.

The first few days will be harder than you think. Feeding can take longer than you expect, as can your baby's daily care. A routine is not always easy to set up, but the guiding and unbreakable rule is to take your lead from your baby.

Parents of special-care babies who need to be nursed in hospital intensive care units don't need to worry about being unable to bond with their babies. As long as parents, under the guidance of the nursing staff, become as intimately involved as possible in the day-to-day care of their baby, they shouldn't suffer any disadvantages.

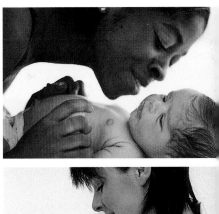

ADJUSTING TO PARENTHOOD

Getting to know your newborn baby is a thrilling experience, but don't be surprised if you feel a slight letdown at times. There are many adjustments to make, and few of them are easy. Somehow you have to coax your baby to fit in with your established family routine, maintain a loving relationship with your partner, and attend to your baby's needs and constant demands for attention.

Many women get bouts of sadness, and not just the "baby blues," which are so common in the first week after delivery. Much more serious is postpartum depression, which needs immediate attention from your doctor.

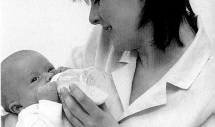

The responsibilities of parenthood may weigh heavily upon you, but watching your baby grow and develop should bring more than enough joy to balance any negative feelings that may occasionally creep in. You'll need some time to yourself to recharge your batteries, while time alone with your partner will help you to keep your relationship alive.

CHAPTER 1

Preparing for pregnancy

As we find out more and more about human eggs and sperm and what makes them healthy, we're realizing how important it is to prepare for pregnancy by taking care of ourselves. Not everything, of course, is always straightforward, but more is known about conception problems, and some can be treated.

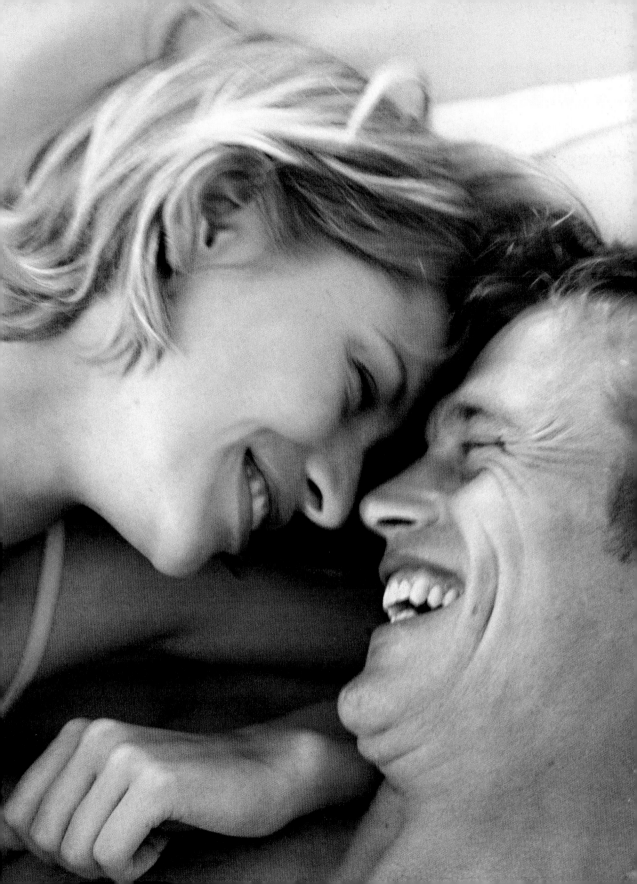

Fit for parenthood

Health really does matter when you're conceiving a baby. The healthier you and your partner are at the time of conception, the better your chances of having a trouble-free pregnancy and labor, and a healthy baby. And the father's health is just as important as the mother's. There's no doubt that becoming a parent will change your life in lots of ways, so it's a good idea to plan ahead as much as you can and think about how these changes might affect you both.

YOUR CHANGING LIFESTYLE

All the things you take for granted about your life and what you do will be affected by the arrival of your baby.

Time Most of us live very busy lives and many new parents think that their new baby will just fit in somehow and life will go on as usual. It won't. Babies and children need a lot of time and attention, and as parents you'll have less time to spend with each other—and other people—than you did before.

Costs Whatever you earn, you'll probably need to spend about 15–25 percent of your income on things related to your child, such as clothing and equipment. But other household costs, such as heating, will rise, too, and you may find you want extra items such as a new washing machine or even a larger car.

Relationships Your relationship with your partner will change when you have a baby, and so will relationships with other people. You may feel closer to your parents—now they're your baby's grandparents—but you might find you have less in common with your childless friends. Make new friendships with other parents if you can—they're going through the same experiences as you.

Smoking This is one of the worst things you can do for the health of your unborn baby, and it's the major cause of avoidable health problems. Risks linked to smoking include miscarriage and still-birth, damage to the placenta, a low-birthweight baby who fails to thrive, and a higher risk of fetal abnormalities. Smoking is one cause of a low sperm count, and a man who smokes while his partner is pregnant may damage his unborn baby's health through passive smoking. And the problems continue. When tested at five, seven, and eleven years old, children of heavy smokers were found to suffer from impaired growth and learning difficulties. Studies have also shown a link between smoking and SIDS (Sudden Infant Death Syndrome).

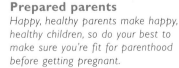

Prepared parents
Happy, healthy parents make happy, healthy children, so do your best to make sure you're fit for parenthood before getting pregnant.

Alcohol This is a poison that can damage the sperm and egg before conception, as well as the developing embryo. The main risks to an unborn baby are mental retardation, retarded growth, and damage to the brain and nervous system—well documented as fetal alcohol syndrome. Alcohol can also cause stillbirth.

Research suggests that the effect of alcohol on pregnant women varies: some are more affected than others. But one thing is certain: if you don't drink during your pregnancy, you'll avoid alcohol-related problems. Women tend to have a lower tolerance to alcohol than men. And because a woman has a higher proportion of fat to water in the body, alcohol can become very highly concentrated in the blood that nourishes the developing baby.

Drugs Only take over-the-counter medicines if you have to, and always check the label. Your pharmacist will advise you about what's safe to take. Illegal drugs should definitely be cut out before trying to conceive. Marijuana interferes with the normal production of male sperm, and the effects can take three to nine months to wear off. Hard drugs such as cocaine, heroin, and morphine can damage the chromosomes in the sperm and egg, leading to abnormalities. When syringes are shared, there's a high risk of contracting HIV, the virus that leads to AIDS. A mother can pass the HIV virus to her baby during pregnancy and the baby can become HIV positive in his own right (see p.19).

Diet and exercise Both are vital to your health and the health of your baby. Do your best to eat a sensible, balanced diet that's low in animal fat and includes at least five portions of fresh fruit and vegetables a day. Make sure you're getting enough folic acid in your diet, because it's known to lower the risk of your baby suffering neural tube defects, such as spina bifida. Folic acid is contained in green leafy vegetables, cereals, and bread, and should also be taken in supplement form for at least three months before conception and three months after. It's a very good idea to get regular exercise, too. Pregnancy puts a strain on your body; the healthier you are beforehand, the better you'll cope.

Age If you're healthy and in shape, your pregnancy should not be any more difficult in your 30s or 40s than in your 20s. Whatever your age, you're likely to have a normal pregnancy and birth, although some problems, such as infertility and chromosomal defects—for example, Down syndrome (see p.24)—do become more common in older parents. Older mothers, and younger women in high-risk groups, are always offered tests for chromosomal abnormalities.

Hazards Be aware of your environment, at home, at work, and elsewhere, and avoid anything that could be dangerous to your own or your baby's health. What we eat, where we work, the places we travel to, and sometimes even the people we meet may be risky for a pregnant woman (see p.169).

STOPPING CONTRACEPTION

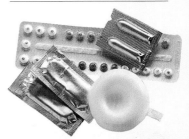

When you decide you want to get pregnant, you can stop barrier methods, such as the diaphragm and sheath, at once. But if you're on the pill or you're using an IUD, a little more planning is needed.

The pill The usual advice is to stop taking the pill a month before trying to conceive, so that you have at least one normal menstrual period before becoming pregnant. But there's evidence to suggest that some women are more fertile immediately after stopping the pill, so this could be the ideal time to try if you've had fertility problems or you have had a miscarriage.

If you suspect that you're pregnant but you're still on the pill, stop taking it. Conceiving on the pill rarely causes any problems, but go to your doctor as soon as you can.

The intrauterine device The IUD works by causing changes in the uterus that prevent fertilized eggs from implanting. A very small number of women get pregnant while using an IUD. Even though removing the IUD carries a risk of miscarriage, it's still generally recommended in order to lower the risk of miscarriage and infection later in the pregnancy. There's a greater risk of having an ectopic pregnancy with some IUDs, so check with your doctor as soon as you know you're pregnant.

TESTING YOUR URINE

If tests show that you have sugar in your urine, it's possible that you have diabetes. However, it's more likely that some sugar has leaked through your kidneys as their threshold for sugar is lowered by pregnancy. You'll need more tests to confirm that this is what has happened.

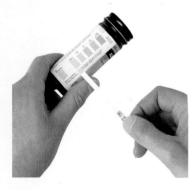

Testing urine
Urine tests are simple to do. A chemically impregnated strip is dipped into a sample of your urine. If sugar is present, the strip changes color and the amount can be compared to a chart that shows glucose levels.

HEALTH CONSIDERATIONS

If you suffer from a chronic long-term condition, such as diabetes mellitus, heart disease, or epilepsy, you can, of course, still have children. It's important, though, to talk with your doctor before you get pregnant so you get the best possible care and help.

Asthma   This is the most common respiratory problem in mothers-to-be and is usually controlled by bronchodilator drugs and inhaled steroids. Asthma drugs don't seem to be a risk to the growing baby, although oral thrush (see p.212), which is often made worse by pregnancy, can be a side effect for the mother.

If you do suffer from asthma, it's important to take extra care of yourself while you're pregnant. Any stress and tension, as well as dust, pollen, and pollution, can cause breathlessness, and this could trigger an asthma attack.

Epilepsy   From a momentary loss of consciousness to grand mal seizures, epilepsy affects one in every 200 people. Research has found that the effect of pregnancy on the frequency and intensity of seizures varies—50 percent of epileptic mothers are unaffected, 40 percent find they are slightly improved, and 10 percent worse. If you do suffer from epilepsy, talk to your doctor well before you hope to conceive. There's a slightly increased risk of neural tube and other defects linked to antiepileptic drugs such as phenytoin and valproate, and your doctor should warn you about this.

Changing the drug treatment can increase the risk of seizures, but women with epilepsy are usually advised—under the supervision of their doctor—to reduce the drugs they take before pregnancy, not during it. While you're pregnant, you'll continue with any drug treatment, but you'll need to be seen frequently by a neurologist who can adjust your drug dosage. Phenytoin prevents absorption of folic acid, so it's very important to take high doses of folic acid supplements before you conceive as well as after, to help lower the risk of birth defects (see p.17). All pregnant women on phenytoin or sodium valproate are also advised to take vitamin K supplements from 36 weeks of pregnancy to help mature the baby's liver.

Diabetes mellitus   Diabetes arises when the pancreas produces insufficient insulin to cope with glucose (sugar) levels in the body. Pregnancy hormones have an anti-insulin effect, which can make diabetes worse, or lead to gestational diabetes in those with an underlying tendency. All pregnant women should have a glucose challenge test at 26–28 weeks to screen for gestational, or pregnancy-induced, diabetes. Diabetes can cause the baby to be large or have heart and respiratory problems, and complications for the mother include chronic thrush, preeclampsia (see p.224), and birth trauma to either the mother or the newborn. So it's important for insulin-dependent diabetic women to have their condition under control before conception, and to monitor blood-sugar levels closely.

Heart disease If you suffer from any kind of heart condition, your doctor will give you special advice about your pregnancy. Generally, you'll be told to get plenty of rest—put your feet up in the afternoon for at least two hours, and spend ten hours in bed at night. Depending on what type of heart condition you have and how severe it is, your doctor or maternal–fetal medicine specialist will make different recommendations. Most women with heart disease can have a safe labor and delivery.

Kidney disease A woman with kidney disease should be able to have children but will need careful monitoring. Women with kidney disease have a higher-than-usual risk of hypertension and preeclampsia. Urinary tract infection is another common problem, but as long as the kidneys remove waste effectively, the pregnancy can continue. If the fetus isn't growing properly, though, doctors may recommend early induction.

Sexually transmitted disease There's a risk of infection to your baby if you have a primary herpes infection at the time your membranes rupture or at labor. Herpes simplex II virus infection may slow your baby's growth, and about half of infants born to a mother with these conditions will develop some form of herpetic infection after birth, possibly affecting the eyes, mouth, and skin. If you have no symptoms, and you're not shedding the virus from your cervix or vagina, the risk that your baby will become infected is less than one in a thousand.

If you have a history of genital herpes, you should still be able to have a normal vaginal delivery, even with an active secondary infection. But if you have herpes ulcers and a primary infection just before labor commences, you'll probably be advised to have a cesarean section to reduce the risk that your baby will catch herpes as he descends the birth canal. Doctors will check for signs of infection at the time of delivery. If you get herpes simplex for the first time when you're pregnant, your doctor may prescribe medication to reduce the severity.

HIV/AIDS The outlook for babies of mothers who have tested HIV-positive is much better than it used to be. The use of oral AZT may protect the developing baby from infection, and the mother will be scanned regularly to check the baby's growth. Doctors may suggest a cesarean delivery to protect the baby, and they will aim for as little invention as possible during labor (for example, no use of scalp electrodes or fetal blood sampling) to lessen the risk that the baby's blood will be contaminated. Although it's not inevitable that the baby of an HIV-positive mother will be HIV-positive and develop AIDS, there's a risk that the baby will be born with HIV antibodies; these are usually maternal antibodies and may disappear within 18 months. Because of the risks, an HIV-positive mother will be given counseling and may be offered the chance to terminate her pregnancy if she wishes.

GERMAN MEASLES

Before you start trying to conceive, ask your doctor to check you for antibodies to the German measles (rubella) virus.

Even if you've been vaccinated in the past, you can't assume you're immune to the disease—the antibodies lose their efficiency after a period of time. Get your doctor to check, and if you're not immune, you'll need to be vaccinated. After vaccination, you'll need to wait at least three months before trying to conceive, because the vaccine is live.

If you're pregnant and you come in contact with someone who has, or is suspected of having, German measles, tell your doctor right away. You'll need to have a blood sample taken and sent sent to a laboratory for antibody testing.

Depending on the result, you might need to have another test 10 days later. If this suggests that you might have German measles, you and your partner will have to decide whether to abort your pregnancy. Some doctors may recommend giving antibodies in the form of gamma globulin to help avoid any damage to the fetus.

TAKE CARE
German measles (rubella) can cause birth defects, particularly if you catch the disease in the first three months of pregnancy. Problems may include deafness, blindness, and heart disease.

The importance of folic acid

Case study

Name   Cressida King
Age   31 years
Past medical history   Nothing abnormal
Obstetric history   One normal delivery

Cressida's first baby, a boy, was born 18 months ago, and now she'd like to have a second child. She had a normal delivery with her son Henry and he was fine, apart from a brown, hairy birthmark at the base of his spine. The doctors explained to Cressida that this kind of birthmark may be linked to spina bifida, but means nothing by itself. Henry has no health problems and he's a robust, loving

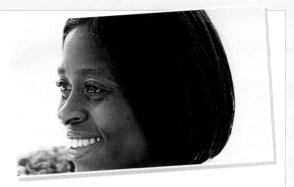

little boy. Cressida is worried that having had one child with this kind of birthmark puts her at greater risk of having a child with spina bifida.

Cressida is thinking about getting pregnant again and has been talking things through with her mother and her sister Oona. Cressida's mother has read about the connection between folic acid deficiency and neural tube defects (spina bifida and hydrocephalus). She thinks Cressida should start taking folic acid supplements now in case she becomes pregnant.

BEING INFORMED

Cressida doesn't like taking pills, even vitamin supplements. Oona thinks that Cressida should speak to her doctor now to help her decide whether she should start taking folic acid, in preparation for conception. Here are a few things for Cressida to think about.

SPINA BIFIDA AND HYDROCEPHALUS

The medical definition of spina bifida is a defect in which part of one or more vertebrae fails to develop completely, leaving part of the spinal cord exposed. Spina bifida can happen anywhere in the spine, but it's most common on the lower back. The severity depends on how much nervous tissue is exposed.

There are different degrees of spina bifida. In one type, the only defect is that the bony arches behind the spinal cord fail to join. When the bone defect is more extensive, there may be neural tube defects such as a *meningocele* with protrusion of the *meninges*, the

membranes surrounding the spinal cord, or, more serious still, a *myelocele* with deformity of the spinal cord. In the developing embryo, the skin, brain, the spinal cord, and the nerves all arise from the same layer of cells. This is why a birthmark over the end of the embryonic neural tube may be the only sign of late closure of the fetal neural tube.

Spina bifida symptoms depend on the severity of the spinal cord exposure; there may be paralysis, incontinence, or hydrocephalus—swelling of the brain.

REDUCING THE RISKS

The spine and the vertebral column develop from a flat layer of cells whose edges come together to form a tube, which is the hollow cavity inside the spinal cord. This closure of the cord and the bones that surround it, the vertebrae, takes place very early in the development of an embryo, usually within four weeks of conception.

Research has shown that a woman needs sufficiently high levels of folic acid in her blood for the neural tube to close normally. Mothers with low blood levels of folic acid have a higher risk of having a baby with spina bifida.

There's something else, too: normally, folic acid is removed from the blood quite quickly, but when you're pregnant the kidneys filter it off from the blood at four times the normal rate. So if you don't eat folic-acid-rich foods or take folic acid supplements regularly, you can become relatively deficient in folic acid, and your levels may drop low enough to put your baby at risk.

It's vital for all pregnant women to take daily supplements of folic acid to keep the blood levels high.

TAKING FOLIC ACID

1. I explained to Cressida that it's not enough to start folic acid when you know you're pregnant. Cressida's mother is right; her folic acid levels need to be topped off at the very moment she conceives, whenever that may be. That means she needs to take folic acid before conception. Experts recommend that all women who're thinking about having a baby start taking folic acid supplements three months before trying to conceive.

2. It's also important to take enough, and experts agree on a daily dose of 400 micrograms.

3. You can get folic acid in several different forms:

• in foods such as liver (eat only about once a week);

• in green leafy vegetables—the darker green the better— and in mushrooms, lima beans, kidney beans, whole-wheat bread, nuts (particularly walnuts), peas, and beans; all women should make these foods part of their diet months before they become pregnant;

• as folic acid capsules in 400-microgram doses, available from pharmacies—take one a day from three months before pregnancy through to term;

• in a nutritious folic acid milk drink available from pharmacies. One carton (about a glass-full) contains your daily folic acid requirements and is ideal if, like Cressida, you don't like taking tablets or capsules.

WOMEN AT RISK

Parents who've had one child with spina bifida are more at risk than parents who've had completely normal children. But having a child with a hairy birthmark (sacral naevus) like Henry has does not mean there's any increased risk in the next pregnancy.

WOMEN WHO ARE NUTRITIONALLY VULNERABLE

As I explained to Cressida, all babies are potentially at some risk of spina bifida and other neural tube defects like hydrocephalus whatever the mother's age—whether she's a first-time mother or already has healthy children—even if she's in the best of health herself. But some women should be especially careful about taking folic acid supplements. So I asked Cressida if she'd ever experienced any of the following:

• allergy to certain key foods, such as cows' milk or wheat;

• being generally run down, underweight, or eating a poor, unbalanced diet;

• a period of overstrict dieting or anorexia nervosa;

• a recent miscarriage or stillbirth;

• drinking or smoking heavily;

• working particularly hard or being subject to a lot of stress.

Women who've had babies close together or given birth to twins or triplets may have vitamin and mineral deficiencies, and so it's particularly important for them to start taking folic acid supplements before falling pregnant again.

Cressida was persuaded by these facts and decided to start on folic acid immediately in the form of the milk drink each morning with breakfast.

Folic acid in food

Foods high in folic acid (50 mcg per serving and above)

Cooked black-eyed beans, Brussels sprouts, beef extract, yeast extract, cooked kidney, kale, spinach, multigrain bread, spring greens, broccoli, and green beans.

Foods with medium folic acid content (15–50 mcg per serving)

Cooked soybeans, cauliflower, cooked chickpeas, potatoes, iceberg lettuce, oranges, peas, orange juice, parsnips, baked beans, whole-wheat bread, cabbage, yogurt, white bread, eggs, brown rice, whole-wheat pasta.

Foods fortified with folic acid

Bread: many supermarkets stock bread that is fortified with folic acid. A two-slice serving of one of these will provide approximately 90 mcg of folic acid.

Cereals: many cereals are fortified, but to very different levels, so always check the label. Some have more than 100 mcg per 30-g serving.

INHERITING GENES

Half of a baby's genes come from his mother, via the egg, and half come from his father, via the sperm.

Each egg and sperm contains a different "mix" of the parents' genes, so each child inherits a different and unique selection of his parents' genetic information.

Most of our individual mix of genes blends together, but some genes are dominant and others recessive. For example, the gene for brown eyes is dominant and the gene for blue eyes is recessive. So a child with one brown-eyed parent and one blue-eyed parent will receive a gene for each, but will have brown eyes because the gene for brown eyes prevails over the gene for blue eyes.

The genetic mix
Your baby will have a unique combination of his parents' genes.

What is a gene?

Genes are chemical codes that control the way every cell in the body works. A gene is a minute unit of DNA (deoxyribonucleic acid) carried on a *chromosome*, which is also made up of DNA. In every body cell, there are at least 50,000 unique genes.

THE "BLUEPRINT" OF THE BODY

Genes influence and direct the growth and working of everything in the human body. They control the pattern for growth, survival, reproduction, and possibly even aging and death for each individual. All cells (except for egg and sperm cells) come from the single egg fertilized by the male's sperm, so the same genetic material is duplicated in every cell in your body. But not all the genes in an individual cell are active; it's where the cell is and what it does that determines which genes are active. For example, different sets of genes are active in bone cells and blood cells.

With the exception of identical twins, there are lots of differences in people's genetic makeup. Genes account for all the little variations in height, hair and eye color, body shape, and gender, for example. Your genetic inheritance also decides how likely you are to have certain diseases.

Chromosomes Genes are carried in pairs along a chromosome (see opposite) and each gene is either dominant or recessive. A recognizable effect is the result of the dominant gene or genes in each pair; the effect of recessive genes will only be seen when there are two recessive genes. Every cell in your body, except egg and sperm cells, normally contains 23 pairs of the threadlike structures called chromosomes. Egg and sperm cells contain only 22 chromosomes plus an X or Y chromosome. Each chromosome contains thousands of genes that are arranged in single file along its length. Chromosomes are made up of two chains of DNA, which are arranged together to form a ladderlike structure, the sides of which are sugar-phosphate molecules. This spirals around on itself and is known as a double helix. DNA has four bases (adenine, cytosine, guanine, and thymine) arranged in different combinations according to the functions of the genes on the different parts of the chromosome. Each combination of bases provides coded instructions that control and regulate the various activities of the body.

CHROMOSOMES, GENES, AND DNA

Chromosomes
There are 23 pairs of chromosomes in the nucleus of every body cell (see left). These thread-like structures consist of 22 general, plus one pair of sex chromosomes (either a pair of X chromosomes, as here, or an X and a Y).

Chromosome

The double helix
The two chains of DNA, which make up each of the 46 chromosomes, are arranged to make a long spiraling ladder.

Each of the four DNA bases—adenine, cytosine, guanine, and thymine—is represented here by a different color

Sugar-phosphate molecules form the sides of the DNA ladder

DNA replication
When a new cell is about to be formed, the DNA in each of the chromosomes "unzips" along the center of the rungs of the ladder, and each half of DNA then duplicates itself. The new DNA chains that are created are genetically identical to the original chromosomes.

Gene

MUTATIONS

Sometimes when a cell divides and duplicates its genetic material, the copying process is not perfect, and there's a fault. This leads to a small change, or *mutation*, in the structure of the genetic material.

Carrying a mutant gene normally has a neutral or harmless effect—most, if not all, of us have a mutant gene as part of our genetic makeup. But it can sometimes have a disadvantageous effect and, more rarely, a beneficial one.

The effects of a mutant gene depend largely upon whether it's carried within the fused egg and sperm, or whether it's a fault in the later copying process of the body cells.

A mutation in the egg or sperm will reproduce itself in all of the body's cells, and can cause genetic disease such as cystic fibrosis (see p.24). A mutated body cell, at worst, will multiply to form a group of abnormal cells in a specific area. These may have only a minor effect in that part of the body, or they could cause deformity or disease. This type of mutation is usually triggered by an outside influence, such as radiation or exposure to cancer-causing agents.

23

DOWN SYNDROME

This chromosomal disorder (see column, right) happens when a fertilized egg has 47 chromosomes instead of the usual 46.

In most cases, the egg itself is defective, because it's formed with the extra chromosome; the sperm may be affected in the same way. This type of Down syndrome is known as *trisomy*. Less commonly, one parent may have a chromosomal abnormality, causing the child to inherit faulty chromosomal material. This is known as *translocation*.

The incidence of Down syndrome rises sharply with the age of the mother, particularly over 35, but various tests can identify the condition in the fetus. Chorionic villus sampling or nuchal scanning (scanning of the fetal neck) can be carried out at 10–12 weeks. At around 20 weeks, amniocentesis can be offered to high-risk mothers.

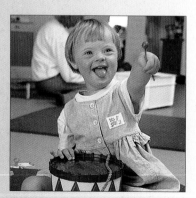

Down syndrome child
One baby in every 1,000 will be born with this disorder. Most cases of Down syndrome occur randomly and aren't passed on. However, one cause—translocation—is inherited, so it's important to explore any family history of Down syndrome.

GENETIC COUNSELING

Inside the nucleus of each cell are the genes and chromosomes that control how the body develops and functions (see also p.22). Genetic disorders happen when genes and chromosomes are abnormal. Genetic diseases can be caused by a single defective gene, several faulty genes, or a fault in the number or shape of chromosomes. There may also be complicating environmental factors. A single defective gene that results in a genetic disorder can be either dominant or recessive, a mutation, or attached to the X chromosome (see below). Abnormal chromosomes that result in genetic disorders are usually new mutations, but may be inherited (see column, left).

If either of you has a history of a genetic disease in your extended family, it's best to ask for genetic counseling (see p.26) before getting pregnant. The number of tests available for genetic diseases is increasing every year, although they can't tell how severe the condition is likely to be. The ultimate decision about whether to attempt to conceive, to go ahead with an existing pregnancy, or to ask for a termination is always up to you, the parents. It's a hard choice, but always remember that although a handicapped child will need lots of special care, many are both affectionate and responsive, and can lead happy, fulfilled lives.

DOMINANT GENETIC DISEASES

Fatal diseases due to dominant genes are rare because affected individuals normally die before they can pass on the genes. However, some, such as familial hypercholesterolemia (see below), can be managed.

Familial hypercholesterolemia FH is the most common dominant genetic disease. Sufferers have such high levels of blood cholesterol that they risk heart attacks and other complications caused by narrowing of the arteries. This condition affects one in 500 people and can be detected by a blood test at birth.

RECESSIVE GENETIC DISEASES

A defective recessive gene is usually masked by a normal dominant one. But if both parents carry a defective recessive gene, each of their children has a one in four chance of inheriting both recessive genes (and therefore one of several disorders) or neither, and a two in four chance of being a carrier. Thus there are always more carriers than sufferers.

Cystic fibrosis CF is the most common recessive gene disorder. One in 20 of the white population carries the CF gene, and one in 2,000 white babies born is affected by the disease. In nonwhites, the incidence is about one in 90,000. This disease mainly affects the lungs and the digestive system. The mucus inside the lungs becomes thick and sticky and builds up, causing chest infections. The mucus also blocks the ducts of various organs, particularly the pancreas, preventing the normal flow of digestive enzymes. If not treated promptly, CF results in malnutrition. Rapid and accurate carrier testing involving analysis of blood or mouth cells is possible. Over 60 percent of sufferers survive into adulthood; some have been helped by heart transplant surgery.

Sickle-cell anemia This is the most common genetic disease among black people (one in 400). It's so called because the red cells are sickle-shaped from defective hemoglobin; this causes them to break down and the small blood vessels to clog, which may result in a stroke. It's usually diagnosed by a blood test, and the mother will be offered chorionic villus sampling (CVS) if both parents are sufferers. People with sickle-cell are susceptible to meningitis and other serious infections but can, with care, live a productive life despite some ill health. Being a carrier of sickle-cell does give protection against malaria.

Thalassemia This is common among Asians and black people, and people of Mediterranean descent. The gene may be dominant or recessive. It causes anemia and chronic ill health, and sufferers may need blood transfusions. If you're at risk, you can have a blood test to check for the disease and find out whether your hemoglobin level is reduced. Thalassemia can be severe, but many cases are mild, allowing people to live more or less normal lives.

Tay–Sachs disease Common among Ashkenazic Jews, this is a fatal condition causing deterioration of the brain because of a deficiency in enzymes. Few children with the disease live beyond three years, and no adequate treatment is known. Tay–Sachs is diagnosed by testing blood for enzyme deficiency.

GENDER-LINKED DISEASES

These are conditions caused by defects on the X chromosome, and only men are affected. If a second normal X chromosome is present, as in a healthy female, it compensates for the abnormal gene. Women, therefore, only carry the disease. Men with the abnormal gene do develop the disease because they have only one X chromosome (the other is a Y chromosome).

Hemophilia This results when the crucial protein involved in blood clotting, Factor VIII, is missing. Sufferers bleed profusely from any injury, external or internal. Effective treatment with factor VIII derived from normal blood is now available, and hemophiliacs can lead relatively normal lives. Diagnosis can be made from a sample of fetal blood at 18–20 weeks of pregnancy.

Duchenne muscular dystrophy This type of muscular dystrophy affects one boy in 5,000. Symptoms are progressive and children become unable to walk. The disease is usually fatal before age 20. It can be detected before birth.

CHROMOSOMAL DISORDERS

These are usually a result of some fault that happens when chromosomes are dividing during the formation of the egg or sperm, or when the fertilized egg is first dividing. More rarely, one parent has an abnormal arrangement of chromosomes.

The type of abnormality and how severe it is depends on whether one or both sex chromosomes, or one of the other 44 chromosomes (autosomes) are affected. The latter are slightly less common than sex chromosomal abnormalities, but can produce more serious, widespread effects. An extra autosome means that one of the 22 pairs of autosomes occurs in triplicate, known as a trisomy (see p.198). The most common trisomy is Down syndrome (see column, far left). In a trisomy, part of a chromosome is missing or an extra piece is joined to a chromosome. Trisomy can cause mental and physical defects.

Occasionally the problem can be caused by translocation. This happens if there is a normal number of chromosomes but they are not arranged correctly (part of one is joined to another). The parent carrier is normal but a child may have an abnormality if he inherits the translocated chromosomes.

Abnormalities of sex chromosomes can cause defects in sexual development, infertility, and even mental retardation. Boys may suffer from Klinefelter syndrome (see p.38), girls from Turner syndrome (they have one X chromosome instead of two). Abnormalities can be diagnosed by chromosome analysis, which may be offered during genetic counseling (see p.26).

CAN YOU BENEFIT?

It's important to seek expert advice if you fall into any of the following groups. Not everyone will be referred for genetic counseling, but it's worth checking with your doctor if any of these factors apply to you:

- if you've had a child with a genetic disorder such as cystic fibrosis, or a chromosomal disorder such as Down syndrome

- if you've had a child with a congenital defect—for example, a club foot (see p.199)

- if there's any history of mental handicap, or abnormal development in your family

- if there's a blood relationship between you and your partner

- if you have a history of repeated miscarriages (see pp. 218 & 222).

Genetic counseling

Very few couples will need genetic counseling, but if you do, the main aim is to discover how great a risk you run of passing on an inheritable disease to your child. Perhaps you're worried because you or your partner have a blood relative (including, perhaps, a previous child) who has suffered from an inheritable disorder. Depending on what you find out, a genetic counselor will also help you decide whether or not to go ahead with trying to conceive.

HOW GENETIC COUNSELING WORKS

When you first meet a genetic counselor, you'll be asked lots of questions about your health, and about your family background. Take along as much information as you can—you may need birth and death certificates of close relatives, for example—and be prepared for the whole project to take some time. The advice you'll be given at the end of it depends on a precise diagnosis of the disease (what it is and why it happened), and on the making of a family tree, with details of all blood relationships and any diseases suffered. Your counselor will assess the degree of risk in your case and help you make an informed decision. If there's a small risk, you may decide to go ahead and try for a baby. If the risks are very great, you may prefer not to take that chance.

For many genetic disorders, such as sickle-cell anaemia or Tay–Sachs (see p.25), prospective parents can be checked to find out if they are carriers. This can be done by seeing evidence of the disease itself, such as sickle-shaped cells, on a blood sample; by looking for the product of the disease, such as the proteins that are present in Tay–Sachs; or by flagging a gene or chromosome. Flagging is a sophisticated technique that is used to find out if a fragment of DNA will attach itself to the patient's chromosome. If it does, the gene, and therefore the disease, is present; if not, it's absent. In most diseases, though, more than one gene is involved, so it can be difficult to check all the elements involved. This is true of cystic fibrosis, although at present the diagnosis can be more than 90 percent certain.

If a couple has already had a child with a congenital defect, the counselor will first rule out any possible causes that aren't inherited—for example, rubella (see p.19). Other possible causes such as exposure to radiation, drugs, or injury will also be looked at. The counselor will examine the child and will arrange for genetic testing to be done.

Sometimes it can be difficult to pinpoint the exact cause of a problem, but you'll be given as thorough a diagnosis as possible, and your chances of having another child with the same disorder outlined. Remember that many disabilities are not genetic and cannot be predicted; genetic evaluation can only reassure you that there's no evidence of an inheritable disease.

THE IMPORTANCE OF YOUR FAMILY HISTORY

A counselor will examine the medical history of both your families to find out if there's any pattern of disease over several generations. For example, James, a six-year-old boy, was suffering with painful, swollen joints. During a conversation with James' parents, the counselor learned that a cousin, and probably a great-uncle as well, suffered from the genetic bleeding disorder known as hemophilia (see family tree, below), which is carried on the female X chromosome.

This information pointed almost immediately to the probable diagnosis—James, too, was suffering from hemophilia. The pain and swelling that he was experiencing was caused by the blood that was leaking into his joints.

HOW GENES ARE INHERITED

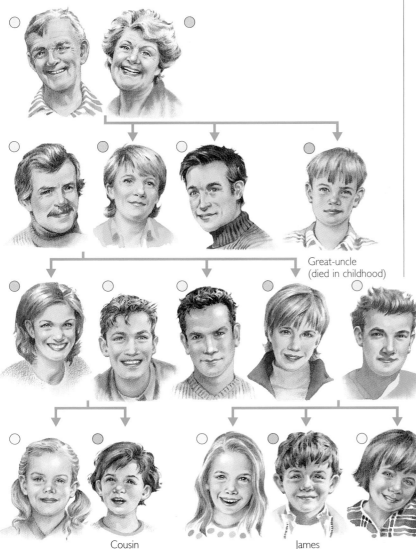

Great-uncle
(died in childhood)

Cousin   James

Family tree
James's mother and some other female relatives are carriers of hemophilia. They don't suffer from the disease themselves, but they do pass on the gene to some of their sons, who develop hemophilia, and to some of their daughters, who become carriers.

⬤ Males with hemophilia

◯ Unaffected males

◉ Probable female carriers of hemophilia gene

◯ Possible female carriers of hemophilia gene

Conceiving a baby

YOUR HORMONES

A woman's ovarian cycle is mostly controlled by the hormones estrogen, progesterone, follicle-stimulating hormone (FSH), and luteinizing hormone (LH).

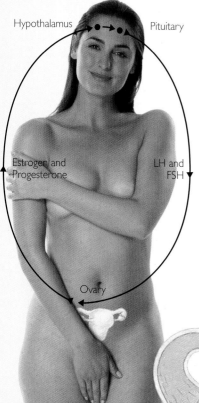

The miracle of birth begins when one of your partner's sperm fuses with one of your eggs to form a single cell. This cell contains its own unique genetic blueprint, which is a mix of genetic material from both parents. The cell then divides and divides again until eventually a new human being is made. The vast majority of normally fertile couples manage to conceive within the first two years of trying.

A woman's entire stock of eggs is made in her two ovaries before her birth. By the fifth month of development, a baby girl's ovaries contain about seven million eggs. Many of these eggs will die before she's born, leaving her with about two million eggs at birth. Eggs continue to die until at puberty most women have between 200,000 and 500,000 eggs. Of these, only 400–500 mature, and they're released by the ovaries during a woman's fertile years at the rate of roughly one a month.

The ovaries are located in the pelvis, close to the trumpetlike endings (*fimbriae*) of the fallopian tubes. The germ cells that eventually develop into a woman's eggs form in the yolk sac that sustains the embryo in the first weeks of development. If the embryo is male, these cells are reabsorbed as the placenta

THE FEMALE REPRODUCTIVE TRACT

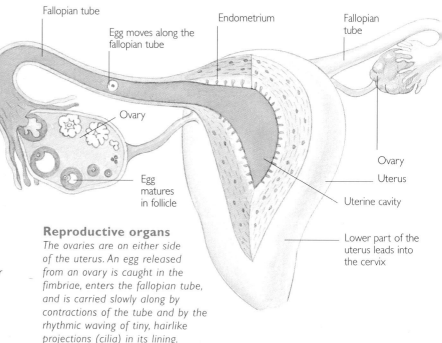

Hormonal control
The development of an ovarian follicle is triggered by FSH from the pituitary gland. The follicles make estrogen, which causes the pituitary to release a burst of LH that cuts FSH production. The LH triggers the release of the egg from the most mature follicle and the corpus luteum, which forms from the follicle after the egg has been released, then produces progesterone.

Reproductive organs
The ovaries are on either side of the uterus. An egg released from an ovary is caught in the fimbriae, enters the fallopian tube, and is carried slowly along by contractions of the tube and by the rhythmic waving of tiny, hairlike projections (cilia) in its lining.

develops. If the embryo is female, about 100 germ cells actually move from the yolk sac, along the umbilical cord, and into the tiny female embryo. Once inside the embryo, the cells migrate to the tissues that will later develop into the ovaries, and there they begin to multiply.

THE OVARIAN CYCLE

During a woman's reproductive life, her ovaries release eggs in cycles. Each of these ovarian cycles lasts about 28 days, and the development and release of an egg ready for fertilization by a sperm is called ovulation. Ovaries usually ovulate alternately. In the first half of each ovarian cycle, about 20 eggs begin to ripen, and occupy fluid-filled sacs (*follicles*). One of these follicles, outgrows the others, matures, and then ruptures, releasing its egg. This happens on or around 14 days before the end of the cycle, whatever the total length of the cycle. The other follicles that had started to ripen then shrivel up and their eggs die.

The ruptured follicle becomes a yellow-colored structure, called the *corpus luteum*. This grows for some days and produces the hormone progesterone, which is essential for the development of an embryo. If the egg is not fertilized, however, the follicle withers away.

A new cycle begins when the lining of the uterus, which is called the *endometrium*, is shed at the beginning of the woman's next period.

FERTILITY FACTS

Fertility varies from person to person and at different stages of life. The following facts are true for most people:

- the fertility of both men and women reaches its peak at about the age of 24

- among couples having intercourse regularly without contraception, 25 percent of women will conceive in the first month, 60 percent within six months, 75 percent within nine months, 80 percent within a year, and 90 percent within 18 months

- after ovulation, an egg can only be fertilized during the next 12–24 hours.

THE MONTHLY CYCLE

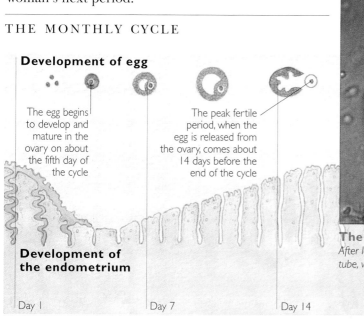

Development of egg

The egg begins to develop and mature in the ovary on about the fifth day of the cycle

The peak fertile period, when the egg is released from the ovary, comes about 14 days before the end of the cycle

Development of the endometrium

Day 1   Day 7   Day 14   Day 21   Day 28

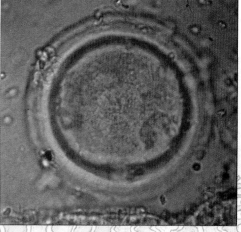

The mature egg
After leaving the ovary, the egg is drawn into the fallopian tube, where it awaits fertilization by a sperm.

The cycle begins
The beginning of the ovarian cycle is signaled by menstruation, the shedding of the endometrium, the lining of the uterus. Estrogen controls the rebuilding of the endometrium.

Fertile period
After ovulation, under the influence of estrogen and progesterone, the endometrium becomes thicker and spongy to receive a fertilized egg.

The cycle ends
If the egg isn't fertilized, the corpus luteum dies and, because estrogen and progesterone levels fall, the endometrium is shed.

MAKING SPERM

The process of making sperm takes place inside a man's testes and is known as spermatogenesis. After puberty, the testicles make sperm continuously at the rate of about 125 million sperm a day. The whole process, from the initial generation of a sperm to its maturing and ejaculation, takes about seven weeks.

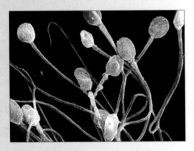

Sperm
Each sperm has a head that contains its genetic material, and a tail for helping it move. A complex network of microscopically tiny tubes within the testes produces spermatids, the forerunners of sperm.

The testes
This cross-section of a testis shows the network of minute tubes that contain the cells from which spermatids are created. These tubes connect with about eight larger tubes; these are the efferent ducts, which carry the developing sperm into the epididymis, where they mature and grow their tails. The testes also produce hormones, the most important being the male sex hormone testosterone, which is the most powerful of the androgens. These hormones are responsible for male secondary sexual characteristics such as facial hair and deepening of the voice, and for male and female sex drives.

The man's role

Sperm, a man's contribution to the conception of his child, are made in his testes (testicles). A man begins making sperm at puberty under the influence of testosterone from the testes, and luteinizing hormone (LH) and follicle-stimulating hormone (FSH) from the pituitary gland. LH and FSH act on the testes as they do on the ovaries. A man goes on making sperm throughout his fertile life and, although the numbers and quality of sperm produced decline from the age of 40, men in their 90s have fathered children. Sperm production speeds up at times of sexual activity, but if ejaculation is very frequent, sperm numbers decrease, lowering a man's fertility.

The mature sperm Each individual sperm is only about $\frac{1}{500}$ in (0.05 mm) long, so it cannot be seen by the naked eye. It's shaped like a tadpole and has a strong tail, five or six times longer than its head, which it uses to move itself along. The tail is attached to the head by a short middle section or body. This contains special cell components called *mitochondria*, which are its energy-producing apparatus. A sperm's head is dark in color because it contains so much genetic material.

The newly formed sperm pass into the *epididymis* at the rear of each testis, where they mature. From the epididymis, matured sperm travel up a tube called the *vas deferens*, which leads to the *seminal vesicle*, a small, saclike structure near the bladder. When a man ejaculates, seminal fluid (semen) is discharged from the penis via the urethra. Semen is made up of sperm, mixed with fluid produced by the seminal vesicle and fluids secreted by the prostate and other glands.

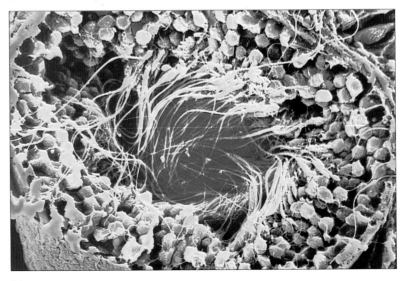

THE MALE REPRODUCTIVE TRACT

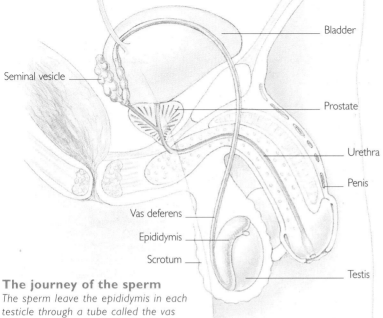

Seminal vesicle

Bladder

Prostate

Urethra

Penis

Vas deferens

Epididymis

Scrotum

Testis

The journey of the sperm
The sperm leave the epididymis in each testicle through a tube called the vas deferens. Each vas deferens, which is about ⅙ in (4 mm) in diameter, runs up the spermatic cord, from which the testis is suspended. From there, each vas deferens loops up around the bladder, down past the seminal vesicle, and into the prostate gland. From the seminal vesicle onward, the vas deferens is known as the ejaculatory duct. At the prostate, each ejaculatory duct joins the urethra, which is the hollow tube inside the penis through which the semen is ejaculated.

EJACULATION
Most men ejaculate about two-thirds of a teaspoon (3.5 ml) of sperm when they make love, but the amount ranges from ½ tsp to 1 tsp (2–6 ml). Each milliliter contains 60–150 million sperm, of which nearly one-quarter are abnormal. Only about three-quarters are *motile* (able to wriggle).

Reaching the egg Although sperm can move ⁄₁₀ inch to ¼ inch (2–3 mm) per minute, their actual speed varies with the acidity of their environment—the higher the acidity, the slower their movement. The vaginal secretions are slightly acidic; so sperm ejaculated into the vagina probably move quite slowly until they reach the more friendly alkaline environment of the uterine cavity. Having gotten through the hostile acidic conditions of the vagina, they then face a longer and more dangerous journey before they reach the egg, far down a fallopian tube. Of about 300 million sperm in an ejaculation, only a few hundred will actually reach the egg. Most of the rest trickle out of the vagina, or are destroyed by vaginal acidity. Others may be swallowed up by cleansing cells within the uterus, enter the wrong fallopian tube, or go into the correct tube but miss the egg altogether.

YOUR BABY'S SEX

The sex of your child depends on whether the fertilizing sperm contains an X chromosome (female) or a Y chromosome (male). The woman's egg always contains an X (female) chromosome.

The X and the Y sperm have different properties. The X sperm (female) are larger, slower, and longer-lived than the Y sperm (male). The X sperm also appears to be favored by the slightly acidic conditions in the vagina.

Some people believe that you can increase your chances of having a male or female baby by when and how often you make love. There's very little scientific evidence to support these ideas, but you may wish to try them if you're eager to choose the gender of your baby.

When For a female baby, make love up to two or three days before ovulation, since only female sperm survive this long. For a male baby, make love on the day of, or just after, ovulation, since the faster male sperm will reach the egg before the female sperm.

How often For a female baby, make love fairly frequently, since this lowers the proportion of male sperm in the semen. For a male baby, make love less often, since this will increase the proportion of male sperm. For most couples, making love every 36 hours around the time of ovulation gives the best chance of conceiving. Making love every day can lower sperm counts. "Saving up" sperm by waiting 10 days is also not a good idea because older sperm don't swim so well.

PENETRATION

This sequence of pictures, taken with an electron microscope, shows fertilization taking place—a sperm penetrating the tough outer membrane of an egg.

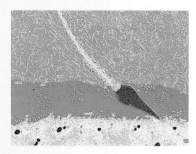

Membrane penetration
The sperm penetrates the membrane of the egg by releasing enzymes that create a hole in it.

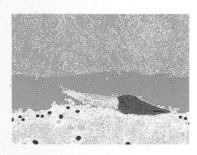

Oocyte penetration
The sperm prepares to penetrate the oocyte, the innermost part of the egg.

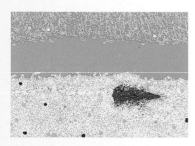

Chromosome transfer
Before joining its chromosomes with those of the egg, the sperm sheds its body and tail.

Fertilization

Fertilization happens when a sperm meets and penetrates an egg. Most human cells contain 46 chromosomes—threadlike structures that carry their genetic information. But sperm cells and egg cells each have only 23 chromosomes. When a sperm and an egg meet and fuse, the resulting fertilized cell has the full 46 chromosomes.

The new cell, which is called a *zygote*, splits first into two identical cells, each with 46 chromosomes. It continues to divide slowly as it travels down the fallopian tube, until it reaches the uterus. By the time it reaches the uterus it is a hollow clump of about 100 cells called a *blastocyst* or *blastula*.

CONCEPTION

Egg meets sperm
The egg is released from its follicle. It travels one-third of the way along the fallopian tube, where it is fertilized.

The fertilized egg keeps dividing as it travels down the fallopian tube

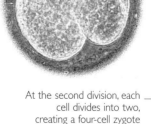

In its first division, the single-cell zygote divides into two identical cells

The third division doubles the cells from four to eight

At the second division, each cell divides into two, creating a four-cell zygote

Cell division
The fertilized egg, now called a zygote, divides repeatedly and eventually forms a solid bundle of cells known as a morula. These cells continue to divide and become a hollow ball of about 100 cells called a blastocyst.

Implantation A week after fertilization has taken place, the blastocyst produces a hormone that helps it to burrow its way into the endometrium. Implantation is usually in the upper one-third of the uterus. The pregnancy is now established and the placenta will start to form.

Twins When a woman releases more than one egg at a time, nonidentical (fraternal) twins may develop from two separate eggs, fertilized by two separate sperm. Each embryo then has its own placenta inside the mother's uterus. Identical twins come from a single egg, fertilized by a single sperm. This egg divides into two, and each develops independently into a genetically identical twin sharing a single placenta. Other multiple pregnancies, such as triplets, start in the same ways as twins and, similarly, the siblings may be identical or fraternal.

Seven days after fertilization, the egg implants itself in the lining of the uterus

Uterus

Embryo development
Once implanted in the uterine lining, the blastocyst then develops into an embryo. It also forms the placenta, the vital link between a baby and its mother. The embryo shown here is about four weeks old.

BOY OR GIRL?

Of the 46 chromosomes that carry the complete human genetic blueprint, the sex of a child is determined by just two, the X and the Y.

The sex chromosomes
A woman's eggs each contain a single X chromosome, while a man's individual sperm carry either an X or a Y chromosome. If an egg is fertilized by an X chromosome sperm, the baby will be a girl (XX). If the sperm has a Y chromosome, the child will be a boy (XY).

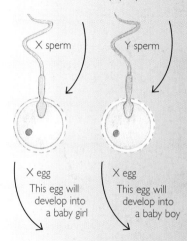

X sperm   Y sperm

X egg
This egg will develop into a baby girl

X egg
This egg will develop into a baby boy

X and Y sperm
A man produces both X sperm and Y sperm. The Y sperm swim faster, but are smaller and live a shorter time than X sperm.

The fully formed baby
By the time a baby is born, repeated cell divisions will have made a highly complex being with several trillion cells from a single cell.

THE AGE FACTOR

The older you are, the longer it can take to conceive, so bear this in mind when you're deciding if you should talk to your doctor about any possible problems. Then again, the older you are, the less time you have, so you might want to get advice early.

- The number of infertile women increases with age: one in 10 women between the ages of 20 and 24 are infertile, but this increases to nearly 30 percent of women age 40–44.

- All treatments for infertility are significantly more successful in couples under 30.

- The overall quality of a woman's eggs diminishes with age, as does the number of healthy eggs produced at any one time.

- A woman's uterus gets less receptive to a fertilized egg as she gets older, so successful implantation is less likely.

THE HORMONE FACTOR

In women, incorrect amounts of luteinizing hormone (LH) and follicle-stimulating hormone (FSH) can affect ovulation (see p.28). In men, these same two hormones, LH and FSH, stimulate the testes to produce sperm, so if a man's pituitary gland does not release enough FSH and LH, his ability to produce sperm will be impaired. In men and women, if the thyroid and adrenal glands are not functioning properly, sperm production and ovulation, respectively, will be affected.

Problems in conceiving

If you're having difficulty getting pregnant, it doesn't necessarily mean you're infertile. Infertility means different things to different people; it certainly means something different to doctors and to couples. Most couples who think they are infertile are only subfertile, and with help they do manage to conceive successfully.

WHAT IS INFERTILITY?

Fertility isn't always a straightforward case of being able, or unable, to conceive. A couple may have no difficulty in conceiving their first child but find they cannot get pregnant a second time; this is called secondary infertility. Another couple, who have both had children with previous partners, may now find that they cannot conceive together.

The fertility of a couple is the sum of their individual fertilities. If both partners have fertility problems, it may be hard for them to conceive. But if one partner's fertility is strong, it may still be possible for the couple to conceive. Most couples do conceive within four to six months of trying. If a couple doesn't manage to get pregnant after six months and they go to their doctor for advice, they're likely to be told to go away, keep trying, and come back after a year if nothing happens.

Age is a factor for women (see column, left). As a woman gets older, the quality of her eggs declines. Statistics show that about 90 percent of women in their twenties will become pregnant within a year of trying, and the rest still have a good chance of becoming pregnant naturally within another year or so. But women in their thirties have a much lower statistical probability of becoming pregnant after a year of trying. They shouldn't wait any longer to get advice.

Ways in which a couple can be helped to conceive a child range from simple advice on sexual technique to drug treatment, surgery, and ultimately the new assisted reproductive technologies (ART) (see p.48). The help is there, but the investigation of infertility can try your patience and resolve. Whichever partner has the fertility problems may feel threatened and even guilty, so be prepared to be generous and supportive.

THE EMOTIONAL IMPACT

Couples who are having problems conceiving may be having other difficulties, too. And if they do go ahead with treatment for infertility, they may find it very stressful—it can mean almost intolerable interference with their sex life and can even erode the love a couple feels for each other. The huge financial costs of investigation and treatment can also be a major source of stress. so it's vital for both partners to be fully committed to this course of action.

Most couples see children as an extension of themselves, as someone to carry on the family name as well as an expansion of their hopes, aims, and ambitions. Being unable to have children can seem like a denial of basic human rights, and an infertile couple can experience feelings of injustice, great disappointment, and grief. The unfulfilled desire for children is a major crisis in the lives of some couples and can made them feel bad about all aspects of life, as well as depressed and guilty. One or both partners may become introspective and antisocial and the relationship may break down under the strain.

THE IMPORTANCE OF COUNSELING

With all the tensions that surround the treatment of infertility, couples need and deserve sound psychological support. If you do decide to start on a course of investigation and treatment, ask your doctor to refer you to a counselor who can help you with the stress of infertility at all stages of its management. Don't feel you have to wait until you find yourselves well into secondary referral; you need help and advice right from the start. Some procedures involve deep self-questioning, which strikes right at the heart of your relationship, and a couple will need a great deal of support. The treatment can also be lengthy and invasive, and there are many ethical issues surrounding assisted reproductive technologies, insemination, and the use of donors.

Psychological factors affecting fertility The way you feel can in itself affect your fertility by causing a hormone disturbance or impotence. So without proper support, fertility treatment may make matters worse. On the other hand, doctors have plenty of anecdotal evidence that some couples suddenly conceive very soon after making the decision to have their infertility investigated. It's as if making the decision to do something about the problem releases the psychological tensions that may have been stopping them from getting pregnant.

UNEXPLAINED INFERTILITY

About 15 percent of couples suffering from fertility problems have to face the fact that their infertility cannot be explained. In those couples, it's tempting to consider radical treatments, but experts generally agree that it's best for them to wait for up to three years, depending on how old the woman is, to see if anything happens naturally. After this there are treatments that can be successful such as GIFT (see p.49) and intrauterine insemination as well as ovarian stimulation by FSH (follicle-stimulating hormone).

Drug treatments with clomiphene, danazol, and bromocriptine are not effective. Investigation to find out whether there could be immunological factors involved may also be fruitful (see p.39).

ISSUES TO CONSIDER

Even before you have professional counseling, it's a good idea to ask yourselves some searching questions, so that some of the issues are out in the open between you from the very beginning.

- If you decided to have fertility treatment, would you tell friends and family, or would you try to keep it a complete secret?

- If you intend to keep it a secret, can you be sure that the truth won't come out, perhaps destructively, at a time of crisis?

- Could you cope with a multiple pregnancy?

- What if one, some, or all of your babies died?

- Having committed so much time and money to having a baby, how easy will you find it to let her go once she grows up?

- How long would you be prepared to persist with infertility treatment?

- Would you consider using donor eggs or sperm?

- Would you think about adoption?

Seeking advice

LIFESTYLE CHANGES

If you are to have the best possible chance of conceiving, you may both have to make some changes in your lifestyle. You're both equally involved and it's important to share the responsibility.

- Stop smoking—both of you.

- Aim for a healthy lifestyle—eat a balanced diet and stay active.

- Do your best to cut down on alcohol (women not more than two units per week, men not more than seven units per week).

- Overweight women can have ovulation problems, so losing weight helps. In one study, 12 out of 13 women who lost 13 lb (6 kg) or more began to ovulate, and 11 out of 12 conceived. Keeping weight within the ideal range is also important for male fertility.

- Don't use temperature charts to find ovulation days (fertile days), and don't confine lovemaking to fertile days; couples used to be advised to time intercourse for these days, but the stress involved can work against you.

- Have penetrative sex two to three times a week.

- Although very frequent sex can diminish the number of sperm in each ejaculate, don't abstain for longer than 10 days or the sperm count will start to fall.

- Women should start taking 0.4 mg of folic acid supplements every day.

- Stop taking illegal drugs. Many of them affect fertility.

First of all, see your family doctor so you can talk about your worries and ask questions. For many couples, the woman seeks advice first, but it's really important for you both to accept that whatever the reasons for your problems, you're both going to need investigation. So try to get off to a good start and make the first visit a joint one.

If you're worried that your doctor won't have time for the kind of detailed, relaxed conversation you need, ask for a longer appointment, perhaps at a time of day when things are less rushed. Or you could try going to the sexual health clinic in your local hospital or a family planning clinic. You don't need a referral from your doctor for either of these, and you should find a team of sympathetic experts able to discuss your problems.

HOW YOUR TREATMENT WILL BE MANAGED

When you first see your doctor, ask how any treatment is likely to be managed. Each stage in the investigation and treatment of infertility should be fully explained to you in a way you can understand, and you'll be given lists of self-help organizations to get in touch with.

Your family doctor may do the initial tests or refer you from the outset. Either way, you'll be referred for all secondary tests and for further treatment to a specialist infertility clinic run by a professional, multiskilled team. Call your insurance company first to find out if your policy covers infertility treatment; many plans do not, and it can be very expensive.

Any infertility treatment is a stressful business, so it's important that the doctors caring for you are relaxed and friendly. The atmosphere of the clinic should be sympathetic so you feel that you'll be listened to properly. The clinic should also provide information on what will be involved, including the pros and cons of any alternative treatments that are relevant.

With this kind of treatment, you have a right to expect that your feelings and preferences are considered by the professionals and that any disagreements will be negotiated between you both. Your doctor and the fertility clinic to which you're referred will want to provide the best possible outcome for you both—that is, for you to conceive and give birth to a healthy baby—but the route to this goal could be rocky, and it's best to be prepared from the outset.

PRIMARY TESTS

Primary tests can be done by your family doctor, although many doctors prefer to refer you. It's important for your partner to be involved, since 30 to 40 percent of infertility is linked to the man's reproductive system. Your doctor will ask about your fertility history as a couple, including your ages, how long you've been trying to conceive, past illnesses or surgery, and any drugs you've been taking that might affect fertility (see column, right). The woman will also be asked about her menstrual cycle, how regular it is, how long her periods last, and whether or not they're painful. You'll also be asked about your job in case either of you could be exposed to dangers at work that may affect fertility. The doctor will also ask about any past sexually transmitted disease in either partner, including chlamydia, and will look at past smear test results.

Primary tests for the woman:
• smear test (if not done recently)
• test for chlamydia (see p.44), which will be treated if found
• physical examination, including an internal examination
• fasting blood glucose and TSH (thyroid stimulating hormone) levels
• a simple blood test for progesterone levels in the second half of the cycle to confirm whether ovulation is taking place.

Primary tests for the man:
• physical examination of the man's penis and testes
• two semen samples to be analyzed by the lab at the clinic where further investigations and secondary tests (see p.41) will be done.

Rapid referral for secondary tests   In some circumstances couples are referred as quickly as possible for secondary investigations at a specialist clinic. These include:
• if either partner is over 35 years of age
• if the woman has a history of *amenorrhea* (absence of periods), or *oligomenorrhea* (sparse or infrequent periods)
• abnormal anatomy on internal examination of the woman or a *varicocele* of the scrotum (see p.39) in the man.

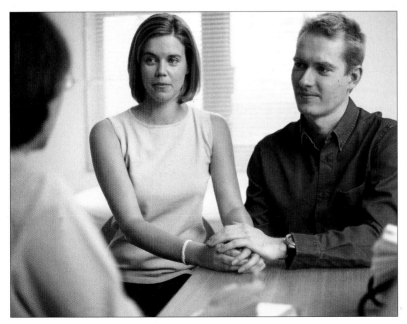

DRUGS THAT CAN AFFECT FERTILITY

Many medications can harm your fertility, affecting sperm, eggs, or sexual activity. Your doctor will want to know if you have been treated with any of the following drugs.

Men
• Sulfasalazine: lowers sperm count

• Nitrofurantoin: lowers sperm count

• Tetracyclines: lower sperm motility

• Cimetidine: causes impotence

• Ketoconazole: causes impotence and lowers sex drive

• Colchicine: lowers fertilization power of sperm

• Antidepressants: cause impotence

• Propranolol: causes impotence

• Chemotherapy: lowers sperm count

• Marijuana and alcohol cause sperm abnormalities; cocaine lowers libido as well as sperm motility and count

Women
• Anti-inflammatories (such as ibuprofen): affect egg follicles

• Chemotherapy: causes ovarian failure

• Marijuana: stops ovulation and interrupts menstruation

Seeing a counselor
It's important to start any investigation of infertility with a thorough talk with your doctor, who'll be able to tell you about the treatment stages and refer you to a specialist fertility clinic where you can see a counselor.

Male infertility

Problems with the sperm themselves are the most common cause of male infertility, although there may also be anatomical problems that affect a man's ability to ejaculate. The study of male fertility is relatively new compared with female fertility, but doctors now know much more about it and about the role of sperm in particular.

PROBLEMS WITH SPERM

Sperm are extremely vulnerable cells. They take seven weeks to form and can be affected by outside influences at any point in their development. Because of this, it's entirely possible for a man to give sperm samples on separate occasions that differ widely both in quality and quantity.

Testicular failure The cause of this is usually hard to establish, but it may be due to a chromosomal problem such as Klinefelter syndrome (when a man has two or more X chromosomes rather than one), testes that did not descend properly after birth, a blow to the testes, such as a sports injury, or the man's having suffered mumps as an adult.

ANATOMICAL PROBLEMS

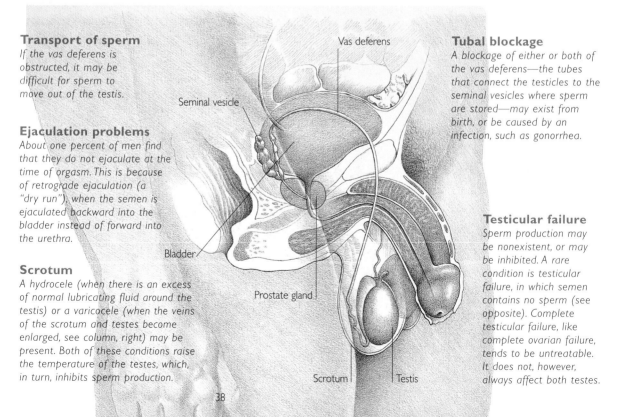

Transport of sperm
If the vas deferens is obstructed, it may be difficult for sperm to move out of the testis.

Ejaculation problems
About one percent of men find that they do not ejaculate at the time of orgasm. This is because of retrograde ejaculation (a "dry run"), when the semen is ejaculated backward into the bladder instead of forward into the urethra.

Scrotum
A hydrocele (when there is an excess of normal lubricating fluid around the testis) or a varicocele (when the veins of the scrotum and testes become enlarged, see column, right) may be present. Both of these conditions raise the temperature of the testes, which, in turn, inhibits sperm production.

Vas deferens

Seminal vesicle

Bladder

Prostate gland

Scrotum | Testis

Tubal blockage
A blockage of either or both of the vas deferens—the tubes that connect the testicles to the seminal vesicles where sperm are stored—may exist from birth, or be caused by an infection, such as gonorrhea.

Testicular failure
Sperm production may be nonexistent, or may be inhibited. A rare condition is testicular failure, in which semen contains no sperm (see opposite). Complete testicular failure, like complete ovarian failure, tends to be untreatable. It does not, however, always affect both testes.

Low sperm counts By itself, a low sperm count does not mean infertility. Many men with low sperm counts father children, but conception tends to take longer. Unfortunately, when there are few sperm, the majority tend to be abnormal or are not very active. Low sperm counts and sperm abnormalities may be caused by hormonal problems, anatomical problems, immunological problems, or even environmental factors.

IMMUNOLOGICAL PROBLEMS

Both men and women may produce antibodies to sperm that can interfere with fertilization, but it's mainly a problem for men. In men, the antibodies are on the surface of sperm, in the semen, or in the blood. In women, antibodies are found in the cervical mucus or in the blood. Antibodies are found in five to 10 percent of infertile couples, but two percent of fertile men also have antibodies.

How antibodies affect fertility The most important antibodies are those that are attached to the sperm themselves: they can affect the way sperm move and their ability to penetrate a woman's cervical mucus and fertilize the egg. Antibodies can also affect the acrosome—the cap on the head of the sperm, which contains enzymes essential for egg penetration (see p.40).

How fertility treatments are affected Antibodies on the surface of the sperm can interfere with IVF (*in vitro fertilization*) and other kinds of ART (assisted reproduction technologies; see p.48). The antibodies can stop sperm from moving and even destroy them. However, the presence of antibodies doesn't necessarily mean that a man can't conceive a child, so many specialists recommend that antibody is not carried only in couples who have "unexplained infertility" (see p.35) and who've already had all the other tests. This is because treatment is difficult and hazardous. The mainstay is moderate to high dosage with steroids, which is known to cause serious fetal side effects in some cases.

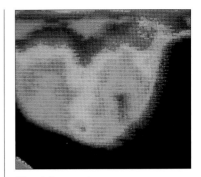

Healthy testes
This thermal photograph shows how healthy testes (blue) are at a lower temperature than the body (orange, top of picture).

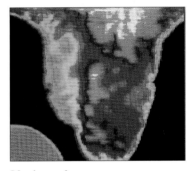

Varicocele
The orange patches on the nearer testis are a varicocele (enlarged veins); the orange color indicates a raised temperature, which can affect normal sperm production.

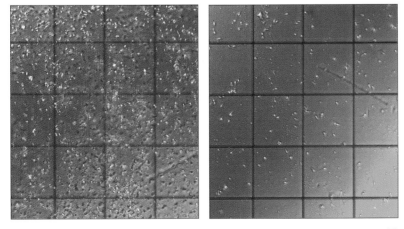

The sperm count
Male fertility is checked by two sperm tests, which also look for any sperm abnormalities. Each milliliter of semen should contain at least 30 million sperm, most of which should be normal. The picture on the left shows a good semen sample. If there are fewer than 20 million sperm per milliliter and there's a high proportion of abnormal sperm, the semen is rated poor. The picture on the right shows an example of poor semen.

Male tests

SEMEN ANALYSIS

If you have to give a semen sample for analysis, follow instructions carefully to make sure that results are accurate and the test won't have to be repeated more than twice.

Taking the sample The man must abstain from sex for three days. He then produces a semen specimen by masturbating into a sterile plastic cup marked with name, date, and the time. The sample is protected from temperature extremes and delivered to the laboratory.

What's healthy? The laboratory would expect the following findings from a healthy semen sample:

Amount: ½ tsp to 1 tsp (2–5ml)

Numbers: more than 20 million sperm per ml

Motility: more than one-half the sperm wriggle

Normality: more than one-third of the sperm are normal

White blood cells: less than 1 million per ml of sperm

When a couple has fertility problems, it's usually the woman who wants to get advice early on, but there's no point in her doing this on her own. If a couple is having difficulty in conceiving, it really doesn't make sense for the man to delay testing. A semen analysis should always be the first test to be done if fertility is to be investigated.

HOW MEN CAN BE HELPED

Studies suggest that sperm counts decreased during the 20th century because of environmental factors such as exposure to estrogens in foodstuffs and chemicals used in the plastics industry that enter the food chain. At one time, much more was known about female infertility than male, but fertility clinics now deal just as much with male problems and diseases. There's a greater chance than ever before that men who have low fertility or are infertile can be helped to achieve natural fatherhood.

Male infertility has nothing to do with virility. A man's sperm may be incapable of fertilizing an egg, yet he may be an excellent lover. In contrast, a man who is unable to make love to a woman may have perfectly viable, fertile sperm.

SEMEN ANALYSIS

One of the first tests for a man is semen analysis. Two samples are usually analyzed, since sperm counts can vary according to circumstances, such as how often he has sexual intercourse. The analysis checks the number of sperm in a sample, how well and how much they move, and their shape. Many specialists believe that even a relatively low sperm count may not affect a man's

ABNORMAL SPERMATOZOA

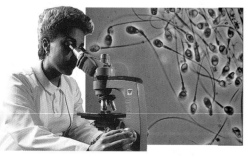

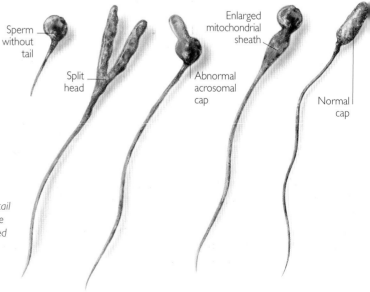

Sperm without tail

Split head

Abnormal acrosomal cap

Enlarged mitochondrial sheath

Normal cap

Examining sperm
If a sperm is to fertilize a female egg successfully, it needs to be properly formed. First, it must have a tail so that it can swim and reach the egg. Second, on the head of the sperm there must be a normal cap, called the acrosome, containing enzymes that play an important part in egg penetration.

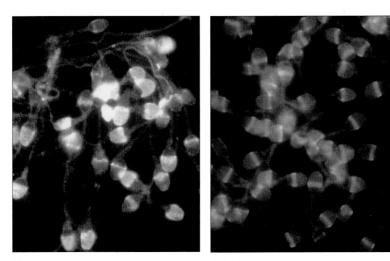

Normal sperm   Defective sperm

Sperm acrosome test
The head of a normal sperm is surrounded by a cap called the acrosome. This contains enzymes that enable the sperm to break through the outer membrane of the egg. If sperm don't have this acrosomal cap, they're incapable of fertilizing an egg. Sperm are tested by using chemicals that glow when they react with the acrosome. These pictures show defective sperm (left) and normal sperm (far left).

fertility. But if he has a low sperm count combined with many sperm that are malformed, move poorly, or both, or if there is a high white blood cell content, then it's likely that his fertility will be affected.

Low sperm counts There are several types of low sperm counts. A semen analysis (see column, left) decides which of the following definitions apply to a particular sperm sample.
• *Azoospermia*: there's no sperm in the semen, either because the man cannot make sperm, he has a blockage affecting the sperm transportation, or he fails to ejaculate
• *Oligospermia*: there are fewer than 20 million sperm per ml of semen. A mild case is fewer than 10–20 million, a moderate case is 5–10 million, and a severe case would be fewer than 5 million
• *Aesthenospermia*: sperm are unable to wriggle even if the count is normal
• *Teratospermia*: a high number of abnormal sperm. This is severe if the man has more than 70 percent abnormal sperm, possibly caused by a chromosomal abnormality or by some kind of environmental damage.

SECONDARY TESTS FOR SPERM FUNCTION

After routine semen analysis (see column, left), microscopic tests of sperm function would be done only at a specialist clinic as part of the secondary stage of investigation of a couple with infertility problems. Special tests examine:
• the ability of sperm to penetrate mucus so they can get through the cervix to the uterus, and from there to the tubes and egg
• the ability of the sperm to recognize the egg and latch on to it—the first step in fertilization (the acrosome test, see above, right)
• the ability to fuse with and fertilize the egg (the egg penetration or hamster test, see column, right).

EGG PENETRATION TEST

A sperm's ability to fertilize an egg can be tested very accurately with the egg penetration test.

The test is done in a laboratory and involves introducing sperm to eggs taken from hamsters and measuring how well the sperm can penetrate and fuse with them.

Hamster eggs are used so that your partner does not have to go through stressful hormone treatment in order to provide eggs for testing. There's no danger of an embryo resulting from the fusion of sperm and these laboratory eggs.

POLYCYSTIC OVARY SYNDROME

Many women have benign ovarian cysts that don't affect fertility. But polycystic ovary syndrome (PCOS) interferes with ovulation and can cause fertility problems.

True PCOS is caused by too much male hormone being produced by the adrenal glands, leading to an abnormally high ratio of LH to FSH. The ovary becomes filled with "cysts"—actually immature follicles that fail to generate eggs. Sufferers have infrequent periods, a tendency to obesity, and excessive body hair.

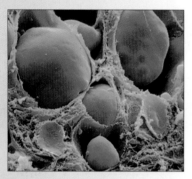

Developing eggs
This hugely magnified picture shows part of a normal ovary, with eggs developing in their follicles.

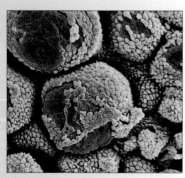

Polycystic ovary
In PCOS, follicles develop into cysts so eggs fail to develop or remain immature.

Female infertility

A huge amount of research has been done over the last few decades into the reasons for female infertility, and great advances have been made in the diagnosis and treatment of problems. The causes of female infertility tend to fall into four main areas, and all of these types can now be treated with varying degrees of success.

FAILURE TO OVULATE

About one-third of female infertility is caused by a woman's failure to release an egg (ovulate). This is usually due to hormonal problems, but occasionally a woman's ovaries are damaged or, more rarely, have run out of eggs.

Hormonal problems   In a woman with a normal ovarian cycle (see p.28), the hormones from the pituitary gland and the ovary are responsible for the healthy growth and maintenance of an egg. In many cases of infertility, too little of one or too much of the other hormone may be present.

For example, at midcycle the hypothalamus should stimulate the pituitary gland to release a massive amount of FSH (follicle-stimulating hormone) and LH (luteinizing hormone) to bring about ovulation, but in 20 percent of cases it fails to do so. So although there may be some FSH and LH, there's not enough for ovulation to take place.

Alternatively, a woman's pituitary gland may be damaged or malfunctioning, causing it to produce either too much FSH and LH or none at all. Or, as a result of too much LH stimulation and not enough FSH, the ovaries may become polycystic (see column, left for more information on this condition) and no longer capable of producing mature eggs.

Problems caused by abnormal hormone levels are often treated with fertility drugs. These include clomiphene, human chorionic gonadotrophin (hCG), and human menopausal gonadotrophin (hMG), in addition to female and pituitary hormones. For 90 percent of women whose infertility is caused by hormonal problems, modern drug therapy can bring about regular ovulation. Unfortunately, for reasons doctors do not yet understand, only about 65 percent of these women will actually get pregnant.

HORMONAL IMBALANCE

Hormones may interfere with conception in other ways than influencing ovulation. For example, a fertilized egg needs progesterone in order to survive. If too little progesterone is produced or it's produced for too short a time, the egg may not survive. Known as *inadequate luteal phase*, this condition can be treated with drugs.

Hyperprolactinemia In this common condition, the body produces too much of the pituitary hormone responsible for milk production. The condition can sometimes be due to a small benign tumor on the pituitary gland called a *prolactinoma*. This leads to an imbalance of FSH and LH, causing infrequent or absent periods in women and lowered sperm production in men.

FIBROIDS AND FERTILITY

Fibroids are benign muscle tumors that can be from the size of pea to a tennis ball. They form within the uterine wall. Fibroids don't necessarily affect fertility, but they can make the uterus misshapen and compress one or both of the fallopian tubes.

Effects on fertility If no other cause for infertility is found, it may be that moderately sized fibroids close to the surface of the uterine lining are interfering with normal implantation of the embryo in the uterus. If they are near the junction of the uterus and the fallopian tubes, they may stop the fertilized egg from reaching the uterus at all.

Fibroids are most common in women over the age of 35, and about one in 45 women develops fibroids by the time she is 45. There's often no cause for concern, since many women with fibroids have no trouble conceiving, but if fibroids do cause problems, they can be removed in an operation called a *myomectomy*. This operation should not be undertaken lightly—it carries a very high risk of bleeding and may require a blood transfusion in as many as 50 percent of cases.

ENDOMETRIOSIS

If you suffer from very painful periods (dysmenorrhea), it's possible that you're suffering from endometriosis, and this will need to be checked.

Endometriosis is a common condition in which cells from the endometrium (the lining of the uterus) spread to other sites in the ovaries, pelvis, and tubes. These respond to the cyclical changes of ovarian hormones, so they bleed when you're menstruating, causing severe abdominal and pelvic pain. Endometriosis interferes with ovulation and, possibly, conception, and causes fertility problems, and should always be looked for in such cases.

STRUCTURAL PROBLEMS

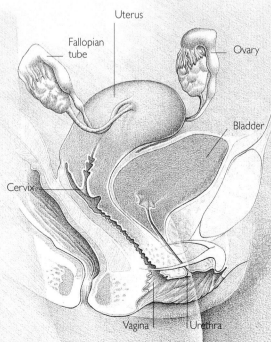

Tubal damage
A previous ectopic pregnancy (see p.225), previous surgery, pelvic inflammation, endometriosis, or an infection, particularly chlamydia (see p.44), may cause blocked or damaged tubes that will prevent natural conception.

Problems with fertilization
In order to reach an egg and fertilize it, sperm must swim through the mucus in the cervix. If there is too little mucus or if it's very thick, sperm cannot get through the cervical canal. If the mucus contains antibodies that attack the sperm directly, the sperm will never reach the egg, so fertilization won't happen.

Uterus
Fallopian tube
Ovary
Bladder
Cervix
Vagina
Urethra

Damage to the ovaries
The ovaries may fail to produce mature eggs. Scarring, caused by surgery, infection, or as a side effect of radiation treatment, can damage the ovary. Or the supply of eggs may become exhausted earlier than normal. This can be due to menopause or its premature onset, surgical damage, or radiation therapy.

Uterine conditions
About 10 percent of infertility cases are caused by problems with the uterus. The uterus may be congenitally abnormal in shape; contain scars, polyps, or fibroids; or be subject to endometriosis (see above).

Female tests

CHLAMYDIA INFECTION

The most common bacterial sexually transmitted infection, chlamydia can cause fertility problems. Up to 70 percent of women have no symptoms, so they don't know they've been infected and aren't treated.

You'll be tested for chlamydia infection as part of your primary investigations because the condition can cause pelvic inflammatory disease (PID). One episode of PID has a 10 percent chance of causing blockage of the fallopian tubes, with the risk rising to 50 percent after three episodes.

The incidence of PID can be reduced by the following:

- selective screening of high-risk women for cervical chlamydia infection, which can be done with a smear test

- screening of all women age 25 years or younger, plus women who have had two or more partners in the last year, who make up nearly 90 percent of infections

- any infertility test involving an instrument being inserted into the uterus can aggravate a cervical infection, so this shouldn't be done without first checking for chlamydia.

Testing for chlamydia infection includes a blood antibody test, cervical swabs for culture, and DNA tests. Sexual partners must be notified, assessed, and treated, since chlamydia may play a part in male infertility, too.

One of the aims of the *primary tests* you'll have is to find out whether or not you are ovulating. If you are, the fertility clinic will start a range of more advanced tests to discover why you haven't been able to conceive. These tests will check the condition of your hormones, ovaries, uterus, and fallopian tubes and look at how well they're functioning.

HORMONE AND OVULATION TESTS

Measuring the levels of hormones in your blood during your menstrual cycle can give useful information. Generally, levels are checked during the first three days of your cycle and again seven days before your period is due. The measurements show how your ovaries, brain, pituitary, and hypothalamus are interacting, and highlight any imbalance in your hormones that may be causing a problem with ovulation. Usually, your estrogen, progesterone, and LH levels are measured and compared to normal ones. Other hormones that can affect ovulation are FSH, testosterone, and prolactin; levels of these in the blood will be checked.

Ultrasound scanning With a simple scan, your fertility specialist can check the development of your ovarian follicles and confirm that you're ovulating. Tracking of the follicle in this way is important if you're taking drugs to stimulate ovulation, as it can help avoid overstimulation, which can be dangerous. Your doctors will also need an accurate assessment of your follicular growth if they need to perform complex assisted conception procedures such as IVF (in vitro fertilization) (see pp.50–1).

Endometrial biopsy Under the influence of estrogen and progesterone, the endometrium (lining of the uterus) changes through the menstrual cycle. There's a definite endometrial thickening and growth during the second half of the menstrual cycle following ovulation, because of the increased amount of progesterone in the body. But if not enough progesterone is made, the endometrium may not be sufficiently developed to allow the embryo to implant successfully. In a biopsy, a tiny sample of your endometrium is taken during the second half of the menstrual cycle. It's examined under a microscope, where any changes due to progesterone levels will be visible.

FALLOPIAN TUBE TESTS

The fallopian tubes are extremely delicate structures. Less than $\frac{5}{32}$ in (4 mm) in diameter at their narrowest, they are easily damaged. Up to one-third of all of the women who attend an infertility clinic are found to have a problem with their fallopian tubes. Once the primary tests have been completed, there are a number of tests that are carried out to check the fallopian tubes. These are among the first investigations made when an infertile couple attends a specialist clinic.

Hysterosalpingogram An HSG is an X-ray picture of the uterus and tubes and can reveal problems inside them. A special dye that can be monitored on an X-ray screen is slowly injected into the uterus and should pass into the fallopian tubes. If it fails to do so, there may be some damage, distortion, or blockage.

Laparoscopy The laparoscope (see below) is a slender telescope—only about the width of a fountain pen—that uses fiber optics to look directly into your abdominal cavity. It gives a superb view of all the organs, allowing your surgeon to assess their health and giving information on adhesions, endometriosis, and ovarian disease. High-quality videos can also be taken through the laparoscope so that your doctors can refer to them later. Although you'll need to have a general anesthetic, laparoscopy can usually be done as an outpatient procedure.

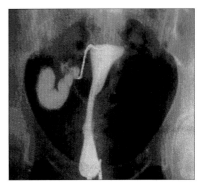

Blocked fallopian tubes
This X-ray image, produced during a hysterosalpingogram, shows that the left fallopian tube is blocked near the uterus. The dye hasn't been able to enter this tube.

USING A LAPAROSCOPE

The laparoscope—a thin viewing tube—is inserted through a tiny incision in the patient's abdomen. This is one of the most important and useful tests for finding out whether a woman's tubes are damaged or blocked.

Healthy ovary
Laparoscopy is useful for showing that organs are healthy, as well as revealing any problems. This picture, taken through a laparoscope, shows a healthy ovary with a mature follicle that will soon burst to release an egg.

Reasons for a laparoscopy
This procedure is commonly used in female infertility treatment. During laparoscopy, eggs may be removed for use in IVF (in vitro fertilization) (see p.50).

An enlarged image, from a tiny camera attached to the tip of the tube, appears on the monitor

A thin tube is inserted into the patient's abdomen

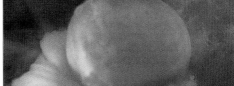

TREATING POLYCYSTIC OVARY SYNDROME

For some women, weight loss is a simple solution to PCOS. If drug treatment is needed, its aim is to stimulate ovulation and produce a healthy egg.

Weight loss

After losing weight, many women with PCOS ovulate normally. A loss of as little as 5 percent has been shown to improve the metabolic and reproductive abnormalities of PCOS. Being obese increases the risks of problems in pregnancy.

Drug treatments

- Clomiphene to induce ovulation

- FSH injection in clomiphene-resistant women.

FIMBRIOPLASTY

A blocked fallopian tube can be opened up with a microsurgical technique known as *fimbrioplasty*. When an egg is released at ovulation, it can then enter the tube and meet the sperm one-third of the way down to bring about fertilization.

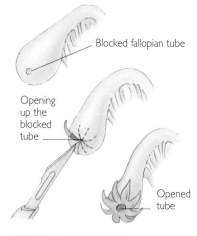

Blocked fallopian tube

Opening up the blocked tube

Opened tube

Treatments for female infertility

If a woman is not ovulating, her ovaries can nearly always be encouraged to produce good-quality eggs by using fertility drugs. These drug treatments used to produce a large number of multiple pregnancies, but much more is now known about the correct dosage, and treatment is very carefully controlled and monitored.

DRUG TREATMENTS

Clomiphene This is the most common fertility drug and is taken for five days at the start of each menstrual cycle. Clomiphene stimulates the release of follicle-stimulating hormone (FSH) by the pituitary gland. This acts on the ovaries and often triggers the ripening of a follicle and then ovulation, usually five to 10 days after the last tablet is taken. Clomiphene's advantages are that it has no major side effects and has a low multiple pregnancy rate— only five to 10 percent. There's a possible association with ovarian cancer after 12 cycles, so if conception isn't achieved after about six cycles, you may be advised to try ART (see p.48).

Clomiphene-resistant PCOS If you're suffering from polycystic ovarian syndrome (PCOS) (see p.42) but you've failed to ovulate or conceive after six months' treatment with clomiphene, your doctors may suggest you have surgery such as ovarian drilling. In this operation, holes are drilled in the surface of your ovary with diathermy or laser in order to stimulate ovulation. If ovulation has not been achieved in three cycles of clomiphene, metformin may be added to reduce insulin levels. This has been found to work best in women who were obese and lost weight during treatment. This drug should be stopped if you become ill, and should not be taken at all if you have renal abnormalities.

Alternatively, you could be given a course of follicle-stimulating hormone (FSH) by injection. The success rates of this treatment are quite high—there's an ovulation rate of about 95 percent per cycle and pregnancy rates of up to 25 percent after three cycles.

Dexamethasone For women with adrenal overactivity as shown by excess hair growth and rising DHEAS levels, dexamethasone may be given to suppress the adrenal gland. It is given in conjunction with clomiphene and has an increased success rate in these women.

Pulsatile GnRH Hypothalamic infertility with amenorrhea is caused by the absence of a hormone called *gonadotrophin releasing factor*, (GnRH), which is made in the part of the brain called the hypothalamus. The role played by GnRH in fertility is to force another part of the brain, the pituitary gland, to release FSH and LH, which in turn stimulate the ovary to ovulate. Women who are deficient in GnRH can be treated with hormone replacements. These are usually given in intravenous "pulses" to mimic normal secretions at 60, 90, and 120 minutes, in an increasing dose per pulse. Ovulation rates as high as 75 percent and pregnancy rates up to 15 percent per cycle can be achieved after GnRH replacement treatment.

Bromocriptine If a woman has high levels of the hormone prolactin in her blood, normal GnRH pulses may be suppressed, so she does not ovulate and cannot conceive. Bromocriptine is the best treatment for this condition—it suppresses prolactin production so the ovaries work properly again, and ovulation rates can be as high as 75 percent. If a woman does get pregnant, bromocriptine treatment should be stopped, but there are no known cases of miscarriage, prematurity, fetal abnormalities, or multiple pregnancies as a result of taking this drug.

SURGICAL PROCEDURES

Microsurgical techniques, involving laparoscopy (see p.45), have greatly improved doctors' ability to repair damaged fallopian tubes.

Tuboplasty (see below, right) Scarred and narrowed fallopian tubes can be unblocked by an operation known as tuboplasty. A small balloon-tipped catheter is inserted into the blocked fallopian tube. The balloon is then inflated to open the damaged tube and create a passage for fertilized or unfertilized eggs to pass through to reach the uterus. The balloon is then deflated and removed.

Fimbrioplasty (see left) Sometimes the frondlike ends of the fallopian tube (known as the fimbriae) fuse together, blocking the opening of the tube and preventing eggs from entering from the ovary. Microsurgical techniques allow the blocked end of the tube to be opened, giving free access for eggs once again.

Reversal of sterilization Reversal of female sterilization is an increasing part of the treatment of infertility. Around three out of every 100 women who are sterilized regret it later and ask for the operation to be reversed, often because they've begun a new relationship and want to have children with their new partner.

If the severed ends of the fallopian tubes are rejoined, the woman has a good chance of achieving a normal pregnancy—rates are as high as 92 percent—but this does depend on the expertise of the surgeons at your particular clinic. Unfortunately, in some clinics, success rates may be less than 50 percent, so it is worth checking this.

Sterilization in which the tubes have been clamped with clips has the highest chance of being successfully reversed. However, IVF (see p.48) may be the treatment of choice for sterilized women, the pregnancy rate being about one in six.

TREATING ENDOMETRIOSIS

Although drug treatments don't help infertility caused by endometriosis (see p.43), the condition can be treated quite successfully by surgery.

Laparoscopic surgery (see p.45) can be used to destroy all visible signs of endometriosis. This increases the chance of conceiving by almost 75 percent in the first 36 weeks after treatment in women under age 40 with mild endometriosis.

Assisted reproduction technology, or ART (see p.48), may be an option for women who don't conceive after laparoscopic surgery, whether or not they have tube problems, and for women with moderate to severe endometriosis.

Some US specialists believe it's better to go straight to ART, without surgical intervention first.

TUBOPLASTY

This procedure is used to open up fallopian tubes that have become scarred or blocked.

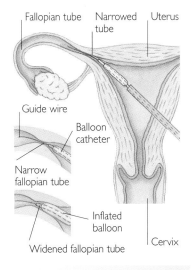

Fallopian tube Narrowed tube Uterus

Guide wire

Balloon catheter

Narrow fallopian tube

Inflated balloon

Cervix

Widened fallopian tube

MEDICAL RISKS OF ART

ART gives many couples new hope, and if all goes well it can result in a healthy pregnancy and a bouncing baby. But it's important to remember that, even if you do conceive, the pregnancy is at a higher risk than usual:

- high miscarriage rate (25 percent)

- high rate of ectopic pregnancies (4 percent)

- high rate of complications (15 percent)

- high rate of premature births (20 percent)

- high rate of cesarean sections (15 percent)

- high rate of multiple pregnancies (15 percent).

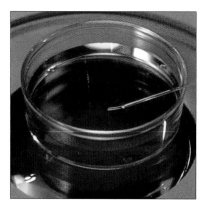

IVF
Harvested eggs are placed in liquid in a petri dish and mixed with sperm. A fertilized egg(s) is then placed in the uterus for implantation.

ART
(assisted reproduction technology)

Assisted reproduction technology has helped many childless couples to become parents. What was once known as in vitro fertilization (IVF) has expanded into a number of different techniques aimed at helping a man and woman conceive and give birth to a healthy child. The rewards are wonderful, but the emotional costs of ART can be high, and any couple considering treatment will need plenty of expert support and counseling.

WHAT IS ART?

ART is a term used to describe a whole range of infertility treatments (see chart, right). Through drugs, laboratory techniques, and even the use of sperm or egg donors, both men and women can be helped to bring about sperm production, ovulation, fertilization, implantation, conception, and birth.

WHY YOU MAY NEED ART

If you or your partner has problems with any stage in the chain of events leading to a healthy baby, you may need ART. Possible difficulties include failure to produce normal, active sperm, failure to ovulate, and failure of healthy sperm to penetrate and fertilize an egg.

ETHICAL CONSIDERATIONS

The science of assisted reproduction technology raises enormous ethical questions that affect the individual, the couple, the family, the community, and society. Most of us would say that if this technology helps a couple who are desperate for a child but have fertility problems, it is morally acceptable. But each situation can be complicated by experience, cultural background, the law, and religious teaching.

Discussing alternatives Each member of a couple has a unique perspective and interest. In addition, there are the interests of the potential child to consider. I don't feel that doctors have the right to question a couple who opt for treatment for infertility. To my mind, the only option is to offer the couple expert counseling so they can discuss alternatives like adoption and the use of donor sperm or eggs.

It's important for specialists to understand that an infertile couple is in a vulnerable position. They bear a heavy responsibility to see that every couple receives impeccable investigation and therapy.

Contentious issues Most people agree that there is no moral problem with ART using the sperm and eggs of partners, the only objection being from the Roman Catholic church. The use of donor eggs, sperm, or even embryos, however, is highly sensitive. Arguments against it include that it violates marriage vows and blurs a child's genetic makeup. On the other hand, all the evidence points to a reassuring track record for such children.

Laws regarding ART vary widely from state to state. In general, donors and surrogates receive some compensation, although this is usually classified as payment for lost wages or inconvenience, rather than direct payment for genetic material or the relinquishing of parental rights. Children conceived through ART have no inherent right to learn the identity of their donors, but provisions for eventual disclosure are often incorporated in the donor's individual contract.

Cryopreservation (freezing of donor sperm or pre-embryos) is another area of concern. Despite religious opposition, cryopreservation has proved to be useful in improving pregnancy rates while avoiding multiple pregnancies. Most moral arguments object only to the fact that some pre-embryos will not survive. In principle, cryopreservation preserves individual human life.

Ethics is not an exact science. There is no absolute moral right and wrong. To impose a moral imperative on another, unwilling person is nothing less than tyranny and flies in the face of enhancing the moral dignity of a couple and their children.

PSYCHOLOGICAL IMPACT

Undergoing any form of ART is stressful. The biggest strains happen at key moments—for example:

- **During ovarian stimulation**
  Anxiety about techniques and the hormonal effects can lead to fear and tension, constraining sexual needs

- **During laboratory investigation**
  Couples fear that embryos might get mixed up or damaged

- **After embryo transfer**
  There may be worry about implantation problems or high order multiple pregnancy.

ART: What the initials mean

IVF	In vitro fertilization (see p.50). Fertilization takes place outside the body, in a glass dish (in vitro means "in glass"), and the fertilized embryo or embryos are replaced into the uterus. Helpful for a woman whose fallopian tubes are damaged, in cases of severe endometriosis, immune problems, unexplained infertility, and older women who have deteriorating egg production.
GIFT	Gamete intra-fallopian transfer. Sperm and ovum are mixed outside the body and immediately transferred back into the fallopian tube so that fertilization can happen "naturally." GIFT is cheaper and has a higher pregnancy rate than IVF, but can only be used for women with healthy fallopian tubes.
ZIFT	Zygote intra-fallopian transfer. As GIFT, except a very young embryo is transferred to the fallopian tube.
SUZI	Subzonal insemination. A type of IVF in which sperm are carefully selected and injected underneath the *zona pellucida* (the outer layer of the egg). This helps men with low sperm counts.
MIST	Micro-insemination sperm transfer. See SUZI above.
ICSI	Intra-cytoplasmic sperm injection. An amazing technique in which a single sperm is selected, specially treated, and injected directly into the egg itself (see p.52). When fertilization has taken place by IVF, the embryo is transferred in the usual way.
MESA	Micro-epididymal sperm aspiration. The surgical extraction of sperm from the epididymis is needed for men who have no sperm in their ejaculate, because of a blocked vas deferens. It precedes ICSI.
TESE	Testicular sperm extraction. As MESA, except the sperm are collected from the testis for ICSI.

The typical pattern of an IVF treatment

Several difficult and complex steps have to be gone through so that you can have your baby: harvesting your eggs; fertilization of the eggs by healthy sperm; implantation of at least one embryo into your uterus; pregnancy to term, and delivery of a healthy baby.

ENSURING A GOOD EGG SUPPLY

So that you have the best chance of a successful pregnancy through IVF treatment, more than one egg at a time is removed for fertilization. Normally a woman will only shed one egg during each ovarian cycle, but a few days after the end of your period your ovaries will be stimulated with drug treatment to make them produce more than one egg. You'll be given drugs, such as clomiphene or hMG (human menopausal gonadotrophin), so that your ovaries produce a number of eggs simultaneously.

RETRIEVING THE MATURE EGGS

Using ultrasound to give a clear picture of the reproductive tract, a gynecologist delicately guides a thin, hollow probe through the vagina and uterus and along a fallopian tube toward the ripened eggs. These eggs are then drawn into the probe by gentle suction.

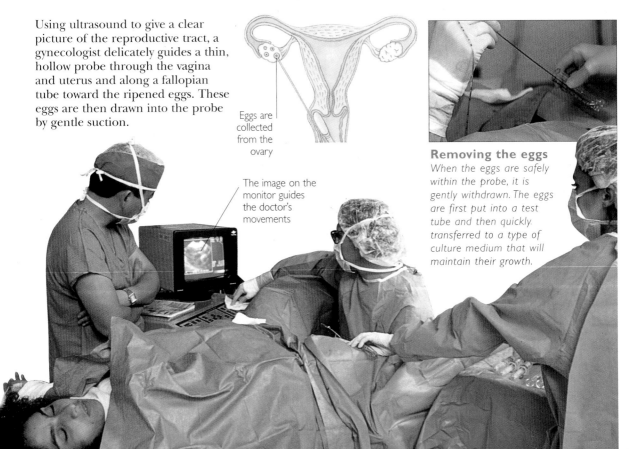

Eggs are collected from the ovary

The image on the monitor guides the doctor's movements

Removing the eggs
When the eggs are safely within the probe, it is gently withdrawn. The eggs are first put into a test tube and then quickly transferred to a type of culture medium that will maintain their growth.

Over the next week or so you'll need to go to the fertility clinic every day so that the development of your eggs can be carefully monitored with ultrasound scans. As the eggs mature, the follicles containing them swell and produce increasing amounts of estrogen. A series of blood tests will detect this increase in estrogen, and the growth of follicles can be precisely measured and tracked by a daily scan.

COLLECTING THE EGGS

When ovulation is imminent, your mature eggs are collected at your clinic under ultrasonic or laparoscopic guidance. Then they're ready for fertilization by your partner's sperm.

Ultrasonic guidance The use of ultrasound pictures to guide the egg retrieval probe is less invasive than using a laparoscope (see below). It can be carried out under light or local anesthetic, instead of a general, and you'll need to spend only a few hours at the fertility clinic.

Laparoscopy (see p.45). This is an another method of viewing your abdominal cavity. The laparoscope, a small, very thin telescope, is passed into your pelvic cavity through a small incision made in your navel. It gives the surgeon direct vision while using a fine, hollow probe to collect ripened eggs from your ovaries. You'll need a general anesthetic for a laparoscopy, and a small amount of carbon dioxide gas will be injected into your abdominal cavity to separate the organs so that the surgeons can see them more easily.

Returning eggs
Once the eggs and sperm have been mixed outside the body, a successfully fertilized egg is injected through the cervix into the uterus for implantation.

CONFIRMING CONCEPTION

The harvested eggs are mixed with your partner's semen, and 18 hours later they're inspected under a microscope to find out if any have been fertilized. It's uncommon for all the eggs to be fertilized and develop into embryos, but two or three usually do. Fertilized eggs are incubated for 48 hours or more, when they will have divided into two to four cells. Provided they show no signs of abnormality, a maximum of three embryos are transferred (see p.53) to your uterus.

The picture on the right shows a sperm approaching an egg.

Advanced ART

Micromanipulation, an extraordinary technique in which not only eggs but individual sperm can be manipulated by a surgeon, makes it possible for a man with a very low sperm count and virtually no active sperm to fertilize his partner's egg and so produce a baby.

MICROMANIPULATION

ICSI (Intracytoplasmic sperm injection, see p.49) is a technique that uses micromanipulation. A prepared egg is placed under a microscope and injected with an individual sperm (see below). Sperm may be collected by masturbation or from the testis itself through surgical techniques such as MESA or TESE (see p.49). Once fertilized, the embryo is incubated and implanted by embryo transfer (see opposite) when it reaches two to four cells in size. ICSI may be offered to couples who fail to conceive by other methods. However, there's some controversy about this

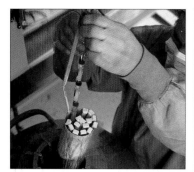

Frozen sperm
Sperm frozen in liquid nitrogen can be used during ICSI procedures. This works particularly well for men with a low sperm count or for sperm with poor movement, since the sperm can be stored and then injected directly into the prepared egg.

ICSI (Intracytoplasmic sperm injection)
In ICSI, an egg is placed under a microscope and then injected with an individual sperm (see right). If the egg is fertilized, it is placed inside the woman's uterus ready for implantation, a process known as "embryo transfer" (see opposite).

Timetable for ICSI
Below is a timeline showing the steps in ICSI through drug treatment to embryo transfer: the principles would be the same for other forms of IVF.

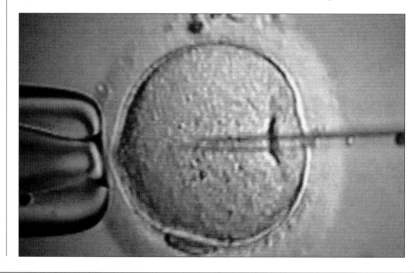

TIMETABLE FOR ICSI (INTRACYTOPLASMIC SPERM INJECTION)

DAY 1	2	3	4	5	6	7	8	9	10	11	12	13	14	15	16	17	18	19

◄———————————————— **DRUG TREATMENT TO ENSURE GOOD EGG SUPPLY** ————————————————►

Days 1-10
Drugs (LH/RH agonists) to suppress menstrual cycle

Days 11-21
Daily gonadotrophin (FSH) injections to stimulate follicle

Day 1
1st day of menstrual cycle

Day 10
Blood test to confirm suppression

Day 14
1st ultrasound scan to check follicle development

Days 18-21
Daily scans to check growth of follicles. On day final scan confirms one follicle is 16–18 mm, oth at least 14 mm, then final FSH injection is give

technique. For example, there's concern that an egg could be fertilized with a substandard sperm, resulting in unhealthy children. But although the pregnancy rate with ICSI is not high, the babies born so far have been normal.

EMBRYO TRANSFER

All forms of IVF (see p.49) mean taking an embryo, usually between two and three days old, from the incubating dish in the laboratory and placing it inside a woman's body. Sadly, two out of three embryo transfers fail to implant. Successful implantation depends on the age of the mother, how receptive her uterus is, and the quality of the embryo. One of the problems is that doctors still don't know when is the best time to transfer an embryo. Studies seem to suggest that delaying the transfer of an embryo to the uterus can increase the chances of implantation. But in one study, there was no difference in pregnancy rates between embryos that were replaced 44 hours after insemination and those that were replaced 68 hours after insemination.

Also, pregnancy rates increase with the numbers of embryos that are replaced: for example, one embryo gives an eight percent chance of becoming pregnant; two embryos give a 25 percent chance. Usually, embryos are transferred at the 8- to 10-cell stage, 72–80 hours after retrieval. Transfer of more than one embryo increases the chance of pregnancy, but the multiple pregnancy rate for IVF is up to 35 percent. This results in an increased likelihood of premature birth, cesarean sections, and newborn illnesses and mortality.

Cryopreserved embryos (see p.49). It's also possible to thaw out cryopreserved (frozen) embryos or eggs from liquid nitrogen (–459°F/–273°C) and transfer them in the same way. The embryo is thawed slowly, at a rate of 46°F (8°C) per minute. However, not all embryos survive this process in a good enough state to implant. Replacement in the womb is done at a point in the menstrual cycle 100 hours after the LH (luteinizing hormone) peak, which is determined by serial blood tests. Pregnancy rates vary from one in six to one in four.

THE FUTURE OF ART

Living proof of the success of this advanced technology are the thousands of ART babies who are now alive and well.

Many doctors feel that ART has gone as far as it can—the pregnancy rate has reached 22 percent, the same as the natural chance to conceive. But there is still much to learn and to do:

- *superovulation* of the ovaries—increasing the number of eggs a woman produces will probably be achieved
- further studies will be made on embryos before transfer
- more research on implantation of the embryo in the uterus
- more research on male infertility, perhaps as the result of refinement of ICSI (see opposite) or the invention of some other method of sperm treatment
- more investigation into cryopreservation techniques, to improve egg-freezing methods and the low pregnancy rate with freeze-thawed embryos
- in vitro maturation of eggs.

	THE STAGES OF FERTILIZATION				26	27	28	29	30	31	32	33	34	35
21	22	23	24	25										
	Day 22 Sperm collected; eggs collected; 6–8 eggs fertilized by ICSI and put in incubator	**Day 23** Eggs checked for initial fertilization	**Day 24** Eggs checked for first cell division	**Day 25** Two 2- or 4-cell embryos transferred to womb					**Days 26–35** Daily progesterone dose to support embryo					
	IVF			EMBRYO TRANSFER										**Day 35** Blood test and scan to confirm pregnancy

If you're thinking of using donors, or a *surrogate* mother, you'll need to have some special counseling to help you through what can be a difficult process.

Using donors can cause tension and disagreement between partners, and it's important to try to be sympathetic to each other's reactions. Sometimes one partner may feel that a donor is being used because of poor sexual performance or procreative failure, and this can cause emotions of guilt or even feelings of subconscious accusation or blame. You also need to think about how you would feel about a child conceived this way. Ask yourself these questions:

- if you were to have a child using donor sperm, or eggs, or both, would the fact that the child wasn't "yours" prevent you from loving her as your own?

- would you feel jealous if a donor conceived a child with your partner when you couldn't?

- would you tell your child about how she was conceived, or would you try to keep it a secret?

- if your child was conceived using donor eggs, or sperm, or both, how would you cope if she wanted to trace her genetic history in later life? And would you be willing to help her?

Using donors

Many childless parents have been helped to become parents by using sperm, eggs, and even embryos given by other people. Surrogacy is also a form of donation—a woman donates her uterus to bear another couple's biological child. Emotional costs can be high for all concerned, and all the issues need to be talked about openly.

DONOR INSEMINATION

The use of donor sperm can be an option in the following situations: when the male partner is sterile or has a very low sperm count that does not respond to treatment; for a couple with a major blood group incompatibility—for example, for a Rhesus-negative woman who has developed antibodies to the Rhesus-positive blood of her partner; when either partner carries a hereditary abnormality; or when a mature, stable, single woman wants a child but not a partner.

Donor insemination (DI) can look like an ideal solution for people in these situations, but there are a number of points that need careful thought. First, the feelings of your partner—some men feel inadequate or even jealous of donors who impregnate their partners. These feelings can affect your life together, and your child once it is born. In addition, some women are repelled by the way they are going to conceive or by the fact that a different man's sperm is used at each visit. Others worry about what kind of man the donor was, or idealize him as a "perfect man." They wonder if their child could unknowingly meet, and perhaps marry, a half-sibling. Using sperm from a donor that you know, or are related to by marriage, can relieve some of these problems, but it can make others worse. It also raises its own problems, such as what happens if the father wants visiting rights.

Most couples feel hesitant about this method of conception, and it's exceedingly stressful, so you do need good counseling. You can insist that there is no mention of DI in your maternity records, and your and your partner's names can be given on the birth certificate. The procedure is covered by law in many, but not all, states. All doctors should be familiar with the donor insemination laws in their state. Currently, donors are anonymous, but it has recently been suggested that their personal information should be kept on file. If children conceived this way want to know their donor's identity once they reach adulthood, they could then be told, provided the donor agrees. Children born from donor insemination have routine pregnancy care and are not at increased risk of pregnancy complications.

EGG DONATION

If a woman is unable to produce an egg herself, donor eggs may be used during IVF treatment. Egg donation does have the advantage that both of you are involved: your partner fertilizes the egg, and you will carry and give birth to the baby. However, it's more complicated than sperm donation—hormonal drugs have to be taken and the eggs collected by surgical techniques (see p.50)—so donor eggs are hard to come by. The main sources are relatives, unknown donors (who, like sperm donors, will no longer have the right to anonymity), and IVF patients who may donate extra eggs produced during their treatment.

There can be problems with egg donation. For example, eggs donated by IVF mothers have an increased risk of chromosomal disorders because IVF patients tend to be older than average. When relatives or friends donate eggs, there can be tensions later.

If you're not producing eggs, you probably won't be menstruating, and this means that the lining of your uterus (endometrium) will be thin and incapable of nourishing a developing embryo. Consequently, you'll need to be given drugs to stimulate it to thicken so that the embryo can implant.

EMBRYO DONATION

A couple who have been through IVF treatment may sometimes wish to donate unused frozen embryos to a childless couple. The embryo is implanted and the woman gives birth to the "adopted" child. Feelings run high on this, and many sensitive issues have been raised. For example, how would the donor parents feel if their own child, or children, die? And what are the chances of the siblings meeting and perhaps having children together?

SELECTING SEMEN AND EMBRYOS

Semen Fresh semen is usually frozen and stored before being used for donor insemination. After collection, the semen is put into a sterile vial and frozen by immersing it in liquid nitrogen. It's then stored while the clinic tests it and the donor for infections. The donor is tested to make sure that he's free of infections, such as hepatitis B or HIV, that could be passed on via his semen. Once it's been determined that the donor was free of infection when he made his donation, the semen is tested for harmful microorganisms, such as bacteria; if these tests prove negative, semen can then be used for insemination.

Up to 50 percent of sperm in the semen do not survive the freezing and thawing. This fall in sperm numbers is partly offset by the fact that it's the healthiest, most robust sperm that do survive. Donor insemination is carried out under the same conditions as artificial insemination with sperm from a partner (see p.49).

Embryos Storage of frozen embryos (see p.53) prevents embryo wastage if several embryos have been fertilized—no more than two are replaced in any cycle because of the risk of multiple pregnancy—and can help another infertile couple. Pregnancies resulting from the use of frozen embryos have raised the success rate of a cycle of IVF treatment from one to 10 percent.

SURROGATE MOTHERS

A surrogate mother is a woman who bears a child on behalf of another. Surrogacy is physically straightforward but fraught with possible moral, legal, and emotional difficulties.

Full surrogacy This is the simplest form of surrogacy: a surrogate mother conceives and carries the child of an infertile woman's partner. Insemination may be indirect (the surrogate is artificially inseminated with the man's sperm) or direct (the man has sexual intercourse with the surrogate).

Partial surrogacy In this arrangement, an egg from the woman who is unable to conceive is fertilized with her partner's sperm and then implanted into the surrogate mother's uterus.

Surrogacy problems When the child is born, it's handed over to the couple who "commissioned" it. They legally adopt the child and the surrogate mother has little or no further involvement. Sometimes, though, the surrogate finds it very hard to part with the child, especially if she is its genetic mother. In some well-publicized cases couples have had to take lengthy and costly legal action in order to get custody of the baby.

There can also be problems if the child is born handicapped or if the surrogate wants to keep up a close relationship with the child and is not allowed to do so. There's also the possibility that either or both of the commissioning parents may find it hard to accept the child fully and lovingly as their own.

Infertility

Case study

Names Peter and Jane
Ages 29 and 27 years
Past medical history Peter had NSU (nonspecific urethritis) three years ago and was treated at a G.U. (genitourinary) clinic. The problem hasn't come back. Peter also had mumps when he was 12 years old. Jane has no relevant medical history
Obstetric history Peter and Jane have been trying for a baby for three years without success

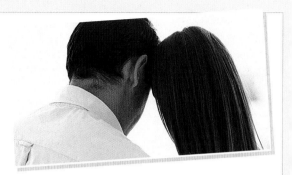

Jane wants some medical advice about what she and Peter should do next, but Peter isn't eager to see the doctor. In the end, Jane visits her doctor on her own.

With 30 approaching fast, Jane is very aware of her biological clock ticking away. She wants a baby and doesn't want to leave conceiving to chance any longer. She knows that men are responsible for half of all infertility and that it's important for her and Peter to tackle the problem together and do whatever is necessary, regardless of sensitivities.

TAKING THE INITIATIVE

Like most women, Jane shoulders the responsibility for starting a family. Like a lot of men, Peter would rather not think about it when they seem to have a problem with conceiving. Women are nearly always the ones who seek advice first about infertility, but quite a lot of men write to me in confidence and independently of their wives to ask advice. Perhaps it's having to face another man in the form of a male doctor that puts men off. In public, many men are defensive.

JOINT RESPONSIBILITIES

For whatever reason, many men don't want to talk about the possibility of being infertile, which in itself is sad. First, infertility is not linked with virility, and men need to understand this and separate these two things in their minds. Second, if a man is found to have less than perfect fertility, there's now a lot that can be done to help him and his partner conceive successfully. Either way, men have to face up to the possibility of

infertility. In half of all infertile couples, the infertile partner is found to be the man. A couple must share the responsibility.

OVERCOMING RESERVATIONS

I explained to Jane that their difficulty with conceiving can't be tackled by her alone. Even if Peter turns out not to be the problem, the investigation of their fertility has to be undertaken as a couple. If he really wants to have children, he must overcome both his embarrassment and any sense of guilt or shame.

PRIMARY TESTS

Jane's doctor said more or less the same, and after about a week of soul-searching, Peter agreed to go along with Jane. Poor Peter—it was only the beginning.

The doctor took Peter's past attack of NSU (nonspecific urethritis) very seriously—any sexually transmitted disease can interfere with fertility. The mumps virus, which may cause inflammation of the testes and damage future sperm production, can also result in problems. Peter had mumps at the age of 12, when his testes were extremely vulnerable. At the end of the first visit to the doctor, things didn't look too bright for Peter. Nor did they improve when the doctor asked him to go to the fertility clinic for semen analysis on two separate occasions.

By this time, Peter felt very much the injured party. But the doctor explained that both Jane and he would need to have primary tests done. Jane's would be in the form of a smear test, a test for chlamydia, an internal examination, and blood tests to confirm that she was ovulating. Peter would have physical examination of his penis and testes and semen analyses.

As the doctor explained, it makes sense to start by checking the form and health of Peter's sperm, It would be a difficult task to examine Jane's eggs, but Peter's sperm are available through the simple method of masturbation (see p.40).

STRAINS ON THE RELATIONSHIP

Things went steadily downhill from this point. Peter hated going to the fertility clinic and having to supply semen samples. He found the process cold, clinical, and inhuman. He felt torn. He wanted to do what was necessary, to please Jane if nothing else, but he felt isolated and persecuted. His morale fell lower and lower at the thought of finding out it was all his fault.

Jane did her best to reassure Peter and show her love for him, but he went deeper and deeper into his shell, refused to talk about the problem, and became very uncommunicative. Jane felt increasingly estranged from Peter. Peter felt unloved and they stopped having sex altogether. Jane, feeling desperate, suggested that they get some counseling. Peter cut short the conversation by leaving the room.

All seemed lost when the results of the semen analysis came back. Peter's sperm count was 5–10 million, and fewer than 30 percent of his sperm were active.

GETTING SUPPORT

At this point I insisted that both Peter and Jane give serious thought to seeing a counselor if only to outline that all was not lost. It was a great struggle, but Peter finally swallowed his male pride and made an appointment to see a fertility counselor with Jane so that they could be prepared for what was to come.

SECONDARY TESTS

The counselor explained that, although a low sperm count with low motility is, of course, a blow, Peter does have some sperm, and some are mobile. This means that even if Peter's sperm fail the egg penetration test, they could use an advanced form of ART (assisted reproduction technology) called ICSI (see p.49). In this an individual sperm would be injected into one of Jane's healthy eggs and could lead to a successful pregnancy and a healthy baby.

This possibility is a cause for rejoicing, not for sadness, nor for Peter's feelings of worthlessness.

EMBARKING ON IVF

An IVF treatment program (see p.50) isn't straightforward for either of them. Jane has to be heavily involved, too, even though her fertility is normal. To increase the chances of having several eggs on which to perform ICSI with Peter's sperm, she'll have to undergo drug treatments and serial tests to make sure her ovaries are goaded into producing several eggs at the same time rather than the usual one. This part of the treatment takes the best part of three weeks, and both Peter and Jane must be prepared for the effect of the fertility hormones on Jane. At the very least she could become moody, irritable, even weepy and tearful. She'll have to make daily visits to the fertility clinic for ultrasound scans during the third week, which will play havoc with her normal life and work. She'll have to make special arrangements, and Peter has to be prepared to help her out.

In fact, the greatest impact of Peter's infertility falls on Jane. Even though Jane is desperate to have a baby, it's easy for resentment to build, especially if the initial treatments aren't successful and she has to undergo several programs. Peter's involvement, by comparison, is very little—all he has to do is provide two specimens of semen each treatment program. That in itself can cause estrangement from Jane. If he's not careful, it's all too easy for Peter to feel shame and guilt and begin to hate Jane (as well as himself) for putting him in this position. It could all backfire.

No couple should face such a painful situation without psychological support, and I think Peter is beginning to accept that. Their fertility clinic has a team of counselors and Peter and Jane have made an appointment to see one next week.

Once they've had all the different steps of the fertility program explained to their satisfaction and all their questions have been answered (I suggest that they sit down and make a list together), I strongly advise them to keep talking about their feelings to each other and to their counselor, every step of the way. If they succeed in conceiving, it'll all be worthwhile.

CHAPTER 2

You and your developing baby

There's nothing as exciting as the month-by-month development of your baby. And the more you understand about how he grows, the better you'll be able to build a relationship with your baby even before he's born.

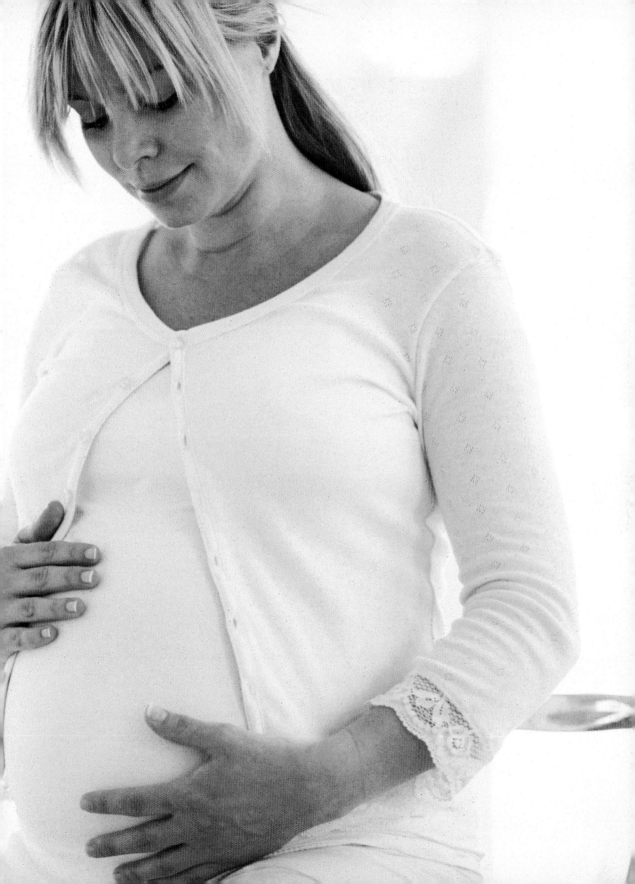

Pregnant!

Many women "know" when they've conceived. This special intuitive feeling is probably due to the very early outpouring of female hormones. First of all, you'll have prolonged high levels of progesterone (which you don't experience unless you're pregnant). Then fetal tissues start to produce *human chorionic gonadotrophin* (hCG) as soon as the embryo is implanted in the uterus, about seven days after fertilization.

SUSPECTING THAT YOU'RE PREGNANT

A few classic signs can make you suspect that you're pregnant before you do a test to make sure.

Missed period You may miss a period within two weeks after conceiving your baby. Although pregnancy is the most common reason for a missed period, it's not the only one, so don't take this as an absolute sign of pregnancy. There are other things, such as jet lag, severe illness, surgery, shock, bereavement, or great stress, that can cause you to miss a period. Periods don't always stop in pregnancy, though. Some women continue having light periods up to the sixth month, and occasionally all the way through their pregnancies.

Urinating more often As soon as your progesterone levels rise and the embryo starts to produce hCG, blood supply to your pelvic area increases, which leads to pelvic congestion. This affects the bladder, which becomes irritable and tries to expel even the smallest quantity of urine. This is why most women feel like they want to pass urine more often than usual, although it may be in only very small quantities. This can happen as early as one week after conception.

Tiredness The very high levels of progesterone in your body have a sedative effect on your body, and this is one of the reasons for tiredness when you're first pregnant. Early in your pregnancy, your metabolism speeds up to support your developing baby and your vital organs, which are having to do so much more work than usual. This can cause you to feel so tired that there's nothing you can do but sleep. If that's how you feel, you must rest—for your sake and your baby's.

Odd tastes and cravings Your saliva often reflects the chemical content of your blood and, as hormone levels rise, the taste in your mouth can change—many women describe it as metallic. You many also notice that certain foods taste different from normal, and that you stop liking things you usually enjoy (coffee is a common example).

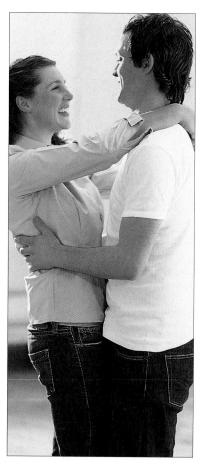

Discovering a new life
Finding out that you're pregnant can be one of the most special moments of your life.

Some women begin to crave certain foods—and occasionally want to eat very strange things, such as coal. There's no real scientific explanation for this, but cravings may be the body's way of trying to make up for a deficiency in certain minerals and trace elements. It's best to control cravings for inedible substances and for high-calorie foods that are low in nutritional value. Otherwise, there's no harm in eating what you feel like, within reason.

Morning sickness Although it's most common in the morning, nausea can come on at any time of day. It's more likely to affect you if you don't eat often enough and your blood sugar level is allowed to drop.

Smell You may notice that your sense of smell becomes more acute when you're pregnant, and everyday odors such as cooking smells make you nauseous. Perfume may also affect you this way, and the way your own perfume smells on you may also change, because your skin's chemistry alters.

Breast changes Even at the start of pregnancy, you may feel changes in your breasts. They may become quite lumpy and sore to the touch; your nipple area may feel tender and sensitive, and will also deepen in color; and veins in your breasts may look larger and more obvious.

CONFIRMING THAT YOU'RE PREGNANT

Once you suspect that you might be pregnant, you'll want to confirm it as soon as possible. There are a number of tests that can be done at different intervals following conception. Some are more accurate than others.

Urine tests The pregnancy hormone known as hCG (human chorionic gonadotrophin) can be detected in your urine. Urine tests can be done at home, at your doctor's office, at family planning clinics, in a hospital, or at a pharmacy. These tests are more than 90 percent reliable. They can be carried out as early as two weeks after conception, although you'll get the most reliable result if you wait four weeks longer before taking them (see also p.62).

Blood test This test has to be carried out by your doctor and is usually only done when there's a problem such as bleeding or pain, or after a cycle of assisted reproduction. The test also accurately detects the hCG in the blood as early as two weeks after conception—about the time your next period is due.

Internal examination At your first prenatal visit, you will probably have blood tests, a pelvic exam, a pap smear, and possibly an ultrasound to confirm fetal viability. A pelvic exam can help the doctor estimate how many weeks pregnant you are.

TELLING THE WORLD

You'll want your partner, and possibly your immediate family, to know the news as soon as you know yourself.

Doctor Your doctor may confirm your pregnancy so you will know immediately. If not, it's important to get in touch with your doctor as soon as you can to talk about birth options and antenatal care.

Employer You may want to talk to your employer before you go to your prenatal clinic (see p.174) for your first visit, probably when you're about three months pregnant. You don't have to tell your employer this early though.

Friends and acquaintances Most miscarriages happen in the first trimester, so you may prefer to wait until the second trimester to tell friends and acquaintances that you're pregnant.

IS YOUR TEST RESULT RIGHT?

There are a number of things that can affect the accuracy of pregnancy tests.

- In older women, hormonal changes caused by approaching menopause can give false positives or negatives.

- If urine is incorrectly collected or stored, there can be errors.

- If the test is performed too early, the concentration of hCG will be too low to detect. It's important to know when your period was due. If your periods are usually irregular or infrequent, this can make it harder to confirm pregnancy.

- If you've taken antidepressant or fertility drugs containing hCG or hMG, these can change the results. Contraceptive pills, antibiotics, and painkillers shouldn't have any effect.

- If the equipment used for a urine test is too hot, the result may be false. Urine must be at room temperature at the time of the test.

HOME TESTING

You'll probably prefer to find out whether or not you're pregnant in the privacy of your own home so you're sure of complete confidentiality. There are a range of pregnancy testing kits available from pharmacies. They're all simple to use and give immediate results that are more than 90 percent accurate.

How the tests work Urine tests check for the presence of hCG (human chorionic gonadotrophin), the hormone that's made by the developing embryo. Two of the main types, the ring and the color tests, involve mixing a chemical solution with a sample of your urine. The chemicals react according to the amount of hCG in your urine. The reaction is shown by a color change in the tube or window strip, or coagulation is prevented, causing a dark ring to appear in the tube. A third test can be done by simply placing the absorbent part of the test in contact with the urine. Signs of hCG may be detected in urine from two weeks after conceiving. Most kits advise using the test between one and four days after the first day of your missed period. If you do perform the test then, repeat it two weeks later when the hCG is more concentrated and the result will be more reliable. Most kits provide two tests so you can confirm the first result.

Take care Use a sample from the first urine you pass in the morning because it will contain a higher concentration of hCG. Don't drink anything before the test, because this will dilute the sample. Make sure you collect your sample in a clean, soap-free container. Follow the kit's instructions very carefully and don't use the test if it's been damaged in any way or is past its expiration date. If you can't do the test immediately, store your urine sample in the refrigerator, but don't keep it for more than 12 hours.

Unexpected result Sometimes you may have a positive first test but a negative second test, followed by your period starting a few days later. Don't worry. Half of all conceptions don't become established pregnancies, as the fertilized egg fails to implant in the lining of the uterus and there's a natural termination. Your first test may have been positive because it was done before the fertilized egg was lost. To avoid this error, do the test around the time of your first missed period. If there's a weak but positive result, repeat the test a few days later with a fresh sample.

EXPECTED ARRIVAL DATE

Once you know you're pregnant, your next question will almost certainly be "When will my baby be born?" There are usually about 266 days or 38 weeks between conception and birth. This is the same as 40 weeks from the start of your last menstrual period (LMP) because ovulation, and therefore conception, is normally two weeks after the start of your period (see chart, right). You can work out the approximate date of your baby's arrival calculating from the first day of your last period. The estimated date of your baby's delivery (EDD) is therefore at 280 days (40 weeks) from the first day of your last period. How accurate this date is depends on whether you have a regular 28-day cycle. If your menstrual cycle is shorter or longer, your delivery date may be earlier or later. If you conceived immediately after coming off the pill, it will be harder for your healthcare provider to give you a firm date, and they will probably have to be guided by your baby's growth.

Medical staff use the EDD when monitoring your baby's development and checking the expected rate of growth. Sometimes too much emphasis is put on this date, leading to unnecessary intervention, and doctors may want to induce labor if they believe your baby is overdue. However, risks to you and your baby don't rise much until after 42 weeks, and most doctors are prepared to let a pregnancy continue, without inducing, if tests show the baby is not at risk (see p.260).

HOW THE EDD CHART WORKS

Find the first day of your last period on the chart by looking for the month in bold type on the left-hand side, then looking along the line until you find the actual date of your LMP. Then look at the figure below it. This is your baby's estimated date of arrival.

YOUR BABY'S ARRIVAL

Don't be anxious if your baby doesn't show signs of arriving on the day you'd expected. About 85 percent of babies born from normal pregnancies are delivered within a week before or after the date predicted.

The EDD is used to give you an approximate idea of when to expect your baby to be born. It's best to be flexible and not to see this as the exact day you'll go into labor and deliver your baby. A healthy pregnancy may last for anything from 38 to 42 weeks.

Your estimated date of delivery

January	1 2 3 4 5 6 7 8 9 10 11 12 13 14 15 16 17 18 19 20 21 22 23 24 25 26 27 28 29 30 31
Oct./Nov.	*8 9 10 11 12 13 14 15 16 17 18 19 20 21 22 23 24 25 26 27 28 29 30 31 1 2 3 4 5 6 7*
February	1 2 3 4 5 6 7 8 9 10 11 12 13 14 15 16 17 18 19 20 21 22 23 24 25 26 27 28
Nov./Dec.	*8 9 10 11 12 13 14 15 16 17 18 19 20 21 22 23 24 25 26 27 28 29 30 1 2 3 4 5*
March	1 2 3 4 5 6 7 8 9 10 11 12 13 14 15 16 17 18 19 20 21 22 23 24 25 26 27 28 29 30 31
Dec./Jan.	*6 7 8 9 10 11 12 13 14 15 16 17 18 19 20 21 22 23 24 25 26 27 28 29 30 31 1 2 3 4 5*
April	1 2 3 4 5 6 7 8 9 10 11 12 13 14 15 16 17 18 19 20 21 22 23 24 25 26 27 28 29 30
Jan./Feb.	*6 7 8 9 10 11 12 13 14 15 16 17 18 19 20 21 22 23 24 25 26 27 28 29 30 31 1 2 3 4*
May	1 2 3 4 5 6 7 8 9 10 11 12 13 14 15 16 17 18 19 20 21 22 23 24 25 26 27 28 29 30 31
Feb./Mar.	*5 6 7 8 9 10 11 12 13 14 15 16 17 18 19 20 21 22 23 24 25 26 27 28 1 2 3 4 5 6 7*
June	1 2 3 4 5 6 7 8 9 10 11 12 13 14 15 16 17 18 19 20 21 22 23 24 25 26 27 28 29 30
Mar./Apr.	*8 9 10 11 12 13 14 15 16 17 18 19 20 21 22 23 24 25 26 27 28 29 30 31 1 2 3 4 5 6*
July	1 2 3 4 5 6 7 8 9 10 11 12 13 14 15 16 17 18 19 20 21 22 23 24 25 26 27 28 29 30 31
Apr./May	*7 8 9 10 11 12 13 14 15 16 17 18 19 20 21 22 23 24 25 26 27 28 29 30 1 2 3 4 5 6 7*
August	1 2 3 4 5 6 7 8 9 10 11 12 13 14 15 16 17 18 19 20 21 22 23 24 25 26 27 28 29 30 31
May/June	*8 9 10 11 12 13 14 15 16 17 18 19 20 21 22 23 24 25 26 27 28 29 30 31 1 2 3 4 5 6 7*
September	1 2 3 4 5 6 7 8 9 10 11 12 13 14 15 16 17 18 19 20 21 22 23 24 25 26 27 28 29 30
June/July	*8 9 10 11 12 13 14 15 16 17 18 19 20 21 22 23 24 25 26 27 28 29 30 1 2 3 4 5 6 7*
October	1 2 3 4 5 6 7 8 9 10 11 12 13 14 15 16 17 18 19 20 21 22 23 24 25 26 27 28 29 30 31
July/Aug.	*8 9 10 11 12 13 14 15 16 17 18 19 20 21 22 23 24 25 26 27 28 29 30 31 1 2 3 4 5 6 7*
November	1 2 3 4 5 6 7 8 9 10 11 12 13 14 15 16 17 18 19 20 21 22 23 24 25 26 27 28 29 30
Aug./Sept.	*8 9 10 11 12 13 14 15 16 17 18 19 20 21 22 23 24 25 26 27 28 29 30 31 1 2 3 4 5 6*
December	1 2 3 4 5 6 7 8 9 10 11 12 13 14 15 16 17 18 19 20 21 22 23 24 25 26 27 28 29 30 31
Sept./Oct.	*7 8 9 10 11 12 13 14 15 16 17 18 19 20 21 22 23 24 25 26 27 28 29 30 1 2 3 4 5 6 7*

PATERNITY LEAVE

Paternity leave is rarely paid in the United States, although a few progressive companies offer new dads paid time off, ranging from a few days to a few weeks. In 2004 California became the first state to offer paid leave. If you work in that state, you may be able to take up to six weeks at partial pay to help care for your new baby.

Paid family leave bills have been introduced in states other than in California as well. In the meantime, however, most fathers take vacation time or sick days when their children are born, and a growing number of dads are taking unpaid family leave from their jobs to spend more time with their newborns.

To find out if you are entitled to unpaid leave, start by asking your company's human resources department. Many employers are required by federal law to allow their employees (both men and women) 12 weeks of unpaid family leave under the Family and Medical Leave Act (FMLA). More information on the provisions of this Act are provided in the main text on this page, under "Working Women."

Your rights

Unfortunately, maternity rights and benefits in the United States lag far behind most other developed nations. In some European countries, for example, new mothers are entitled to partial or full salary, extended leave, and prescription coverage. In the US, it is important to negotiate with your employer well before you deliver and to take full advantage of what the law allows. The human resources department at your workplace can help point you in the right direction.

MINIMUM RIGHTS

Regardless of how many hours you work or how long you've been employed, you are entitled to working conditions that are safe for you and your unborn child. The Occupational Safety and Health Administration (OSHA) requires employers to provide a workplace free of known hazards, while the Pregnancy Discrimination Act (PDA) requires employers to treat pregnancy as they would any other medical condition. This means that they must offer the same disability leave and pay. The PDA also makes it illegal to hire, fire, or refuse to promote a woman because she is pregnant. Your human resources department can provide you with additional information.

WORKING WOMEN

Another major federal law in the United States that protects the health, safey, and employment rights of pregnant working women, is the Family and Medical Leave Act (FMLA), which requires employers with 50 or more employees to allow up to 12 weeks of unpaid leave for certain family and medical reasons, including childbirth, the adoption of a child or assuming the care of a foster child, during any 12–month period. In addition, the FMLA makes provision for the care of a spouse, child, or a parent with a serious health condition, and it protects a worker who is not able to do her job because of her own serous health condition, including a pregnancy- or birth-related disability. To take disability leave, a woman must have worked for at least 1,250 hours for her empoloyer, and for at least 12 months. Certain kinds of paid leave, such as vacation time or sick leave, may be substituted for unpaid leave, depending on whatever you and your employer negotiate.

Under the provision of the FMLA, you are entitled to the same position or to a similar one that provides equivalent benefits, salary, and other terms of employment, when you return to work. Although you can't lose benefits that you have already earned, salary and seniority benefits can't be accrued during your maternity leave. State family leave laws may be more or less restrictive than the federal statute. Local laws, as well as any collective bargaining agreements, may supercede federal regulations.

When	What you need to do	Why you need to do it
Before you are pregnant	Check with your employer to determine the company's maternity leave policies. If you are unemployed or sick, you may be entitled to government assistance. Check with your local health department.	To maximize your employee benefits.
After 12 weeks or after you receive amniocentesis results	If you are working, inform your employer.	To maximize your employee benefits.
About 12 weeks before your baby is due	Discuss your maternity-leave plans with your employer	To negotiate the best maternity-leave package possible
About 10 weeks before your baby is due	Give your employer a letter summarizing your maternity-leave plans and what you have agreed upon.	To clarify your expectations and your employer's. This gives both of you time to fine-tune points.
At least 30 days before going on maternity leave	Inform your employer in writing.	To protect your rights under the Family and Medical Leave Act.
One month before due date, or later (or earlier for a multiple birth)	Leave work.	To give you time to rest and prepare for birth.
1–2 days after birth	Submit information for birth certificate; apply for baby's Social Security number.	More straightforward than waiting until after the birth.
2–3 weeks after birth	Purchase copy (copies) of baby's birth certificate.	For easy recordkeeping.
6–8 weeks after birth	Receive baby's Social Security card.	For tax purposes.
6–8 weeks after birth	Tell your employer whether you expect to return to work on the date agreed upon.	To keep good relations and hold your job for your return.

First trimester

In the first three months you'll probably put on about 2–4 lb (1–2 kg), if you haven't had too much trouble with nausea.

Your baby will weigh only 1.7 oz (48 g). The rest of the weight is made up of your baby's support system (the placenta and amniotic fluid), your enlarged uterus and breasts, and the extra amount of blood in your body. Your own fat stores will make up about the same weight gain as your baby.

When you're pregnant, the three trimesters are your major milestones. The trimesters aren't three periods of exactly three months each—they're of different lengths, defined by the way a baby grows and develops. The first trimester starts with the presumed date of conception (two weeks after your last period), and represents the first twelve weeks of your baby's life in the womb. The second trimester ends at 28 weeks, and the third trimester is the rest of your pregnancy.

In the first trimester, your body adjusts to being pregnant. At first you won't look any different, and you might not feel different, either, but the activities of your hormones will soon start to affect you in various ways. You might experience lots of mood swings, you may want to make love more or less often, and you may find that your appetite changes and you start choosing simpler, blander food than usual.

PHYSICAL CHANGES

Your pregnant body is having to work very hard to accommodate your developing embryo and the placenta. When you're pregnant, your body's metabolic rate increases and is between 10 and 25 percent higher than normal. This means that all the body's functions are stepped up. Your cardiac output rises steeply, almost to the maximum level that will be kept up throughout the rest of your pregnancy. Your heart rate rises, too, and will go on doing so until the middle of the second trimester. Your breathing becomes more rapid because you now need to send more oxygen to your baby and breathe out more carbon dioxide.

Because of the action of increased levels of estrogen and progesterone in your body, your breasts quickly become larger and heavier. They're usually tender to the touch from very early on, too. There's an increase in fatty deposits in your breasts, and new milk ducts grow. The areola around your nipple becomes darker and develops little nodules called Montgomery's tubercles. Underneath your skin, you'll notice a network of bluish lines appearing as blood supply to your breasts increases.

Your uterus becomes larger even in early pregnancy, but you won't feel it through the abdominal wall until the end of the first trimester, when it begins to rise above your pelvic brim. While the uterus is still low in your pelvis, it'll start to press on your bladder as it get bigger, so you'll almost certainly find that you need to urinate more often.

The muscle fibers of your uterus begin to thicken until it becomes very solid. Even so, you probably won't notice your waistline changing until the end of this first trimester.

TAKING CARE OF YOURSELF

When you're pregnant, you need extra carbohydrates and protein to supply your growing baby and the placenta, as well as your uterus and breasts, so it's vital to eat healthily right from the start. If you have difficulty keeping meals down, eat little and often throughout the day. Many women feel most nauseous when their stomach is empty, like in the morning. You'll need extra fluids, too, so drink at least eight glasses of liquid a day. You should avoid drugs, caffeine, junk food, alcohol, and smoking throughout your whole pregnancy, but it's particularly important at this time, when fetal organs are forming. Make sure you get plenty of rest, too.

Clothes You'll feel happier in comfortable clothes. You won't need to buy maternity clothes yet, but there's nothing worse than wearing something tight and uncomfortable, so try to stay a step ahead of your increasing size. You'll probably need a larger bra almost right away, preferably a properly fitted maternity bra (see **Maternity wear**, p.163).

YOUR PRENATAL CARE

Your doctor may confirm that you're pregnant, or you may make an appointment with the prenatal clinic as soon as you've had a positive test result. If this is the case, you may not be seen until your next trimester. At the first visit to the clinic, your healthcare provider will ask you about your own and your family's medical histories. You'll also have a thorough physical examination, including urine and blood tests.

MAKING PLANS

Your doctor will talk to you about choices for childbirth in your area—what hospitals you could go to and what arrangements could be made for a home birth. Some practices may offer prenatal care, whether complete or shared with your hospital. Now is the time to start thinking about the type of delivery you want and where you're most likely to get it. Books like this one can help you decide what kind of birth you would prefer to have, as well as give you in-depth information on everything related to pregnancy, birth, and baby care.

Some women buy their unborn baby a little gift, such as a teddy bear, as soon as they know they're pregnant, but many feel that anything more than this is tempting fate. You might like to start keeping a daily journal of your health and feelings during the first trimester, so you'll have a complete record of your pregnancy.

YOUR PREGNANCY

Finding out that you're pregnant is very exciting, especially if it's the first time. Here are some of the early physical signs that will confirm the pregnancy test.

- Your breasts will grow larger, heavier, and feel more sensitive.

- You'll notice more pigmentation on your nipples, and any moles and freckles will get bigger.

- You may feel very tired and may even feel depressed. This may be difficult to accept at such a happy time, but it is caused by hormonal changes.

- You'll probably have some feelings of nausea, especially first thing in the morning.

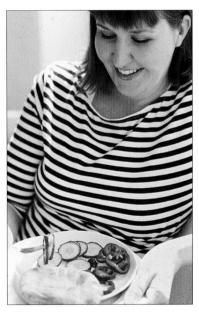

Your appetite in pregnancy
You may feel like eating some unusual foods or lose your taste for foods that you normally enjoy.

Second trimester

By this time your pregnancy will be well established and many of the little problems you may have had in early pregnancy will have disappeared. It's the time you may need to have certain tests. If you're over 35 years old or have a family history of congenital abnormalities, for example, you'll be offered amniocentesis. You may also need an amniocentesis if other tests, such as the nuchal scan, show there's a need for more detailed analysis.

PHYSICAL CHANGES

Your nipples may begin to make colostrum—your baby's first food—and leak slightly from time to time. Your waistline gradually starts to disappear and you'll now "look" pregnant. You may notice you have more pigmentation on your areolae and on freckles and moles (see p.158). Your gums may become slightly spongy, probably because of the action of pregnancy hormones. There's no reason why you should have more dental decay during pregnancy, though, and there's no truth in the saying "a tooth lost for every child."

Digestion The hormone that helps your cervix stretch to allow your baby to be born also affects other muscles in your body. All the muscles of your intestinal tract will be relaxed and this can cause many of the minor discomforts during your pregnancy.

You may suffer heartburn because the sphincter, or muscular, ring at the top of the stomach is more relaxed than usual. This allows the acid contents of your stomach to come back into your esophagus, causing discomfort. Your gastric secretions are also reduced, so food remains for longer in the stomach.

Because your intestinal muscles are relaxed, you'll also have fewer bowel movements, and although this does allow your food to be absorbed more completely, it can also lead to constipation in pregnancy.

Your increasing size Once your uterus has grown above your pelvis, you'll notice that your waistline is beginning to disappear. You'll probably want to start wearing larger, more comfortable clothing (see p.162).

On the other hand, many women are told they look small-for-dates during the second trimester. If this happens to you, don't worry. How big you'll look at this time depends on many different things, including your particular height and build; whether this is your first pregnancy or not, because uterine muscle tends to get stretched after the first child; and the size of your baby. If your doctor is happy with the way your pregnancy is progressing, then you can be, too.

TAKING CARE OF YOURSELF

During this trimester you'll gain the most weight of your pregnancy (about 13 lb/6 kg), and it's vital to keep eating well (see p.128). You may find that your posture changes as the muscles of your abdominal wall become more and more stretched to make room for your growing uterus. As your uterus gets bigger, your center of gravity changes because you're carrying more weight in front. Try not to start leaning backward or you may get a backache (see also p.160).

Backaches You may have some backaches because the increased blood flow to your whole pelvis causes some softening and relaxation of the ligaments of the sacrum, which attach your pelvic bones to your spine at the back. Also, the ligaments and the cartilage at the front of your pelvis loosen and the mobility of these joints is slightly increased.

To help prevent backaches, sit with a straight back and try not to slouch. You'll find it best to sit on a hard chair or the floor. Always bend with a straight back. Don't lift anything heavy if you can help it (see also p.160), but if you do need to, bend from your knees and lift from a crouching position.

YOUR PRENATAL CARE

You'll have regular urine, weight, and blood pressure checks. If necessary, you'll have tests for chromosomal defects. From this time, too, your healthcare providers will want to measure that your baby is growing enough. They will feel your abdomen to check the size and shape of your uterus and the height of the fundus (see p.178), and they'll listen for your baby's heartbeat. During the fourth month you'll probably have an ultrasound scan, and you'll have the special thrill of seeing your baby for the first time. You'll be able to hear your baby's incredibly fast heartbeat, too, (see column, p.178) and you may see your baby moving.

PREPARING FOR YOUR BABY

Toward the end of this second trimester, you'll probably be feeling well and full of energy, so it's a good time to make most of the preparations for your baby. For example, you could set up your baby's room and start shopping for some of the equipment you'll need. It's a good idea to do at least some of these things now rather than to wait until the third trimester. By then, you'll rapidly be getting bigger, and you might not feel like going shopping. You may also find that you start feeling very tired again.

YOUR PREGNANCY

In the second trimester you'll start to feel more comfortable with being pregnant. You'll love the feeling of your baby moving inside you, and you'll be energetic and full of life.

- You'll feel like making love again—or more often. Some women experience their first orgasm or multiple orgasm at this time.

- Your abdomen will become rounded. You'll lose your waistline and "look" pregnant.

- Your pigmentation will increase, and you may notice a darker line developing down the center of your abdomen—the linea nigra (see p.158).

- You might suffer from indigestion and rib pain.

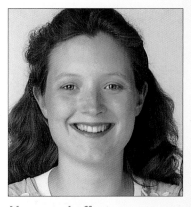

Hormonal effects
As the placenta takes over the production of pregnancy hormones, your hormone levels should begin to balance out. As this happens you'll feel calmer and more positive than you did in the first trimester. You'll look better, too—your hair will be thicker and shinier and your complexion clear and glowing.

Third trimester

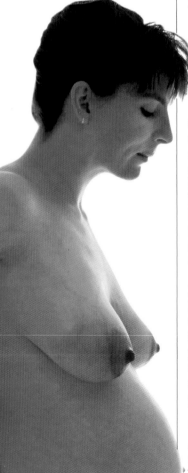

At this time you might start to feel anxious about labor and wish you could have your baby now. Don't worry—this doesn't mean there's anything wrong. Your feelings of urgency are caused by metabolic changes in your brain. Subtle shifts happen in each trimester, bringing about the tiredness of the first, the elation and energy of the second, and now the anxiety of the third.

PHYSICAL CHANGES

You're rapidly getting bigger now, and you're bound to feel tired. You may not be sleeping as well as usual at night, and you'll need to rest more and take naps during the day (see opposite). As your ligaments stretch and give way, you might start to find walking around uncomfortable. Once your baby has settled into your pelvis, you'll find you won't feel so breathless because there's less pressure on your diaphragm.

Breathing Because your diaphragm can't move as much when your baby grows bigger, you breathe more deeply when you're pregnant. You take in more air with each breath, which allows for better mixing of gases and the more efficient consumption of oxygen. This lifts your ventilation rate from the normal seven quarts (liters) of air per minute to 10 quarts (liters) per minute, an increase of more than 40 percent. However, your oxygen requirements are only 20 percent more. This leads to overbreathing, which means that you breathe out more carbon dioxide per breath than is normally the case. The low level of CO_2 in the blood causes a shortness of breath, which you may find bothersome during this trimester. Relief from this shortness of breath should come when your baby engages in your pelvis and there's less pressure on your diaphragm. Meanwhile, it'll help to sit in a semi-propped-up position whenever you can and try not to overdo things.

Possible problems Some women suffer from hypertension (high blood pressure—see p.178) in later pregnancy. Some major warning signs of this are swollen and puffy hands, wrists, ankles, feet, and face. Your healthcare provider will check for these at your prenatal visits. Preeclampsia (see p.224) may interfere with the functioning of your placenta and prevent it from carrying nutrients to your baby efficiently. If you do develop preeclampsia, you may have to go into the hospital.

CARING FOR YOURSELF

As the third trimester goes on, the extra weight you're carrying may cause more backaches and make you feel tired all the time. You'll probably find it difficult to sleep in the last weeks, because it's hard to get comfortable in bed. Don't take sleeping pills—they'll make your baby sleepy, too. Take your time with everything and make sure you get enough rest. Take catnaps during the day and be sure to give yourself some quiet times when you can relax. If you don't feel like making love or it's difficult because of your increasing size, you may find that massage helps you relax. Eat lots of fresh fruit and vegetables and drink at least eight glasses of fluid per day, as you'll probably pass urine more often. You may be constipated at times.

YOUR PRENATAL CARE

You'll have more frequent checkups during this trimester. Your doctor may use different tests to judge your baby's health and well-being, such as ultrasound, fetal heart rate monitoring, and hormonal measurements. At each stage you should be told what's being done and why. Unlike the special tests in the first and second trimester—chorionic villus sampling, amniocentesis, and cordocentesis (see pp.184–187)—none of the tests at this time are invasive of your uterus. You'll have regular urine and blood pressure tests and your feet and hands will be checked for possible swelling, although such swelling may be normal if there aren't any other symptoms. From your thirty-sixth week up to the start of labor, you'll visit your caregiver more often you did in the earlier months of your pregnancy.

PREPARING FOR YOUR BABY

By the time you're nearing the end of your third trimester, you'll need to have prepared your baby's room and have the essential items of clothing and equipment ready—you never know, your baby might arrive early.

You may find yourself thinking more and more about the labor, and some women find that they worry obsessively about it. Try not to be too anxious. No one can predict what will happen during your labor, since everyone's experience is unique, but most births go without a hitch.

YOUR PREGNANCY

In this trimester, practical matters such as going to childbirth classes and getting your baby's clothes and room ready will vie with daydreaming and fantasizing about the new arrival.

- You'll probably get tired easily, although you may find it hard to rest.
- You'll notice Braxton-Hicks contractions (see p.270) more and more.
- You'll have visited the hospital where you're going to give birth and met the staff. If you're planning a home birth, you'll need to get everything ready.
- You might worry about whether you can tell when you're in labor or not. Even for an experienced obstetrician or midwife, it can be difficult to know when labor has really started. Don't be afraid to call your healthcare provider for advice if you're in any doubt.

Baby's clothes and accessories
Before your baby's birth, you'll need to have a selection of bedding, baby clothes, diapers, and diaper-changing equipment ready.

01
02
03
04
05
06
07
08
09
10
11
12
13
14
15
16
17
18
19
20
21
22
23
24
25
26
27
28
29
30
31
32
33
34
35
36
37
38
39
40

MOTHER

At the end of the first month of pregnancy, you probably won't be sure that you're pregnant, although you may have your suspicions. Some pregnancy kits can give you a positive result even at this stage.

Symptoms You'll notice few, if any, symptoms at this stage, although you may feel mild PMS-type symptoms and pass urine more often than usual. Your breasts may feel sore and heavy and your nipples may tingle. You may even feel sick at this stage.

Ovulation cycle Once the embryo has implanted on the lining of your uterus, your normal ovulation cycle stops. The *corpus luteum* (see p.28) in the ovary continues to make progesterone, which prevents you from having periods and keeps the pregnancy healthy and viable.

Cervix The hormone progesterone makes your cervical mucus dense and thick, forming a plug. This plug stays in place until the end of your pregnancy, when it comes out (the show).

Uterus The wall of your uterus softens so that the embryo can become firmly embedded. Your uterus starts to get bigger almost from the moment of implantation.

First 6 weeks

Your fertilized egg becomes a ball of cells (*blastocyst*), which floats into your uterus and implants itself in the lining. The basis for your baby's future development is now laid down.

YOUR BABY'S PROGRESS

Once it has implanted, the embryo begins to make chemicals that have two functions. First, they signal to your body that the embryo has arrived, and this triggers changes in your body: your ovulation cycle stops; the mucus in your cervix thickens; your uterine wall softens; and your breasts begin to grow. Second, your immune system is suppressed so that the embryo is not treated as foreign and rejected, but is allowed to grow. Also, an outer layer of the ball of cells becomes a protective cocoon around the embryo. This cocoon will create the beginnings of the placenta and the support system in which the embryo will grow—the *amniotic sac* (the watery balloon in which it will float), the *chorion* (a safety cushion around the amniotic sac), and the yolk sac (which will make blood cells until the liver takes over). The chorion then grows fingerlike projections, the *chorionic villi*, with which the cocoon burrows firmly into your uterine lining.

The cells specialize Throughout these early weeks, the embryo's cells become more specialized. There are now three layers of

YOUR BABY AT SIX WEEKS OF PREGNANCY

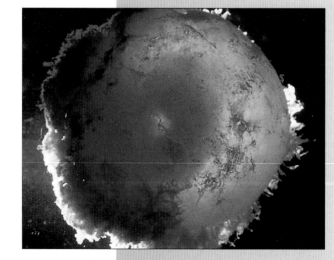

The sixth week
Surrounding layers of chorion and amnion protect the embryo, and blocks of tissue that will become the vertebrae can be seen to have started forming. Between these grow bunches of nerves.

Baby's vital statistics
By the end of the sixth week of life, the embryo will be about ⅛ in (4 mm) long. It will weigh less than 0.03 oz (1 g).

them. Each layer will create different organs of your baby's body. The innermost layer makes a primitive tube that later develops into the lungs, liver, thyroid gland, pancreas, urinary tract, and bladder. The middle layer will become the skeleton, muscles (including the heart muscle), testes (or ovaries), kidneys, spleen, blood vessels, blood cells, and the deepest layer of skin, the dermis. The outer layer will provide the skin, sweat glands, nipples (and breasts, if your baby is a girl), hair, nails, tooth enamel, and the lenses of the eyes.

THE EMBRYO'S SUPPORT SYSTEM

The villi, fingerlike projections, of the growing placenta intermingle with the mother's blood vessels of the uterine wall in such a way that they eventually become surrounded by "lakes" of blood. The mother's blood flows in and around these spaces and, because it is divided by only a cell or two from fetal blood, exchange of nutrients and waste between fetus and mother can take place in these blood spaces. The placenta is a hormone factory pumping out hormones, such as human *chorionic gonadotrophin* (hCG), that are designed to support a healthy pregnancy. Until the sixth week, the embryo's blood cells are supplied by the yolk sac. After the end of the third week, the blood circulation is pumped by the baby's own heart.

BABY

Probably even before you know you're pregnant, the embryo reaches a critical stage in development so it's vital to plan for pregnancy.

Spinal cord During the second week of life, a dark mark appears on the back of the embryo. This marks the position of the spinal cord.

Heart By the end of the third week, the embryo has a heart that's now beginning to beat.

Sensitivity In the third week, the embryo enters a sensitive phase of development when all the major organs are forming. Embryos are generally robust but can be harmed by drugs, alcohol, smoking, infections, and so on. Many don't survive, largely because of serious chromosomal defects.

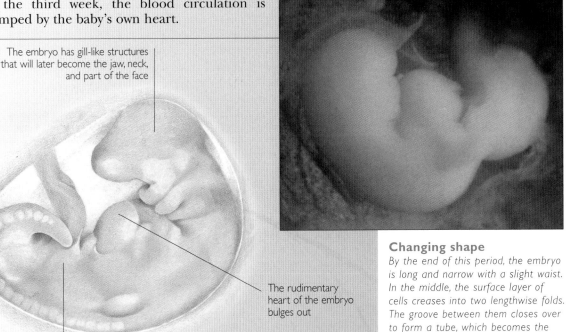

The embryo has gill-like structures that will later become the jaw, neck, and part of the face

The rudimentary heart of the embryo bulges out

The beginnings of the spinal cord appear

Changing shape

By the end of this period, the embryo is long and narrow with a slight waist. In the middle, the surface layer of cells creases into two lengthwise folds. The groove between them closes over to form a tube, which becomes the spinal cord. The tube grows at the top; this will become the brain.

MOTHER

Some women find that morning sickness is one of the first signs of pregnancy. Other changes happen that may not be as noticeable.

Metabolic changes Very early in your pregnancy, your metabolic rate begins to increase, so you need to take in more protein and calories.

Circulatory changes Your total blood volume begins to rise. About 25 percent of this is being used by the placental system.

Genitals The blood supply to your vagina and vulva increases quite rapidly, and they both become a purplish color. Your vaginal walls become softened and relaxed, and an increasing amount of a watery substance is made, so you'll have more discharge while you're pregnant.

Breasts Your breasts may start to swell or feel tender and heavier than usual. The skin around your areola begins to develop a softer, lighter area known as the secondary areola.

Tiredness You are likely to get tired more easily than usual.

Skin problems If your face tends to break out before your period, it's also likely to happen again now.

Up to 10 weeks

This is a time of very rapid and crucial development—your baby quadruples in size. The embryo is lying in the center of a large placental cocoon, and is still very tiny. As it develops, its cells are constantly changing to make new structures.

YOUR BABY'S PROGRESS

Inside the tube that will eventually become your baby's brain and spinal cord, the cells multiply at an amazing rate, then move away to the areas where they will become active. Nerve cells that will form the brain travel along pathways that are being laid down by *glial* (glue) cells. These cells allow the nerve cells to move toward each other, connect, and become active.

Your baby's head is growing rapidly in order to make room for the enlarging brain, and the body is becoming less curved. A neck begins to develop and the primitive tail disappears.

The skin now starts to develop into its two layers, and the sweat glands and sebaceous (oil-producing) glands begin to form. Hair then starts to grow from the hair follicles so that the skin becomes downy. All the major organs develop. The heart achieves its final form and beats strongly. The stomach, liver, spleen, appendix, and intestine develop. The intestine becomes so long it forms a loop, the circulatory system is established, and most muscles begin to take on their final form.

YOUR BABY AT 10 WEEKS OF PREGNANCY

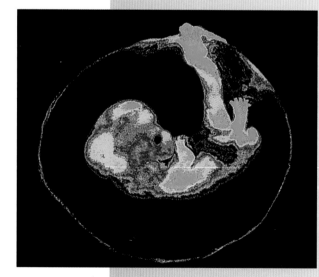

Color-enhanced scan
The developing umbilical cord and placenta can be clearly seen in the top right-hand corner of the ultrasound scan.

Baby's vital statistics
By the end of this month your baby's crown-to-rump length will be 1 in (2.5 cm). Your baby will weigh about 0.1 oz (3 g).

Facial features Under the skin on the baby's face, a primitive bone structure has developed, and these bones are now fusing together. One of these goes down between the eyes and ends on either side of the nostrils, thus forming the nose and the middle of the upper lip. Two others appear under the eyes, forming the cheeks and sides of the upper lip. Two more grow under the mouth, fusing to form the lower lip and chin. All this provides the framework to which the facial muscles become attached, which then allows the face to move.

There's already some pigment in the eyes, which are covered and very far apart. The inside and outside parts of the ears begin to form and the taste buds start developing. The tooth buds of all nonpermanent teeth are now in place.

Arms and legs Embryonic limbs continue to develop. Wrists and fingers appear on the arm buds, which become longer and project forward. The arms become bent at the elbow. Touch-pads form on the fingertips. Leg buds sprout, then develop three distinct sections—thigh, calf, and foot. Toes start to appear. At this stage, your baby's arms and hands grow faster than her legs and feet.

This trend will continue after your baby's been born—she'll be able to grasp objects long before she's starts walking.

BABY

Nutrients pass from your body into the placenta and the umbilical cord to feed your baby, who needs more and more nourishment to support the rapid growth.

Heart rate The baby's heart beats at 140–150 per minute, which is about twice the rate of yours.

Body shape The baby's head is still very large in comparison with the body and is bent forward on the chest. The body begins to straighten and get longer.

Internal organs All organs are now in place and most major structures will have been formed.

Reflexes Your baby can respond to touch, although you won't be able to feel any movements yet.

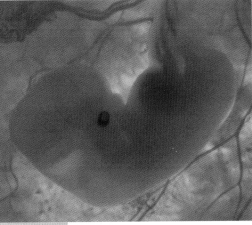

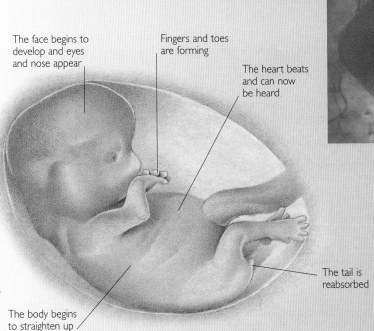

The face begins to develop and eyes and nose appear

Fingers and toes are forming

The heart beats and can now be heard

The tail is reabsorbed

The body begins to straighten up

External features
At this stage the embryo's eyes have some pigment and there are visible signs of nostrils, lips, and ears. The rudimentary ears now divide into inner and outer sections, the eyelids form, and the tip of the nose can be seen. The embryo's muscles start to build, and by the seventh week of life the first embryonic movement can be detected using ultrasound. This picture shows the embryo at six weeks after conception.

01
02
03
04
05
06
07
08
09
10
11
12
13
14
15
16
17
18
19
20
21
22
23
24
25
26
27
28
29
30
31
32
33
34
35
36
37
38
39
40

Up to 14 weeks

By 14 weeks after your last period, all of your baby's major organs have formed and his intestines are sealed in his abdominal cavity. He now starts to grow and mature.

YOUR BABY'S PROGRESS

By the eleventh week of pregnancy, your baby is recognizable as a human being, and he's now called a fetus (offspring) rather than an embryo. His head is very large compared with the rest of his body—by 14 weeks, it's about one-third of his whole length. His eyes are completely formed, although his eyelids are still developing and remain closed. His face, too, is completely formed. His trunk has straightened out and the first bone tissue and ribs appear. He has nails on his fingers and toes, and he may have some hair. The external genital organs are now growing, and doctors may able to tell your baby's sex by ultrasound. His heart is beating between 110 and 160 times per minute and his circulatory system is continuing to develop. He swallows amniotic fluid and excretes it as urine.

His sucking reflex is getting established—he purses his lips, turns his head, and wrinkles his forehead. The muscles he'll use

YOUR BABY AT 14 WEEKS OF PREGNANCY

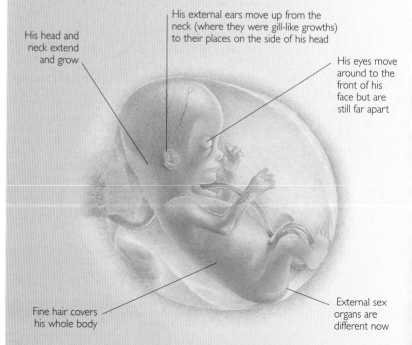

His head and neck extend and grow

His external ears move up from the neck (where they were gill-like growths) to their places on the side of his head

His eyes move around to the front of his face but are still far apart

Fine hair covers his whole body

External sex organs are different now

after he's born for breathing and swallowing are also being exercised. In fact, by the end of this month, your baby will have discovered movement. He now begins to move around vigorously, but you probably won't be able to feel his movements until the fourth month.

Blood-cell production While your baby will go on relying on the placenta for his nourishment, oxygen, and the clearance of waste until he is born, he has to have a system of blood-cell formation that will eventually support life outside the womb. Toward the end of this month, the yolk sac becomes superfluous as its task of producing blood cells is taken over by your baby's developing bone marrow, liver, and spleen.

HIS SUPPORT SYSTEM

The placenta is developing very quickly, making sure that there's a rich network of blood vessels to provide your baby with vital nourishment. Now the layers thicken and grow until the chorion and membranes cover the entire inner surface area of the uterus. The umbilical cord is now completely mature and is made up of three intertwined blood vessels wrapped in a fatty sheath. The large vein carries nutrients and oxygen-rich blood to your baby, while the two, smaller, arteries carry waste products and oxygen-poor blood from your baby to the placenta. The umbilical cord is coiled like a spring because the sheath is longer than the blood vessels. This allows your baby plenty of room to move around without the risk of damaging his lifeline.

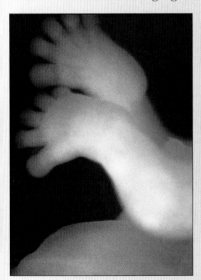

Feet and hands
Your baby's fingers and toes are growing rapidly and becoming fully formed.

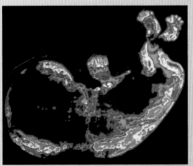

12-week-old fetus
Your baby's profile has become more human and his features are much more clearly defined. He now has a definite chin, a large forehead, and a button nose. His eyelids have begun to develop across his fully formed eyes, and he's beginning to respond to what happens outside the womb—if his mother's abdomen is poked, he'll try to wriggle away. An ultrasound scan would show that he's moving at this stage, but you can't feel his movements until next month at the earliest.

MOTHER

You'll probably start to feel better during this month, particularly if you've been suffering badly from nausea and vomiting.

Weight You'll probably begin to put on weight as your baby and his support system grow rapidly.

Hormones Your hormones begin to settle down and you'll probably feel much less emotionally unbalanced and vulnerable.

Fundal height Your developing baby is causing the fundus (see External examination, p.178) of your uterus to rise through the pelvic brim where it can be felt. You'll probably have an ultrasound scan at this time to confirm the stage of pregnancy.

Outlook If you've been anxious about your pregnancy, you'll probably feel more relaxed now as the risk of miscarriage diminishes to practically nothing.

Circulatory system Your cardiac output has reached almost the maximum level that will be kept up throughout the rest of your pregnancy. To lower your blood pressure, the arteries and veins in your extremities relax, so your hands and feet are nearly always warm.

BABY

Your baby is fully formed; now he needs to mature. He's very active at this stage, although you won't feel him yet.

Bones In the form of flexible cartilage, the bones in his body are rapidly growing.

Movements He jerks his body, bends his arms and legs, and has hiccups.

Jaws These already show 32 permanent tooth buds.

Amniotic sac He floats in a warm bath of amniotic fluid (at 99.5°F/ 37.5°C, the temperature of the amniotic fluid is higher than your body temperature). He has plenty of room to move.

> **Baby's vital statistics**
> *By the end of this month his crown- to-rump length will be 3½ in (9 cm), and he'll weigh 1.7 oz (48 g).*

01
02
03
04
05
06
07
08
09
10
11
12
13
14
15
16
17
18
19
20
21
22
23
24
25
26
27
28
29
30
31
32
33
34
35
36
37
38
39
40

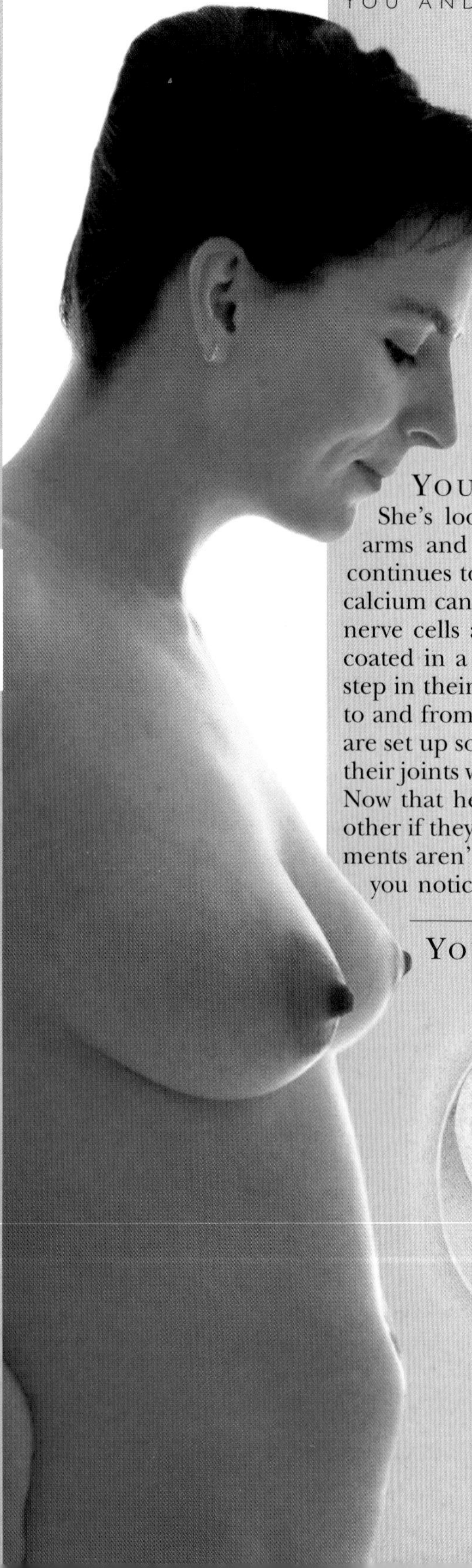

Up to 18 weeks

The second trimester starts from the fourteenth week of pregnancy. Your baby is steadily growing, and if you have a scan now, it'll be possible to tell your baby's sex. If your doctors think it necessary, they may suggest you have various tests around this time to rule out any abnormalities. The length of your baby's thighbone will be measured, as well as the diameter of her head. The head measurement will be used to confirm the EDD.

YOUR BABY'S PROGRESS

She's looking more human now, with legs longer than her arms and the parts of her legs in proportion. Her skeleton continues to produce more bone, and those parts with sufficient calcium can be seen on X-rays. She now has the same number of nerve cells as an adult. The nerves from her brain begin to be coated in a layer of *myelin* (protective fat). This is an important step in their maturation because it helps the passage of messages to and from the brain. Connections between nerves and muscles are set up so that your baby's well-formed limbs can move around their joints when the muscles are stimulated to contract and relax. Now that her arms are long enough, her hands can grasp each other if they touch accidentally, and she can form fists. Her movements aren't yet under the control of her brain, though. Nor do you notice them yet because she's not big enough to activate

YOUR BABY AT 18 WEEKS OF PREGNANCY

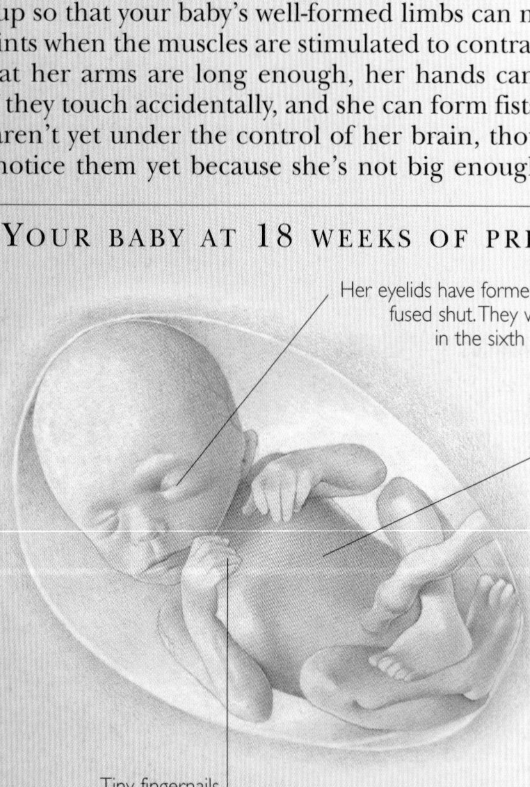

Her eyelids have formed and are fused shut. They will open in the sixth month

Breathing movements can now be detected, as can the protective "brown fat"

Tiny fingernails can be seen

nerve endings on your uterine wall. Second-time mothers tend to feel their baby's movements sooner (see p.194).

Your baby's external genital organs are taking on a more distinctive appearance. A girl's vaginal plate, the beginnings of her vagina, is clearly developing, and a boy's testes are well on their way to descending into the scrotum.

HER SUPPORT SYSTEM

The placenta is making the increasing amounts of hormones (chorionic gonadotrophin, estrogen, and progesterone) that are needed throughout pregnancy. It's also making an assortment of other hormones that keep your uterus healthy and play an essential part in the growth and development of your breasts in preparation for feeding your baby. The placenta forms a barrier against general infection, although not against viruses such as rubella (German measles) and AIDS, and poisons such as alcohol and nicotine. By the end of the sixteenth week, the placenta has grown in thickness to about half an inch (1 cm) and three-and-a-half inches (7–8 cm) across.

The placenta continues to grow until, at term, it weighs a pound (500 g), and measures an inch and a half (3 cm) thick and 8–10 inches (20–25 cm) across. It's firmly attached to the uterine wall (usually the upper part).

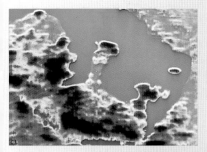

Ultrasound scan
At this time, your baby's nose, fingers, and toes can be seen clearly on a scan. Her head is still large compared with her body.

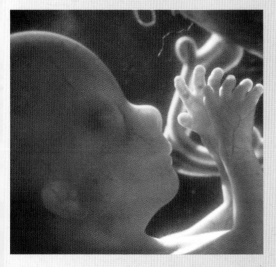

Head and face
Her face is looking more human and she's starting to frown and squint. Eyebrows and eyelashes start to grow, and the hair on her head is colored by pigment cells. Her eyes look straight ahead, although they're still widely spaced. The retinas of her eyes are sensitive to light, although they're still covered by her eyelids, and she's aware of bright light outside of her mother's body.

MOTHER

You're showing many signs that pregnancy is advancing well, although you may not have gained much weight. You'll probably have extra vitality and energy.

Nipples They're darkening in color as your skin becomes more deeply pigmented. They may tingle and feel sore, and the surface veins are becoming more prominent.

Heart This is working twice as hard as before, moving enough blood (six quarts/liters per minute) to meet the increasing needs of your vital organs. Your uterus and skin need twice as much blood as usual and your kidneys 25 percent more.

Abdomen You may develop a dark line, called the linea nigra, down the center of your abdomen. Your uterus has been forced out of the pelvic cavity into your abdomen by your growing baby and can be felt on examination.

Quickening Toward the end of this month, you'll probably feel your baby moving—a bubbling, fluttering sensation like butterflies, little fish, or wind! First-time mothers feel movements later than women in subsequent pregnancies (see also p.194).

BABY

Your baby's skin is transparent and her blood vessels can be seen clearly. Her bones, which are beginning to harden throughout her body, can also be seen.

Taste buds They've begun to develop on her tongue.

Ears As the tiny bones inside her ears harden, she begins to hear sounds—your voice, your heart, and your digestion rumbling.

Lungs They are developing, and she "breathes" the amniotic fluid. She'll continue to receive oxygen via the placenta until she's born.

Baby's vital statistics
By the end of this month her crown-to-rump length will be 5½ in (13.5 cm), and she'll weigh 6 oz (180 g).

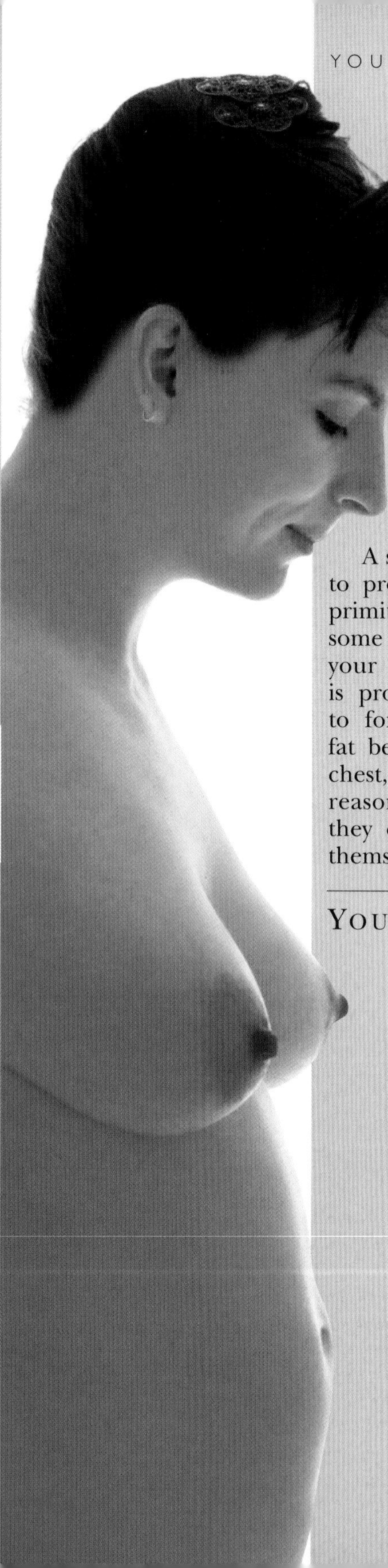

01
02
03
04
05
06
07
08
09
10
11
12
13
14
15
16
17
18
19
20
21
22
23
24
25
26
27
28
29
30
31
32
33
34
35
36
37
38
39
40

Up to 22 weeks

By this time your baby has grown enough to have developed a nervous system and muscles that allow him to move around in your womb. Because he's still so small, he can swim up and down and be in any position at any time.

YOUR BABY'S PROGRESS

Up until about 19 weeks after your last period, your baby grows very rapidly. Now this growth rate slows down, apart from his weight gain, and he matures in other ways. He begins to build up his defense systems.

A sheath begins to form around the nerves in his spinal cord to protect them from possible damage. He also has his own primitive immune system, which will help to defend him from some infections. To make body heat and keep up his temperature, your baby needs some specialized fatty tissue. This is provided by a substance called "brown fat," which began to form during the fourth month. Now, deposits of brown fat begin to build up in areas of his body such as his neck, chest, and crotch. This will continue until term. One of the reasons that premature babies are so vulnerable is that they don't yet have enough brown fat, and so cannot keep themselves warm.

YOUR BABY AT 22 WEEKS OF PREGNANCY

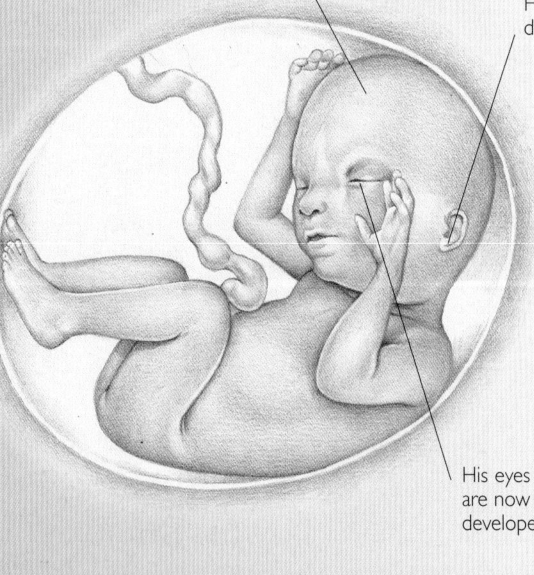

Fine hair (lanugo) covers his body

His ears have developed

His eyes and eyelids are now well developed

His skin will continue to grow, although it'll be red and wrinkled because there's so little fat underneath it. His body begins to get plumper from now on. The sebaceous glands (oil-producing glands in the skin) become active and make a waxy, greasy substance called *vernix caseosa*. This protects his skin during its long immersion in the amniotic fluid.

Your baby's body is also covered with fine hair called *lanugo*. Nobody is quite sure why babies have this hair, but it may help to regulate the body temperature, or it may help hold the protective vernix caseosa in place.

His movements   As his nerve fibers become connected and his muscles continue to develop and grow stronger, his movements become more purposeful and coordinated. He embarks on his own gymnastics program—stretching, grasping, turning—to build up his muscles, improve his motor ability, and strengthen his bones. These movements can make your abdomen sore.

Sex organs   A boy's scrotum is solid at this stage. A girl's vagina starts to become hollow and her ovaries contain about seven million eggs, which will be reduced to about two million at birth. By the time she reaches puberty, she'll have between 200,000 and 500,000 eggs, and she'll release only 400–500 of these during her adult life—around one per month until menopause. Nipples and underlying mammary glands develop in both sexes.

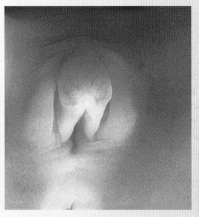

Your baby's genitalia
Your baby's sex was determined at conception. Ultrasound or fetoscopy can only reveal what sex your baby is if there's a direct view of the external genitals. The picture above shows the genitalia of a 17-week-old male fetus.

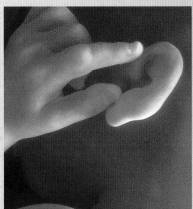

His hearing
Your baby can hear the sounds of your blood flowing through your blood vessels, your heart beating, and your stomach rumbling. He can hear sounds from outside the uterus and will respond to sound, rhythm, and melody from now on. It's a good idea to sing and talk to your unborn child. After birth, he'll probably be soothed by the same songs, finding them reassuring, and he'll feel safe and secure when he hears his parents' voices.

MOTHER

Around this time, well into your second trimester, you'll probably notice a mood change. You'll feel that your energy, and sense of fun have come back and any nausea should have disappeared.

Movements   If you didn't feel your baby move earlier, you'll certainly feel him now. The experience of your baby "quickening" inside you is wonderful.

Abdomen   Your waistline has disappeared and you may notice stretch marks.

Skin   Dilated blood vessels may cause tiny red marks (spider naevi) to appear on your face, arms, and shoulders. These should fade after the birth.

Minor complaints   Your gums may become spongy, probably because of hormonal influences. You may have some constipation and heartburn. You're more likely to get bladder infections because of the relaxation of the smooth muscle in the urinary tract.

Metabolic changes   Your thyroid gland becomes more active, and this can cause you to perspire more heavily than usual. Your breathing will get deeper and you may feel short of breath when you take your exercise.

BABY

Although he's well developed, your baby cannot yet survive outside your womb. His lungs and digestive system aren't fully formed, nor can he maintain his own body heat properly.

Vernix caseosa   This waxy coating made by his skin glands keeps his skin supple.

Taste   He can now tell sweet from bitter.

Touch   His skin is now sensitive to touch, and he will move in response to any pressure that is put on your abdomen.

Teeth   Hidden in his gums, many of his "baby" teeth have already been formed.

Heartbeat   This can now be heard by less sensitive stethoscopes.

> **Baby's vital statistics**
> *By the end of this month his crown- to-rump length will be 7 in (18.5 cm) and he'll weigh 1 lb (0.5 kg).*

01
02
03
04
05
06
07
08
09
10
11
12
13
14
15
16
17
18
19
20
21
22
23
24
25
26
27
28
29
30
31
32
33
34
35
36
37
38
39
40

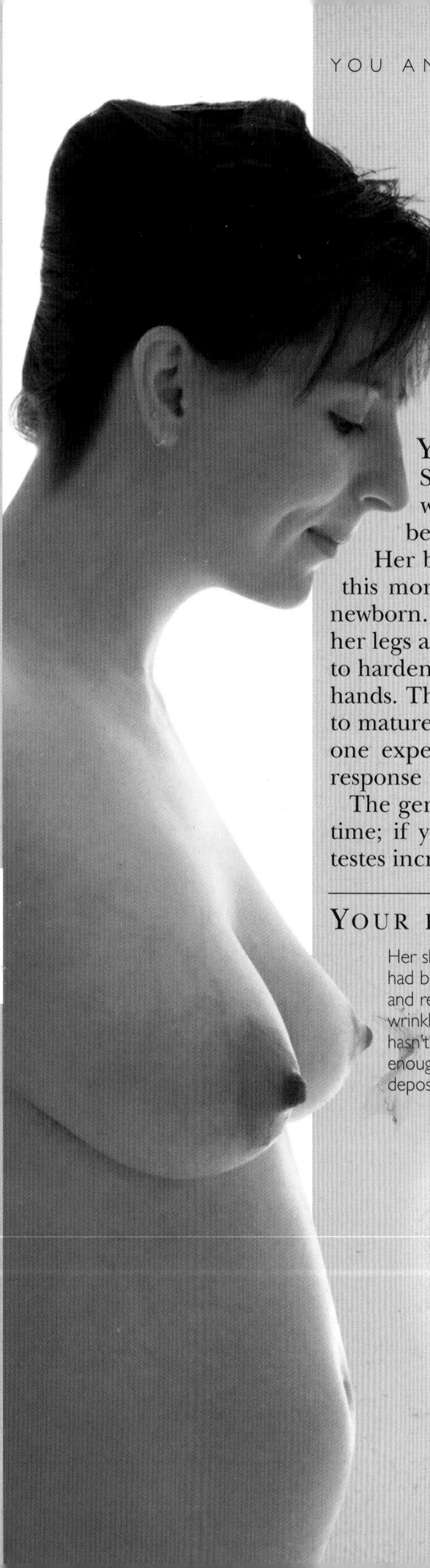

Up to 26 weeks

Your baby is growing taller and stronger, and her movements are becoming more complex. She's also showing signs of sensitivity, awareness, and intelligence. A baby born after 24 weeks of pregnancy could survive with specialized intensive care in a neonatal unit.

YOUR BABY'S PROGRESS

She's still red and skinny, but she'll soon start to put on weight. Her skin may look very wrinkled, but this is because she doesn't yet have much fat to plump it out.

Her body is growing faster than her head, and by the end of this month her proportions are about the same as those of a newborn. Her arms and legs have their normal amount of muscle, her legs and body are in proportion, and her bone are beginning to harden in the center. Lines start to appear on the palms of her hands. The brain cells she'll use for conscious thought now start to mature, and she begins to be able to remember and learn. (In one experiment, babies in the womb were trained to kick in response to a particular vibration.)

The genitals of a boy and girl look completely different by this time; if your baby is a boy, testosterone-producing cells in the testes increase in number.

YOUR BABY AT 26 WEEKS OF PREGNANCY

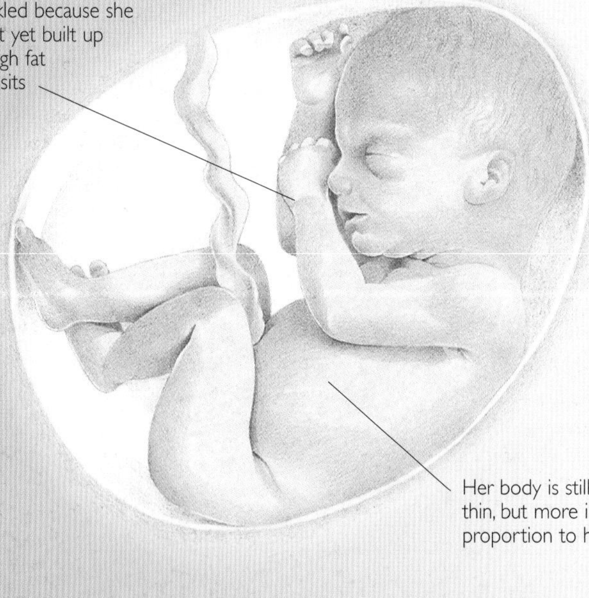

Her skin has lost the translucent look it had before and has become opaque and reddish-looking. It's still wrinkled because she hasn't yet built up enough fat deposits

Her body is still thin, but more in proportion to her head

Her hearing Your baby can hear sound frequencies that you can't hear. She'll move more in response to high frequencies than to low ones and she'll move her body in rhythm with your speech. From this month she will begin to respond to drum beats by jumping up and down. Some mothers say they've had to leave concerts because their unborn babies wouldn't keep still.

If she hears a piece of music often, she may realize it's familiar to her when she grows up – even if she can't remember ever hearing it. Some musicians have said that they "knew" unseen pieces of music, and later found out that their mothers played these to them while they were in the womb.

She'll also learn to recognize her father's voice from this month onward. A baby whose father talks to her while she's in the womb can pick out her father's voice in a roomful of people immediately after she is born. She'll respond to it emotionally. For example, if she's upset, she'll stop crying when she hears her father talking and calm down.

Her breathing Inside her lungs, more and more air sacs are forming. They'll continue to increase in number until she's about eight years old. Around them, the blood vessels that will help her to absorb oxygen and expel carbon dioxide are multiplying. Her nostrils have opened, too, and she's beginning to make breathing movements with her muscles, so that her system has plenty of breathing practice before she's born.

MOTHER

Your baby's movements are well established now, and you'll feel some every day. When she hiccups, for example, you'll feel a sudden jerk.

Weight You'll be putting on weight at the rate of about 1 lb (0.5 kg) per week. Don't worry if you are told you look "small for dates." Your size will depend on many things, such as your build, how tall you are, the way you move, and the amount of amniotic fluid inside. It's the size of your growing baby that counts, and that will be checked by ultrasound scanning.

Aches and pains As your baby grows, and your uterus along with her, they push upward against your rib cage. It'll rise by about 2 in (5 cm) and your lower ribs will spread outward. This can give you rib pain and, because your baby is now beginning to press upon your stomach, you may also start to have bouts of indigestion and heartburn (see p.208). As your uterine muscle stretches, you may get stitchlike pains down the sides of your abdomen.

BABY

She continues to grow slowly and steadily. If she's born prematurely, she'd have a slim chance of survival now.

Lungs The *bronchi* (the main tubes leading from her windpipe to her lungs) are growing, although they aren't yet mature.

Brain The patterns of her brain waves are now like those of a full-term newborn child. The source of these brain waves is thought to be the cortex, the highly evolved part of the brain. She's now developed patterns of sleeping and waking.

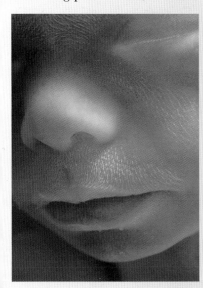

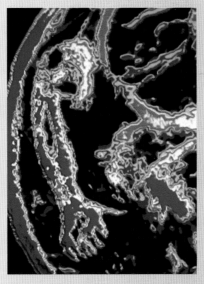

Your baby's face
The features of this six-month-old fetus are much like those of a newborn baby. Lanugo, the downy hair on a baby's skin, forms patterns because of the oblique way in which the hair roots are positioned in the skin.

Ultrasound
Your baby is growing bigger, gaining weight, and taking up more space in your womb. The picture above has been taken by ultrasound and then color-enhanced. You can see the baby's fully formed arm, hand, and shoulder.

Baby's vital statistics
By the end of this month her crown-to-rump length will be 10 in (25 cm) and she will weigh just under 2 lb (1 kg).

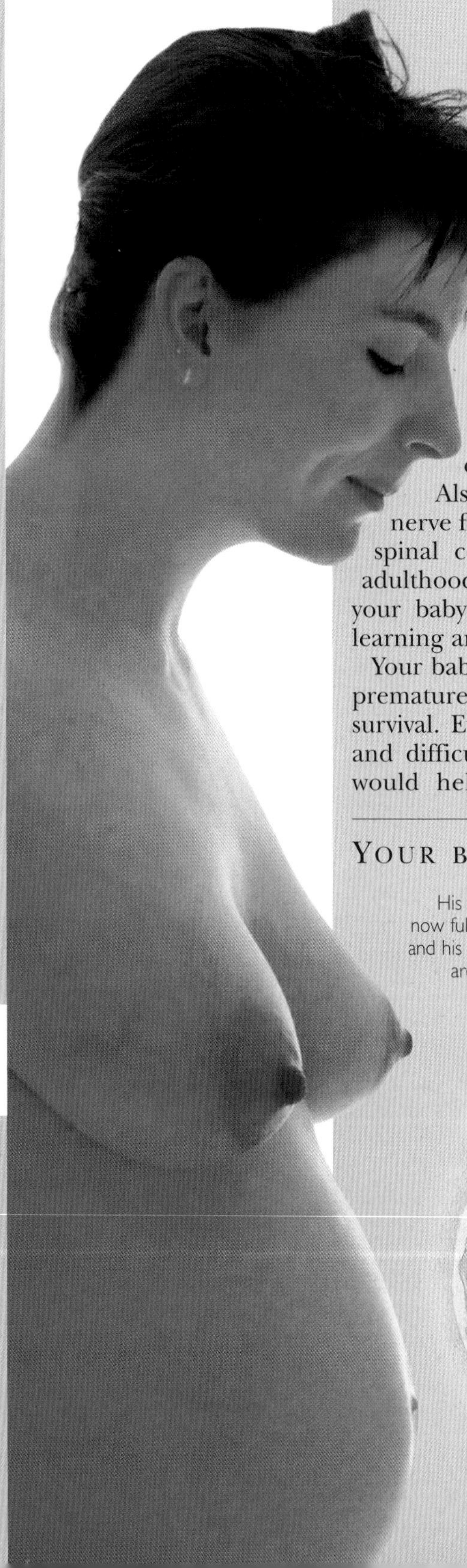

Up to 30 weeks

Your baby's now so big that when your doctor or midwife examines you, they can check his position and the way he's lying. This is the last month he can do a somersault.

YOUR BABY'S PROGRESS

Great changes take place in your baby's nervous system this month. His brain grows larger (to fit inside the skull, it has to fold over and wrinkle up until it looks like a walnut), and his brain cells and nerve circuits are all fully linked and active.

Also, a protective fatty sheath begins to form around his nerve fibers, just as a similar sheath formed earlier around his spinal cord. This fatty sheath keeps developing until early adulthood. Thanks to this, nerve impulses can travel faster and your baby is now able to cope with more complex types of learning and movement.

Your baby starts getting ready for birth. (If he were to be born prematurely at this stage, he'd have an excellent chance of survival. Even though he might have some breathing problems and difficulty in keeping himself warm, modern care facilities would help him thrive.) He's beginning to gain some fat

YOUR BABY AT 30 WEEKS OF PREGNANCY

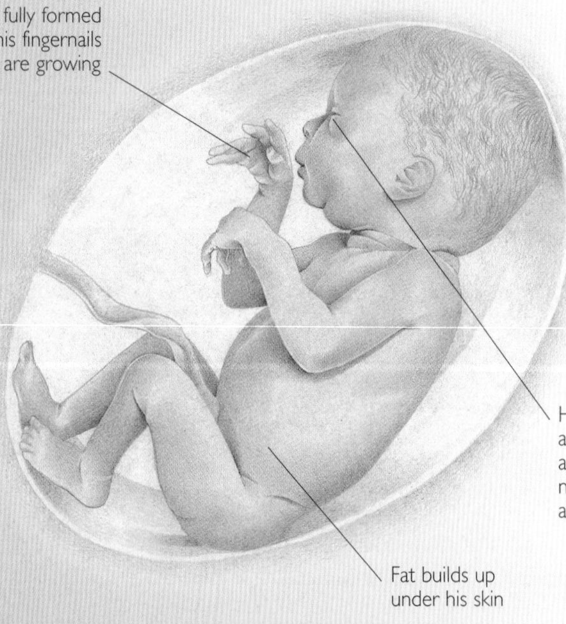

His hands are now fully formed and his fingernails are growing

His eyelids are open and he can now see and focus

Fat builds up under his skin

01
02
03
04
05
06
07
08
09
10
11
12
13
14
15
16
17
18
19
20
21
22
23
24
25
26
27
28
29
30
31
32
33
34
35
36
37
38
39
40

underneath his skin, which starts to smooth out, lose its wrinkles, and look more rounded. His coat of hairy lanugo may reduce to just a patch on his back and shoulders. The membranes that sealed and protected his eyes while they were growing will have fulfilled their function by the beginning of this month. His eyes are now fully formed and his eyelids have separated, allowing his eyes to open. He continues to develop the swallowing and sucking skills he'll need as soon as he's born.

His breathing By now he's developed his mature breathing rhythm, and the air sacs in his lungs start to get ready for the first breath he'll take in the world outside your womb. The air sacs line themselves with a coating of special cells and a fluid (surfactant) that will prevent them from collapsing.

His movements He'll find he has less room to move around and may move less. He'll wriggle uncomfortably if you're in a position that doesn't feel good to him (see p.194).

Orientation During his weeks of "gymnastics practice," your baby has done more than increase his muscle tone—he's developed the ability to position himself in space. He'll probably continue to lie with his head upward during this month, although if he's maturing fast he may turn upside down and settle into place for delivery (engage) earlier than usual. This is more common in first babies. Babies can continue turning up to 36 weeks.

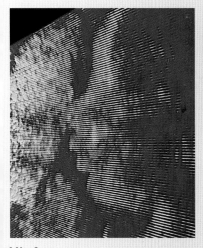

His face
The baby's maturing profile can be seen clearly in the ultrasound scan above.

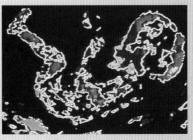

Your baby grows
His body is now growing plumper as fat builds up under his skin, filling out the wrinkles. His eyebrows and eyelashes are fully developed, and the hair on his scalp is growing longer. His eyelids have now opened, and he begins to practice seeing and focusing; the limitations of his field of vision (8–9 in/20–25 cm) at birth are thought to be related to how far he's able to see while in the uterus. As the ultrasound above shows, his head and body look more balanced in size. He now has the proportions of a newborn baby.

MOTHER

This ends your second trimester. You may start to feel tired and, knowing that your baby just needs to mature, you may begin to think more about his birth.

Colostrum Your breasts will probably have made this sweet, watery fluid, which is less rich than breast milk and easier to digest. It will provide your baby with his first few meals before your milk comes through (see also p.326).

Urination Your growing baby will now be pressing against your bladder and you'll feel like passing urine more often. You may occasionally leak urine unexpectedly if you cough or sneeze.

Sleeping problems You'll find it hard to get comfortable if you're big. Lying on your side with one knee to your chest and the other stretched out will probably be most comfortable position.

Low back pain You may get backaches because of a shift of your center of gravity caused by the enlarged uterus, plus the slight loosening of the pelvic joints. Wearing low-heeled shoes and sitting with a straight back on a hard chair or the floor will help. Don't lift heavy objects if you can help it.

BABY

Your baby continues to gain weight and mature. He keeps in touch with you by wriggling and kicking.

Temperature He now begins to control his own body temperature.

Fat White fat begins to build up under his skin.

Red blood cells His bone marrow has now completely taken over responsibility for the making of red blood cells.

Urine He passes about 1 pint (0.5 liters) of urine into the amniotic fluid every day.

Genitals The testes of boy babies descend first into the groin and then into the scrotum. Premature boy babies will usually have undescended testicles.

> **Baby's vital statistics**
> *By the end of this month his crown- to-rump length will be 11 in (28 cm), and he'll weigh about 3 lb (1.5 kg).*

01
02
03
04
05
06
07
08
09
10
11
12
13
14
15
16
17
18
19
20
21
22
23
24
25
26
27
28
29
30
31
32
33
34
35
36
37
38
39
40

Up to 34 weeks

Thirty-four weeks after your last period, your baby is perfectly formed. All her proportions are exactly as you'd expect them to be at birth. She still has some maturing to do, though, and some more weight to gain before she's ready to be born.

YOUR BABY'S PROGRESS

Her organs are now almost fully mature, except for her lungs. These aren't yet completely developed, although they're making increasing quantities of *surfactant*, the fluid that will stop them from collapsing once she begins to breathe air. She makes strong movements that can be felt on the surface of your abdomen. Almost all babies born at this time survive.

Her skin, nails, and hair Her skin is now pink rather than red, because of the deposits of white fat underneath it. Fat deposits build up under her skin to provide energy and regulate her body temperature after she's born. The protective vernix caseosa that covers her skin is now very thick. Her fingernails now reach the ends of her fingers but her toenails are not yet fully grown. She may have quite a lot of hair on her head.

Her eyes Her irises can now dilate and contract. They'll contract in response to bright light, and also to allow her to focus,

YOUR BABY AT 34 WEEKS OF PREGNANCY

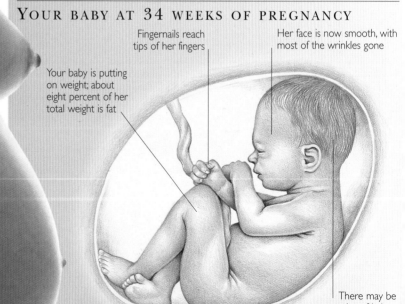

Fingernails reach
tips of her fingers

Her face is now smooth, with
most of the wrinkles gone

Your baby is putting
on weight; about
eight percent of her
total weight is fat

There may be
a lot of hair
on her head

although she won't need to develop this skill until after she's born. She can close her eyelids, and she has begun to blink.

Her position Some babies take up the head-downward position about now, but there's still plenty of time—most don't engage until after 36 weeks. She may remain in the breech (bottom-down) position (see p.307) until birth, although most babies do turn on their own.

HER SUPPORT SYSTEM

From this month the placenta layers may start to thin. To make estrogen, the placenta converts a testosterone-like hormone that's made by your baby's adrenal glands. By this month these glands are as big as those of an adolescent, and every day they produce 10 times as much hormone as an adult's adrenal glands. They'll shrink rapidly after birth.

The amniotic sac, or bag of waters, contains a large amount of fluid, most of which is the baby's urine—she can produce as much as a pint (half a liter) of urine every day. Excess vernix caseosa, nutrients, and products necessary for the maturing of her lungs are also in the amniotic sac. The umbilical cord is large, strong, and tough. A firm, gelatinous substance surrounds the blood vessels and prevents kinks or knots in the cord that could affect your baby's blood supply.

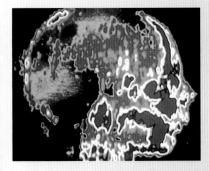

Her head and face
The ultrasound on the left shows very clearly how both the shape of her head and her profile have developed, so she now looks like a "real baby,"

Your baby's size
It's now becoming a tight fit in the uterus, especially if your baby is large. Because of this, she may start to move less, although you should still be able to feel her moving (see pp.194 & 195). Her body, like that of the baby in the ultrasound scan on the right, will now start to become tightly curled as her elbow and knee space is restricted. Quite a few babies are bottom-down (breech) at the start of this month (see column, p.259), but most will have tipped head-down by term.

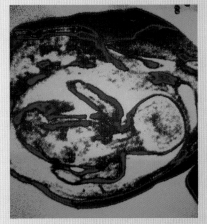

MOTHER

You'll probably be having prenatal checks more often now. Your doctor will monitor your blood pressure and urine and check your baby's position.

Contractions Your uterus hardens and contracts as practice for labor. These are known as Braxton-Hicks contractions. They last only about 30 seconds, and you may not even be aware of them.

Pelvis Your pelvis has now expanded and may ache, especially at the back.

Blood Some women may have a low hemoglobin level at this stage of pregnancy. Make sure you are taking your iron to prepare for the blood loss you will experience at delivery.

Abdomen Your baby is getting bigger, so your uterus is pushed hard against your lower ribs, and your rib cage may become quite sore. Your abdomen is so stretched that your navel sticks out, and the increased pigmentation of the linea nigra can make it look very prominent.

BABY

Your baby's main activity now is to settle into a head-down position and adjust to her lack of space in the uterus.

Eyes She can now focus and blink.

Weight gain She'll have gained at least 2 lb (about 1 kg) since last month. Most of this is increased muscle tissue and fat.

Lungs Her lungs are still developing so that she can adjust to breathing outside the uterus. If she were to be born at this stage, she'd almost certainly have breathing difficulties, although she would have an excellent chance of survival.

Baby's vital statistics
By the end of this month her crown-to-rump length will be about 12 in (32 cm), and she'll weigh about 5 lb (2.5 kg).

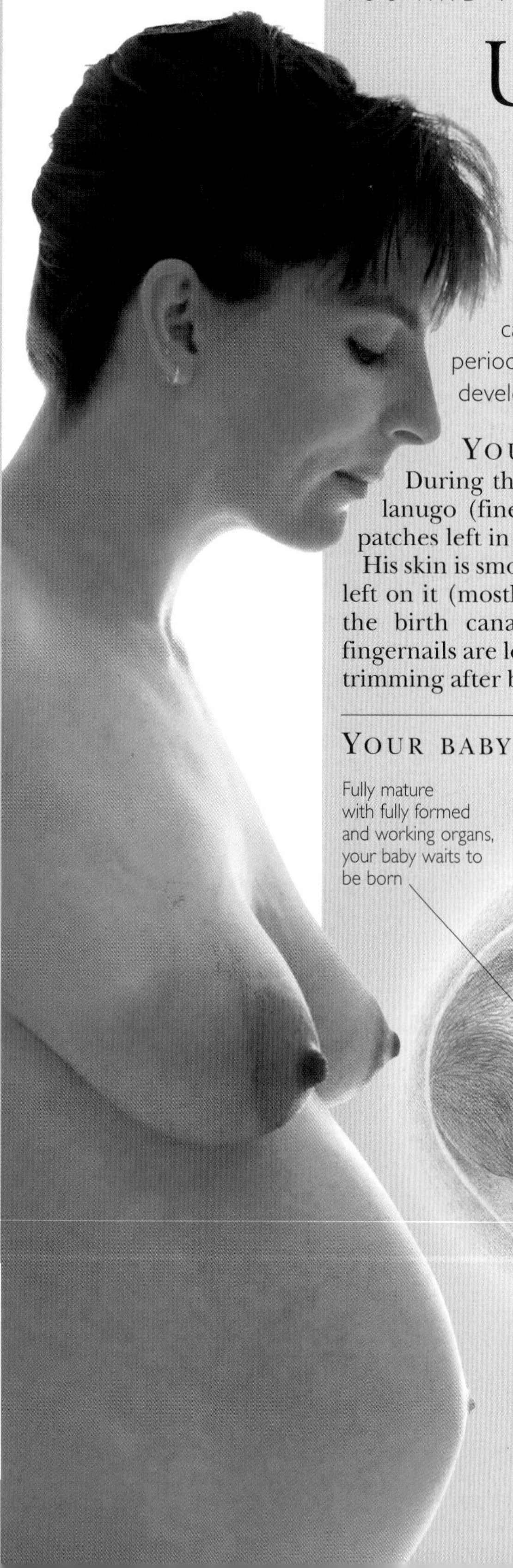

Up to 40 weeks

It can be hard to calculate the exact date of conception, although most women have their fertile time about 14 days after the first day of their menstrual period. Because of this, doctors use an artificial but convenient time scale of 40 weeks, calculated from the date of your last menstrual period. A baby actually reaches "full term," meaning it's fully developed, after about 38 weeks.

YOUR BABY'S PROGRESS

During this month your baby will usually shed most of the lanugo (fine hair) from his body. There may be some small patches left in odd places and perhaps some in his body creases. His skin is smooth and soft, and there is still some vernix caseosa left on it (mostly on his back), which will help his passage down the birth canal. He'll be almost chubby before birth. His fingernails are long and may have scratched his face—they'll need trimming after birth. His eyes are blue, although they may change

YOUR BABY AT 40 WEEKS OF PREGNANCY

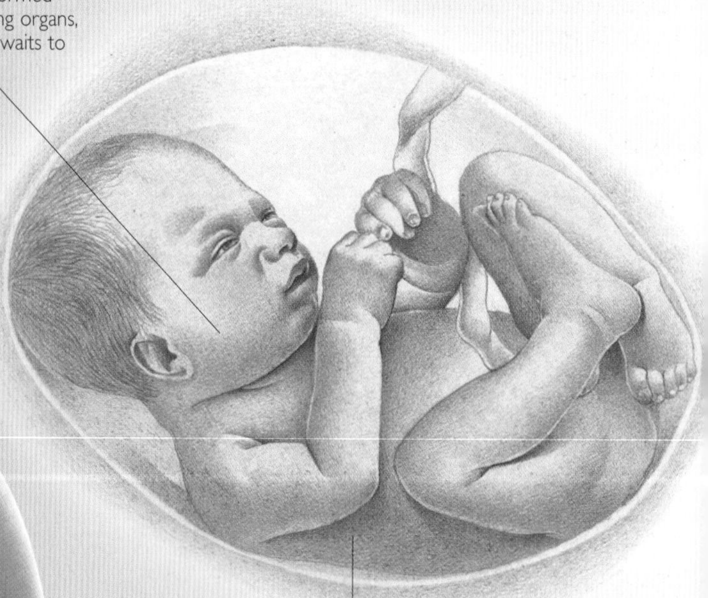

Fully mature with fully formed and working organs, your baby waits to be born

His body is plump and round. By the last week of pregnancy, he just barely fits inside your uterus and has to curl up very tightly

01
02
03
04
05
06
07
08
09
10
11
12
13
14
15
16
17
18
19
20
21
22
23
24
25
26
27
28
29
30
31
32
33
34
35
36
37
38
39
40

in the weeks after birth. When he's awake, his eyes are open. In these last weeks, your baby produces increasing amounts of a hormone called *cortisone* from his adrenal glands. This helps his lungs to mature and prepare for his first breath.

Meconium Your baby's intestines are filled with a dark green, almost black, substance called *meconium.* This is a mixture of the secretions from his alimentary glands together with the lanugo that's been shed from his body, pigment, and cells from the wall of his bowel. It'll be the first bowel motion he'll pass after birth, but he may pass it during delivery.

Immune system His own system is still immature, so to make up for this he receives antibodies from you via the placenta. These protect him against anything that you have antibodies for, such as flu, mumps, and German measles. After he's born, he'll keep getting antibodies from you via your breast milk.

HIS SUPPORT SYSTEM

The placenta now measures 8–10 inches (20–25 cm) in diameter and is just over an inch (3 cm) thick, thus creating a wide area for the exchange of nourishment and waste products between your system and your baby's. There's now more than a quart (liter) of water in the amniotic sac.

The hormones made by the placenta are stimulating your breasts to swell and fill with milk. This also causes swelling in your baby's breasts, whether it is a boy or a girl. This will go down after birth. If your baby is a girl, the stopping of these same hormones following delivery may cause her to have a light bleeding from her vagina (like a period) a few days after her birth.

MOTHER

When you see your doctor or midwife at this stage, they'll be checking to make sure everything is going well.

Engagement In most first-time mothers, the baby's head drops down into the pelvis at about 36 weeks. You'll feel more comfortable then and it'll be easier to breathe. It's normal for your baby's head not to engage until later, sometimes not until labor has started.

Posture You may tend to make up for extra weight at the front by leaning backward. This throws your head back so that your line of vision is different from usual. Your center of gravity has altered, so you may bump into things or drop them.

Sleeping and resting It may be more and more difficult for you to get a good night's sleep as your large abdomen makes it hard to get comfortable. Put your feet up and rest as much as you can, though.

Nesting instinct This usually happens during prelabor (see p.270) and often seems to make you want to do things like cleaning the oven! Try to resist it—you'll need all your energy for giving birth.

BABY

Your baby prepares to be born; his lungs mature and the last of his brown fat is laid down.

Reproductive organs The testes of most boy babies will have descended by now. In a girl baby, the ovaries are still above the pelvic brim and don't reach their final position until after birth.

Movements Although your baby's movements will be much less than they were earlier, you should still be able to feel him kick.

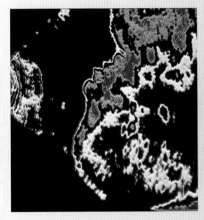

Engaged head
The ultrasound scan above shows the baby lying head down, with his head against his mother's cervix (bottom right-hand corner).

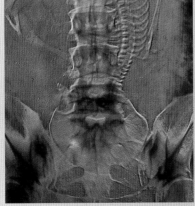

Prepared for birth
As your baby gets heavier and matures, he'll tip head-down in your uterus. In the color-enhanced X-ray above, the baby's head can be seen settled deeply into the mother's pelvis.

Baby's vital statistics
By the end of this month his crown-to-rump length will be about 14–15 in (35–37 cm), and he'll weigh about 6½–9 lb (3–4 kg).

CHAPTER 3

Preparing for fatherhood

Most men have strong nurturing instincts, and most, given half a chance, make excellent fathers. No one feels confident about parenthood, and the prospect of becoming a father can be daunting. A little thought and preparation in advance can go a long way toward boosting morale and giving a man a sense of fulfillment.

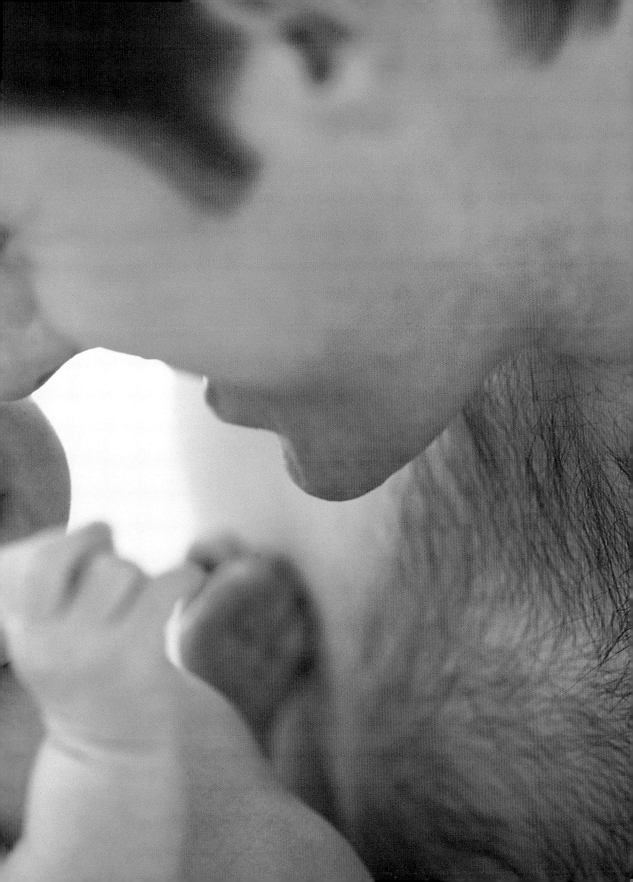

Becoming a dad

THE MODERN FATHER

Most men are happy to share the tasks that used to be seen more as a mother's responsibility. They are just as capable as women of bathing the baby, doing the grocery shopping, and taking children to and from school.

- More men are becoming stay-at-home dads and the main caregivers of their children.

- Many fathers are fitting family matters, like walking children to school, helping in the classroom, or taking their child to the doctor, into their working day.

- Most fathers love to share the bedtime bath and story routine, especially if they've been away from their children all day.

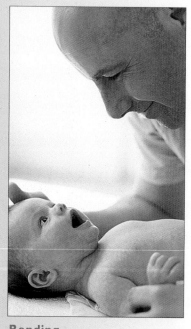

Bonding
A father starts to form lifelong bonds with his baby during the first weeks of life, so he needs plenty of contact.

This chapter is for dads. Even though getting pregnant and having a baby is very much a joint venture for a couple, fathers usually take a back seat in books like this. I'd like to correct that bias. Your baby doesn't have any notion about the difference between mothers and fathers. She just wants to be loved and cared for. Men can do these things just as well as women, and caring for your baby helps build your relationship with her for the future. That fact alone makes a powerful argument for parenting being equal and shared.

MAKING ROOM FOR FATHERS

Don't worry—getting involved with parenting needn't be a problem. With a little planning and a generous heart, both of you can enjoy sharing all the aspects of caring for your baby. After all, baby care means loving your baby, encouraging your baby, teaching your baby, watching your baby grow and develop, and establishing bonds with your baby that will probably be the strongest you ever make with anyone. Being a parent is perhaps the most important job any of us do. Who in their right mind would not want to be a part of all that?

As a father, try not to allow yourself to miss out on this unique relationship. And you'll find that when you're fully involved with your baby, a little miracle happens along the way: your relationship with your baby's mother flourishes, too.

No one has trouble defining a mother's role. Mothers care for children: they feed, comfort, dress, and bathe; they encourage, teach, carry, undress, put to bed, and maybe sing to sleep. We all know this because it's what our mothers did for us when we were children. Defining a father's role is more difficult, and many men are struggling to come to terms with what it means to be a modern father.

Finding a role model Much as you may love your own father, you may want your own relationship with your children to be different. Men today are encouraged to have a much more hands-on approach to caring for their children, but few have a role model to show them what this actually means. What's really needed is for fathers to be much more involved with the day-to-day business of child care—for them to be more like mothers.

Your baby doesn't mind Babies and young children are happy to be cared for by their father or mother. What your baby needs is comfort, warmth, and security from her parents. Although she'll soon learn to tell her mother and father apart, she's not going to make value judgments based on what mothers and fathers ought to do. Apart from breastfeeding, there's nothing a woman can do for a baby that can't be done by a man.

The need for parenting Babies don't need mothering and fathering, they need parenting. They need the most important adults in their lives to be models of what parents do for their children. When this happens, the next generation of fathers will not be at a loss to know what a father's role should be. A child will only start to look to one parent rather than the other for her needs if this is what she learns she should do from her experiences. If you, as a father, never change her diaper, hold her when she cries, or play and laugh with her, of course she'll relate more to the parent who does do all those things.

YOUR FEELINGS ABOUT HAVING A FAMILY

However much you long for a family, the decision to go ahead and have a child needs the same reasoned, clear-eyed evaluation you'd give to any other major change in your life, such as buying a house or a new car. It helps to be open with one another about your feelings and to put into words some of the thoughts and questions that may be lurking in the back of your mind. Even if you think you both really want a baby because you love each other and it seems like the natural thing to do, it's still a good idea to talk about all the issues involved. Have you thought about how a baby will affect your way of life? Does having a child seem like the right thing for you as a couple, or are you just reacting to pressure from others, such as the potential grandparents? Do you both have the same desire for a baby?

The caring father
Once you start getting involved in the care of your baby, you'll find that you enjoy it—and you can be good at it.

A NEW KIND OF PARENTING

Family life has changed in recent years, and people have different expectations. A father used to be a protector, out at work all day and with little direct involvement in the care of children. Now, fathers and mothers are equal partners at home. Both may be working, full- or part-time, and sharing the financial responsibilities and the juggling of caring for home and family. Some couples may decide they don't want to use any form of child care and so one of them takes a career break to stay at home. In an increasing number of couples, it's the father who opts to be the caregiver while his wife earns the money, overturning traditional patterns of family life. One reason why such families are often strong and successful units is because they make their plans carefully and take account of both partners' talents. But whatever practical arrangements you make, providing a stable, loving, and open environment in which to bring up children is what matters the most.

BONDING WITH YOUR BABY

It's never too early to start bonding with your baby. Babies can hear sounds outside the womb by five or six months. If you talk to your baby, he'll get to know your voice even before he's born—in fact, he'll be able to hear your low-pitched voice more clearly than his mother's. To help you bond with your baby:

- gently massage your partner's tummy and feel your baby move

- talk and coo softly to your baby, and kiss and nuzzle him through your partner's skin

- listen to your baby's heartbeat—a cardboard tube, such as a toilet paper roll, can make a good amplifier

- go to scans with your partner and watch your baby develop (see p.180)

- read as much about pregnancy and birth as you can—at least as much as your partner does—so that you can talk things over together

- talk over names for your baby together—this gives your unborn baby a personality and you can start relating to him or to her

- check the dates of prenatal checkups and any childbirth classes your partner goes to, and plan ahead so you can go along, too.

The expectant father

The moment you find out that you're going to be a father is one of the most exciting of your life, and you'll probably feel just as emotional about the news as your partner does. You may find, though, that most people will assume it doesn't affect you much, and once the first excitement has worn off, they'll stop asking you how you're feeling. Don't let this stop you from talking to your partner about the pregnancy and getting involved in plans for the birth. Allow your unborn baby to become as big a part of your life as you can. After all, this great event is something that's happening to both of you, not just to your partner.

UNDERSTANDING YOUR FEELINGS

For the first couple of months, your partner will look much the same as usual and you may find the fact that you're expecting a baby hard to take in. Don't worry if your feelings about the pregnancy aren't the same as hers at first; your experiences are very different. A couple doesn't suddenly become one person with one set of feelings just because they're having a baby together. Later on, when you see your partner's body beginning to change and you've seen your baby on a scan and felt his first movements, the idea of having a child of your own will become more real.

You may find at this time that your feelings of joy and excitement are mixed with fears and worries about how your life will be affected and whether you'll be able to cope financially. There's no doubt that having a child can be an extra financial burden, especially if one of you is going to give up your job to care for your baby, but don't rush into making life-changing decisions. It may be tempting to start looking for a new job or seek a promotion that might bring in some more money, but it's difficult to know how you'll feel about extra responsibility a year down the line, once you're a parent. You may find that having time to spend with your child is more important to you than offering material possessions.

GETTING INVOLVED

When you're an expectant father, you're likely to feel not quite in control of things. You may feel like an outsider, and well-meaning female friends and relatives may assume you're not really involved and seem to push you out of what they see as their territory. Medical professionals, such as obstetricians and midwives, will understandably direct their conversations at your partner more than at you.

Take the initiative Don't just step back and allow your female relatives and friends to become more involved than you. Talk to your own friends and colleagues: some may tease you at first, but you'll probably find other fathers will be eager to share their experiences with you. Try to find out as much as you can about the pregnancy so that you can understand what's happening in your partner's body. Go with her to the scans so that you can see your baby developing, talk about the fact you're going to be a father, and ask as many questions as you want.

PLAN FOR THE BIRTH TOGETHER

Talk to your partner about the type of birth she wants (see p.106) and how you can best be involved. Plan to talk to your employer about taking time off for prenatal appointments as well as for the birth and afterward, so that you can spend some time at home with your partner after your baby is born.

The birth plan Go through the birth plan together (see p.122), but don't impose your views. If she feels strongly about certain aspects, such as trying for a drug-free labor (see p.282), respect her feelings but make sure you both know the pros and cons. Some men worry that they'll feel squeamish at the birth, but few do. Witnessing the birth of your child is probably one of the most moving things that will ever happen to you, and holding your baby in the first few seconds of life not only helps bond the two of you but is a tremendous emotional experience.

IT'S YOUR BABY, TOO

There's no need to hold back any of your feelings or thoughts. Feel free to:

- be open about your feelings

- express your concerns

- talk frankly to your partner about sex so it doesn't become an issue

- be involved in all arrangements and plans for the birth

- go to childbirth classes

- go to prenatal appointments to hear your baby's heartbeat and see him move on the ultrasound

- visit the hospital and delivery room with your partner and meet any professionals involved

- be present at the birth.

What to do	How it can help you
Talk to your partner	The best way to understand how your partner is feeling and what's going on in her body is to talk to her. Ask her what it feels like when your baby moves; go over your plans for the birth together; find out if she has particular discomforts. She'll be pleased to share her experiences with you.
Go to childbirth classes	If you go to childbirth classes (especially father-only sessions) you'll have a chance to learn about what will happen at the birth and talk through your own worries. This will help you to work out the best way to support your partner and allow you to be more involved in making decisions about the birth.
Talk to other fathers	Get to know the other expectant fathers at childbirth classes—they'll probably be feeling much the same as you and be glad to have someone to talk to. Talk to friends and colleagues who have babies; find out what their experience was like and ask their advice.
Read about pregnancy	Read pregnancy and parenting books and any leaflets you're given. The more you understand about what's going on during the pregnancy, the more familiar it will become, and you'll appreciate more how your partner is feeling. You'll also be able to give your partner support if she's worried or anxious about anything.
Ask questions	Go to prenatal appointments with your partner so that you can meet the professionals and be present at the examinations. If you're a first-time parent, there'll be things you don't understand and need to know more about. If you ask questions of professionals, they're more likely to involve you.

Fathers at the birth

COPING WITH THE UNEXPECTED

A labor that doesn't go as planned can be scary for both of you. It helps to be prepared in advance and accept the fact that unexpected interventions may be necessary.

- Well before your baby is due, talk to your partner about what she feels about any special situation that could come up. Make sure you know her views and preferences for anything that might happen. Bear in mind, though, that she may change her mind if a situation does arise.

- Unless it's an absolute emergency, make sure that you and your partner get a chance to talk through any interventions suggested and ask questions if anything isn't clear. But remember that the final decision is hers.

- If your medical attendants suggest something you know your partner wants to avoid, try to buy time. For instance, if labor has slowed, suggest a change of position before starting measures to accelerate labor.

- If the medical team decides the labor needs monitoring with high-tech equipment, try not to be distracted by it. Concentrate on your partner, not the machines.

- If something unexpected happens, and the medical team has to intervene, it's not your partner's fault. These things happen.

- Whatever happens, talk about it afterward with your partner, but also with friends and, if necessary, health professionals. You'll have a lot of feelings to work through.

When the due date is near, make sure your partner can always get in touch with you easily. If you have a cell phone, keep it switched on. Your support during the labor and birth will be a huge comfort to your partner, and you have a practical role, too. Trust your intuition and judgment as to what's needed and ask for feedback.

DURING LABOR

Your partner will need you with her once labor starts. You may feel that the medical staff have everything under control and there's not a lot you can do, but there is, and it's important for you to be there and to be loving and intimate with your partner. However you're feeling yourself, try to be slow and gentle, quiet and reassuring. Don't try to do too much and get in the way of the medical staff or become an irritation to your partner; always give her space when she wants it. Be positive and don't criticize her; she needs plenty of praise, encouragement, and sympathy to keep her going.

Practical help There are lots of things you can do to help your partner cope with the discomfort and the pain of giving birth. Offer practical help such getting her a warm hot-water bottle if she's got a backache, refreshing her with sprays of water or a cool washcloth if she's too hot, and giving her sips of water if her mouth is dry. If she wants to go without pain relief, encourage her while it seems reasonable, but if she asks for it, don't try to talk her out of it. She's the one who's in pain. You'll certainly have talked about it beforehand as part of your planning, and she may at that time have been quite adamant that she didn't want pain relief. But if she changes her mind in labor, don't argue with her; nobody can possibly know how they're going to feel when giving birth until it actually happens.

Seeking explanations Talk to the doctor or midwife if you don't understand what's happening, or if you're worried. They're there to help both of you, and they are professionals who have your partner's and your baby's best interests at heart. At the same time, don't let the hospital staff and their machines become the focus of your attention. Your job is to support your partner.

Your partner's moods Keep your sense of humor; if your partner shouts—or swears—at you, or seems to get angry or overwrought, take it in stride. It's her way of coping with a very stressful situation and quite often happens, particularly at the transition phase of the first stage of labor (see p.273). Treat it as a positive step toward the birth—it's a sign that the second stage of labor isn't far off.

SECOND STAGE AND BIRTH

Helping your partner and watching your baby being born is an overwhelming experience for all fathers. The second stage is hard work for mothers, but there are ways you can really help your partner during this stage, so that you can feel as involved in your baby's birth as possible.

Practical help If you've been going to childbirth classes together, you'll already have worked out together the positions that your partner thinks will be best for her when giving birth. Help her to get into the position she feels is right, and support her there. Of course, this may not be the one she thought of using, nor even be among the ones you've practiced. That doesn't matter; just support her in whatever position she feels comfortable in at the time. Keep talking to her and encouraging her all the time throughout the second stage, and stay in physical contact so she knows you're with her all the way.

The moment of birth If you can see your baby's head as it crowns, describe it to your partner or hold a mirror for her so she can see the head, too—this will be a huge encouragement to her. Don't get in the midwife's way, though—she'll need to be able to monitor your baby's progress second by second. Once your baby is fully out, let your partner know what sex it is, even if you'd been told this during the pregnancy. It's a good idea to say that you have a son or a daughter, not just "it's a boy" or "it's a girl"; the words "son" and "daughter" express family feelings. If the midwife agrees, clamp and cut your baby's cord yourself. It's a fantastic moment—the moment your baby really becomes an individual being.

Sharing feelings When your baby is born, share the first minutes of your child's life with your partner. If you feel like crying, don't hold back. This is one of the most emotional moments of your life. By all means photograph or film your partner and baby, but don't do this instead of helping them if they need you. They are more important than anything else.

MEETING YOUR BABY

This is the moment you've waited nine months for, the moment when you can take your baby in your arms together for the first time. Everything you've just gone through will feel worthwhile. Your doctor will probably lay the baby on your partner's tummy or give him to one of you to hold while the cord is clamped and cut; take your shirt off so your baby can feel and smell your skin. Hold him close to your face and let him look up into yours. Share this moment and savor it; this is a meeting that will change both your lives forever. It's also the moment when you claim your new status as parents. You'll never forget this experience. It's so emotional that you'll probably both find yourselves weeping with joy and relief.

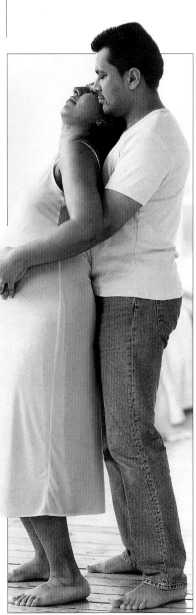

Positions for labor
Support your partner in whatever position she finds most comfortable for giving birth. Many women like to stand or squat, and being held by their partner provides warmth and loving reassurance.

AFTER THE BIRTH

After the birth, you may feel as emotionally exhausted as your partner, but don't forget how physically exhausting labor and birth is for a woman. Because your partner is so tired, she may not appear to experience quite the same emotions as you.

Your partner's reactions You'll probably feel a wave of euphoria now that your baby is born, but, particularly if labor has been long and arduous, your partner may be just too tired to enjoy this same "buzz" immediately. It doesn't mean she isn't as excited and delighted as you are, but after a lengthy labor, it's not surprising if she finds it difficult to express her enthusiasm right away. Just hold her close and let her know how proud you are of her and of your new son or daughter. Stay with them both for as long as possible after the birth, and help get them settled into the postnatal ward.

Valuing your role Be ready to congratulate your partner on her achievement, and let her know how much you appreciate her. But although all your thoughts will be with her, don't belittle your own contribution and the support you've been able to give. You may think you haven't really been much help—this is a common feeling for fathers who've seen their partners struggling through labor, particularly if it was a long one. Most mothers, though, say just how important it was to have the emotional support and encouragement from their partner throughout labor and at the baby's birth.

Saying hello Take the chance to hold your baby while your partner is being stitched, or checked. Go to a quiet corner of the room and get to know the new member of your family. Let her look into your eyes. and hold her close, just 8–10 in (20–25 cm) from your face. She'll be able to see you and smell you, and she'll learn to recognize you from the very beginning (see p.316). Remember, too, that sight is not her only way of experiencing this new world, and that the sense of touch is very important to babies. Take your shirt off and hold her against your skin or gently stroke her—both are strong ways of bonding with your new baby.

CESAREAN DELIVERIES

Even if your partner has chosen in advance to have a cesarean delivery (see p.308) she'll still be anxious, because it's quite a major operation. But if she has to have an emergency cesarean after labor has started, she may feel distressed, bewildered, and helpless. There's much you can do to smooth the way for her. If she's finding it difficult to talk to the doctors, make sure you find out exactly why they want her to have a cesarean. Although she has to give her permission for the operation, she may still not be quite clear afterward what the reasons were, so it's important for you to help her understand them.

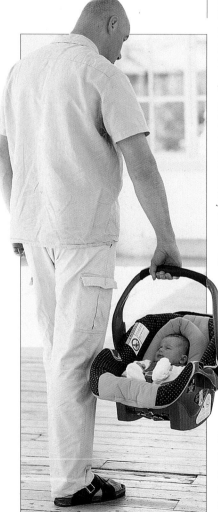

Helping after a cesarean
If your partner has had a cesarean delivery, she'll need plenty of rest so she can heal and recover. She'll need your help with lifting and carrying in the first weeks after the birth.

Cesarean under local anesthesia Unless your partner particularly wants a general anesthetic or the operation is too urgent, ask if it can be done under epidural anesthesia. This means you can share the experience and meet your new baby together. During the operation, you can sit by your partner's head and reassure her that all is well. You don't have to watch what's going on; you'll both be shielded by the surgical drapes. But if you find the operation distressing or you feel faint—and many people do, even nurses—leave the room quickly. Don't hang on—the medical staff have enough to do without caring for you.

Cesarean under general anesthetic If the cesarean is being done under general anesthetic, your partner may not regain consciousness for an hour or more, and you'll probably be given your baby to hold for much of this time. Do cherish this very special time with your baby: father–child bonding can often be at its best following a cesarean section birth, because the early time you have together is so precious.

SUDDEN BIRTH—THE FATHER'S ROLE

Occasionally labor comes on with such speed that a mother is overwhelmed by the desire to push before her partner can get professional help, let alone take her to the hospital! Although the second stage can take a couple of hours, it may not, and babies have been known to be born after a couple of pushes. If it looks as if this is about to happen, there's no need to worry—babies who come quickly are almost always strong and vigorous, and most emergency births are perfectly straightforward, with no complications.

What to do first Don't leave your partner alone for more than a minute or two; she needs to know that you are right there. Help her get into a comfortable position, then call the doctor or midwife and explain the situation. If you can't get hold of them, call the emergency services and ask for an ambulance to come as soon as possible. Wash your hands well and get a heap of clean towels ready. Fold one and put it to one side for the baby. If you've got time, find some old sheets or plastic sheeting to cover the floor and furniture.

During the birth Watch for the top of your baby's head appearing at the vaginal opening. When you see it, ask your partner to stop pushing if she can and just pant. This will give her vagina a chance to stretch fully without tearing. Feel around your baby's neck to check if the cord is looped around it. If it is, hook your finger under the cord and draw it over her head. Hold your baby firmly as she emerges—she'll be slippery—and give her straight to her mother to hold. Wrap her immediately in the spare towel so she doesn't get cold. Don't touch the cord. If the placenta is delivered before medical help arrives, put it in a dish or plastic bowl so it can be checked by the midwife or doctor.

HOME ALONE

When you go home after the birth, leaving your partner in the hospital, you may feel lonely and possibly a bit "flat." Don't worry—there's plenty that you can do.

- Get on the phone and share the good news with everyone. Your friends and relatives will want all the details, so have them ready.

- Take the chance to catch up on sleep. You've had an exhausting time, too, during the labor, and you'll be better able to support your partner when she comes home if you've had some rest.

- Fit straps in your car for the baby seat, if you haven't already gotten around to this.

- Catch up with the laundry and cleaning at home and stock up on food, so that everything is ready and welcoming when your partner and your new baby come home.

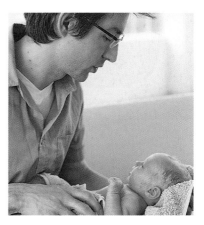

Caring for your baby
Take every chance to care for your baby. Tasks such as bathing her and changing her diapers give you time to bond with her, and you'll find it very rewarding.

WHAT A NEW DAD NEEDS

As a new father, you may feel that your relationship with your partner is one-way traffic at this time, with you giving all the support. It's reasonable to expect something back, and your partner should try to:

- recognize your difficulties. It'll help both of you if she can accept that this is a confusing and emotional time for you, too

- give you some of her time. Caring for your baby will be time-consuming, but it's good for you as a couple and as new parents if she can try to devote some time to your relationship

- allow you to make mistakes. If your partner gave birth in the hospital, she'll have had more time to get used to your baby. She'll need to let you get used to handling and caring for your baby—and not criticize if you're a little clumsy at first

- be open about when to resume sex. You may feel like it before she does, but be understanding. If your partner is breastfeeding, sex may be uncomfortable for her because the hormones that produce breast milk tend to make the vagina dry. There's also a risk of conceiving—some women become pregnant within three months of delivery. Accept that it's better to be content with loving, nonpenetrative sex until after she's had her six-week postnatal visit and she's had a chance to discuss contraception with her doctor.

Learning about your new baby

The first few weeks with your baby are very important for getting to know him and for you to start feeling comfortable in your new role as a father. Your contribution is vital, so try to set aside some time each day to be with your baby.

IN THE FIRST FEW DAYS

If your partner and your new baby spend a few days in the hospital after the birth, you may feel cut off from them. At the same time, you may be feeling an intense joy and elation that you want to share, while your partner seems a bit distant as her body recovers from the birth and she tries to get breastfeeding started. Don't worry—there's plenty you can do that will involve you with both mother and baby.

Take the initiative Don't wait to be asked to share your baby's care. Take the chance to learn how to do all the practical things your baby needs while your partner is still in the hospital.

Get to know your baby Use these early days to establish a close relationship. Even if your partner is in the hospital, change your baby's diapers and get used to handling him. Talk to him, hold him close so that he can focus on your face, or simply hold him if he's asleep. Bring him to your partner when he needs to be fed, and try to be there when he has his first bath.

Be ready for your partner's mood swings Sometime during the first week, your partner may get the "baby blues." They can happen as a reaction to the sudden withdrawal of the pregnancy hormones and to all her new responsibilities. These "baby blues" are temporary and shouldn't last more than a week to 10 days. Your partner may try to hide her feelings so as not to worry you or because she fears you won't take her seriously. Don't belittle her or make light of her state of mind—she has a lot to cope with. If her baby blues last more than two weeks, speak to your doctor about the possibility that your partner has postpartum depression (see p.361).

THE NEW RELATIONSHIP

Concentrate on building your relationship with your baby from the start, and spend as much time as possible with him. Don't isolate yourself or just see yourself as the breadwinner. Being an equal partner in your baby's care will be enormously rewarding to you and will help your family as a whole.

Give your baby love Babies need as much love and cuddling as they can get, and there's no difference between a mother's love and a father's love, except, of course, when your baby is hungry and needs breastfeeding. At all other times, he'll be just as happy with your closeness and attention. Being close and loving with your baby will mean that he learns to feel secure and content with both of you. This will help him settle down and also take some pressure off your partner.

Support your partner Your partner will be very tired in the early weeks after the hard work of the labor and birth, and from the physical and emotional responsibility of breastfeeding. Give her as much time and space as you can for coping with the feeding ,and reassure her constantly that she's doing a great job. Your support can make all the difference. If you've gone back to work, call home during the day, and do as much as you can for your partner and your baby in the evenings and at weekends. Perhaps you could develop your own special routine with your baby.

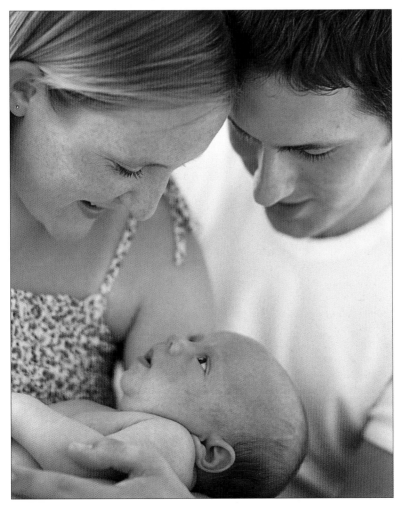

WHAT A NEW MOM NEEDS

As a new father, you may be tempted to concentrate only on the day-to-day business of caring for the baby. Remember that your partner has strong emotional needs, too. Try to:

- recognize her vulnerability. A new mother feels very exposed, both physically and emotionally, in the days after the birth

- appreciate the depth of her feelings. Try to accept the strength of a mother's overwhelming involvement in your baby. Even if this seems to exclude everyone else, don't see it as a rejection of yourself

- protect her privacy. One of your most important roles is to make sure your partner isn't overwhelmed by visitors. Help her get enough time and space to get used to breastfeeding and to recover from the labor and birth.

Spending time together
Time spent with your new baby and your partner is irreplaceable. Even if you have to go back to work, try to spend as much time together as you can, especially in the early days.

SLEEP ROUTINES

Understanding the way your baby's sleep patterns work will help you to tune in to his needs, particularly at night.

Your baby's sleep needs I'm afraid they're probably less than you think. He'll spend 50–80 percent of the time in light sleep, when he wakes very easily. His sleep cycle—light, deep, light—is shorter than an adult's, and he's vulnerable to waking each time he passes from one sleep state to another. Your baby isn't waking to spite you. He's programmed to wake up for all kinds of reasons—when he's wet, hot, cold, sick—because his survival depends on it.

Having a sleep routine Your baby has to be deeply asleep before he'll settle down, so try a soothing sleep routine—gentle rocking, quiet songs, and talking softly. When he first falls asleep, lay him down and gently pat his shoulder at about 60 beats a minute for a few minutes. He's deeply asleep when his eyelids don't twitch and his limbs feel limp.

Getting home late If you're back at work and you find your baby's usually asleep by the time you get home, ask your partner if he can nap more in the afternoon so that he's awake when you arrive. This might not work, so don't blame your partner. Instead, try getting up earlier to spend time with your baby before work.

Night duty

WHAT TO DO	HOW IT CAN HELP
Prepare yourselves for broken nights	Many babies continue to wake once or twice during the night well beyond 12 months. If you're both prepared for this, you'll find it easier to cope.
Share the burden	Take turns getting up when your baby wakes. You may both be back at work, or one of you may be staying at home while the other goes to work, but remember that caring for a baby is also a full-time job.
Adjust your sleep pattern	Broken nights are not necessarily sleepless nights. By adjusting to a new sleep pattern, you'll find that you're able to wake, attend to your baby, and then go back to sleep immediately.
Keep your baby close	Have your baby's crib by the side of your bed so you don't have to disturb yourselves too much when he wakes for a feeding. Put him back in his crib when you're ready to go back to sleep.
Stay together	Sleeping apart so only one of you is disturbed may seem to be a tempting solution but could undermine your relationship with each other and with your baby. Keep as a last resort—if one of you is ill or particularly tired.
Avoid sleep deprivation	Long-term sleep deprivation can affect your health. It's better for you both to lose some sleep than for one of you to take all the burden and become completely exhausted.

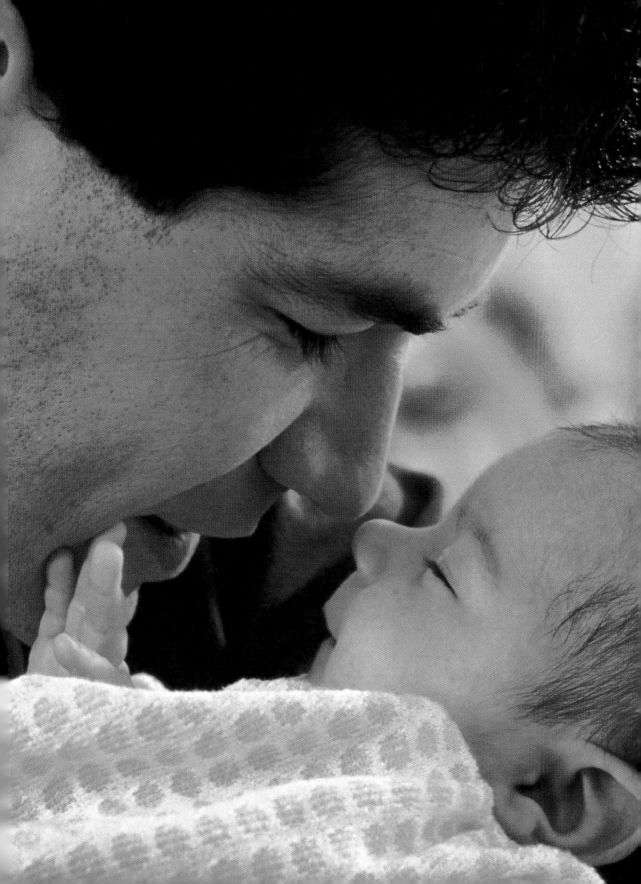

CHAPTER 4

The birth of your choice

There are many choices to make about the way you'll give birth to your child, and it's important to know all the options. In theory, there's no reason why you shouldn't have exactly the kind of birth you want, but it's up to you and your partner to make sure you're able to take an assertive, informed role in the way your labor and delivery will be handled.

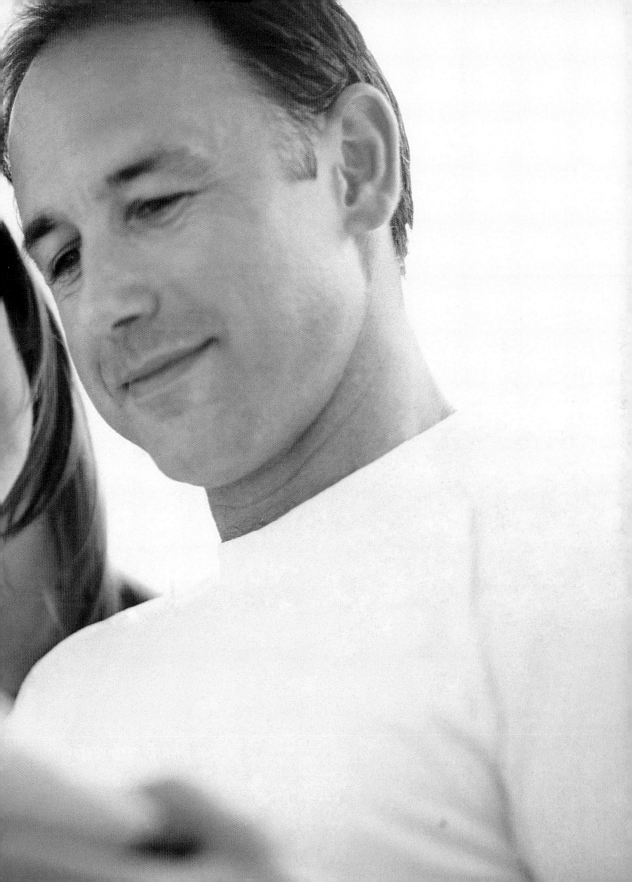

The choices in childbirth

ACTIVE BIRTH

Whether you opt to have your baby in a hospital or a birthing center, you'll be encouraged to have an active birth, in which your partner or birth coach is also involved.

An active birth means that you're not lying down in bed for the labor and delivery. Mothers are encouraged to move around, supported by their partners, and get actively involved in the process of childbirth in whatever positions feel most comfortable.

Most childbirth classes include guidance on preparing yourself for an active birth and there's no doubt that movements and positions that help aim contractions downwards, pushing the baby toward the floor, make labor more efficient. Squatting, kneeling, sitting, or standing can all help reduce pain and make labor easier, shorter, and more comfortable. A mother who's free to move around as she wishes may be less likely to need an episiotomy or a Cesarean section.

Women today want to be more in control of their health, including the birth of their children, and the medical profession has generally responded enthusiastically to the changing desires and needs of women. Choices in childbirth have never been greater, nor women's wishes more paramount. Most mothers want to have their children more naturally, either in a birthing center or a hospital.

THE MODERN NATURAL BIRTH

Most women would like childbirth to be as natural as possible: they want the process of birth and delivery to be familiar so they don't feel nervous or afraid; they like to have a calm, friendly atmosphere, in which they're allowed to take up the positions that are most comfortable for them and there's no undue pressure to take pain-relieving drugs; and they prefer to avoid any unnecessary medical intervention. Female bodies are well designed for giving birth; the soft tissues of the birth passage open so that a baby can pass through. Breathing and relaxation techniques can make birth even easier to manage, and most women now have opportunities to learn these techniques.

Your birth assistant
Every woman going into labor should have someone other than medical and nursing professionals to help and encourage her. Your best supporter is your partner, especially if he's gone to prenatal classes with you. A sister or a best friend could also be great, particularly if they've had children themselves. Research shows that good emotional and physical support from a trusted helper can reduce a laboring woman's need for pain-relieving drugs.

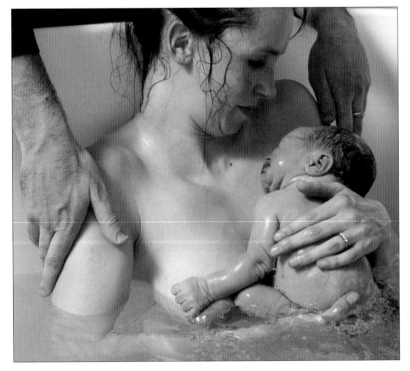

Most of the natural childbirth philosophies include some form of psychological re-learning to help you reduce your expectation of pain and raise your pain threshold. Learning special breathing techniques is usually central to the philosophy. There are slight variations in the different types, but all teach you intense concentration on breathing patterns and the ability to relax your body at will. The best way to experience a totally natural birth is in a dedicated center or at home (see below). But most general hospitals now accept that women want to give birth in whatever position they find most comfortable. Some hospitals have birthing pools and other helpful aids to make labor less painful.

THE MODERN MANAGED BIRTH

Normal pregnancies and uncomplicated births are managed, many times, by teams of midwives and, although they may take place in a hospital, the trend is toward less medical intervention. In a managed birth, labor is actively controlled for the safety of both mother and baby. A highly controlled birth in a hospital is essential for some women who may have complications during pregnancy, labor, and birth.

In a hospital setting all the modern obstetric procedures are available, whether your birth is complicated or not. Epidural anesthesia is literally on tap and electronic fetal monitoring may be necessary. Consequently, medical intervention is more common in a hospital than at a birthing center, and you can expect more inductions and Cesarian sections there. Although these practices are of course helpful in the percentage of births where intervention is needed, it's now recognized that the routine use of them isn't justified (see Contentious issues in childbirth, p.108). However, many women find a hospital setting makes childbirth the event they expect it to be, and they feel more secure there. If there were a true emergency, a few minutes could have a major impact on the outcome.

BIRTHING CENTERS

In many communities, there has been a movement away from traditional hospital deliveries, especially for women whose pregnancies are at low risk of birth complications. Birthing centers are now a popular option for these moms-to-be and, conveniently, they are often located in or nearby a hospital. Over the past few years, hospitals have made efforts to provide a comfortable homelike environment where you can labor, deliver, and recover without having to move between rooms. Also, many hospitals are now encouraging women to keep their baby at their bedside, if they choose.

Certified nurse midwives, who work as a team with an obstetrician or a family physician, attend an increasing number of deliveries in birthing centers and hospitals around the country, and are able to provide much of your prenatal care. Your midwife generally spends more time with you during labor than the average doctor and may be more flexible about birthing options.

WATER LABOR

More and more women like to spend at least some of their labor in water.

Being in water, whether it is a birthing poor or a shower, has become increasingly popular as a means of managing pain during the first stage of labor.

Most birthing centers and an increasing number of hospitals now have water-birthing rooms. Ideally, the water in a birthing pool should be at body temperature (98.6°F/37°C). If the water is any hotter, the mother may be at a risk of dehydration and a rise in blood pressure. A study of the use of water in labor indicated that labor is more efficient if the mother enters the water only after she's reached 5cm dilation.

Although the American College of Obstetrics and Gynecology has not yet endorsed water births nor issued guidelines, most doctors and midwives advise that you leave the pool for the third stage of labor because the relaxing effects of the water could theoretically increase bleeding after delivery or encourage the placenta to be retained.

CONTENTIOUS ISSUES IN CHILDBIRTH

Some of the procedures that used to happen almost automatically during labor and childbirth are being looked at afresh. Some are now thought unnecessary or unjustified. On the other hand, most of today's obstetricians believe that they can make childbirth a safer and happier experience for mother and baby with the help of the modern technology available. For women in the first stage of labor, this may include the use of effective pain relief, including epidurals; monitoring of the baby's heart with a rate meter and the uterine contractions with a *tocograph*; recording how much the cervix has dilated on a *partogram* to make sure that progress is being made, and the occasional use of an *oxytocin* drip to make sure that uterine contractions are strong enough, frequent, and regular.

There's more detailed information on the following subjects in other parts of this book, but this might a good time to start thinking about certain issues. If you're aware of the arguments against some of these medical practices, you'll be more confident about questioning them, if you need to, with your medical and nursing attendants. Generally, they should be happy to go along with your wishes, but occasionally you may be told that to continue with a particular option will put your baby and you at serious risk— for instance, if your baby is showing signs of distress and you're still determined to continue with a totally natural childbirth. In this situation, it's good to have an alternative birth plan ready (see column, p.123) and to be prepared to change it if need be.

This doesn't happen very often, though, so don't give in to medical intervention you're not happy about until you feel you've had thorough answers to your question. There can sometimes be intervention because doctors want to get a baby out quickly. An episiotomy, for instance, may be made necessary when you're encouraged to deliver your baby's head before the skin and muscles in your perineum have been given a chance to stretch. Given time, very few women need an episiotomy—as Michel Odent has proved.

Nothing by mouth There's no medical nor scientific rationale for starving a woman during labor—in fact, quite the opposite. Sometimes a laboring woman has a sudden need for energy and wants sugar. Other women don't feel like eating anything, but they certainly need fluids; labor is hard work and uses up lots of energy, which causes sweating, and a woman must replace the fluids that she's lost through her skin. That said, if there's a high risk of a woman having an emergency cesarean, it's safer to give anesthetic on an empty stomach.

Switching rooms In most hospitals, you should be able to labor and deliver your baby in the same room, without having to move. Depending on the hospital, you may need to be moved to an operating room if you have to have an emergency cesarean.

Otherwise, you should have peaceful surroundings, in a room equipped with good lighting, oxygen, and a suction apparatus to clear out the baby's air passages.

Induction Starting labor artificially isn't a new idea, but it only became an easy procedure in the second half of the twentieth century. Labor should only be induced for medical reasons such as preeclampsia, high blood pressure, or post-maturity, when induction can save the lives of mothers and babies.

Amniotomy This means that the membranes (the bag of waters) surrounding the baby are artificially ruptured. It's not a routine procedure and is generally only done early in labor if the baby's heart rate is abnormal. Amniotomy is done for three reasons. The first is so that electronic fetal monitoring equipment can be set in place; the second is to check if the amniotic fluid contains *meconium* (this is the baby's first bowel movement and its presence may indicate fetal distress); the third reason is that once the bag of waters has been removed, the baby's head can then press hard on the mother's cervix, so helping along the dilatation of the cervix and completion of the first stage of labor.

Fetal monitoring For this, a heart-rate sensor is strapped to the mother's abdomen. A low-risk mother is monitored only intermittently through her labor, although some hospitals prefer to monitor for about 20 minutes on admission so there's a permanent record of the baby's heart rate in case there are any problems later on. Some hospitals use continuous fetal monitoring that is watched from a central station—a clear advantage for women with high-risk pregnancies. Fetal monitoring should not mean a woman has to keep still. Although movement is limited, you can sit on the bed and even stand up if you want to change position. Obviously, having a "window" into the uterus during labor is of great value, but if the monitors aren't working properly and data is misinterpreted by untrained staff, it ceases to be an advantage. Using a monitor may also switch attention from the mother to a machine, which can be disconcerting for a laboring woman.

Forceps These tong-shaped instruments are used to ease the baby's head out of the birth canal. Forceps have saved the lives of many babies and their mothers, and can reduce the need for a cesarean section for a baby that is stuck up in the pelvis. The use of forceps does mean that an episiotomy is likely but not inevitable. Vacuum extraction (see pp.306 & 307), in which a cup is attached to the baby's head by suction, is increasingly being used instead of forceps.

Episiotomy This is a surgical cut to enlarge the vaginal outlet at delivery, and is the most commonly performed operation in the

THE UNKINDEST CUT?

An episiotomy is an incision that helps deliver a baby's head, but isn't always needed (see p.110).

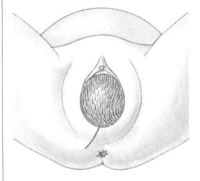

The mediolateral cut
This cut is angled down and away from the vagina and the perineum into the muscle.

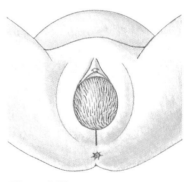

The midline cut
This cut is made straight down into the perineum, between the vagina and anus.

If you've already had an epidural, you probably won't need any further anesthetic before an episiotomy. If you haven't had an epidural, you'll need a local anesthetic in your perineum, known as a pudendal block.

WHEN YOU NEED AN EPISIOTOMY

There are times when an episiotomy is needed to make sure that your baby can be delivered safely.

- If the birth is imminent and your perineum hasn't had time to stretch slowly.

- If your baby's head is too large for your vaginal opening.

- When you aren't able to control your pushing and you can't stop when you need to and then push gradually and smoothly.

- When your baby is in distress.

- If you need a forceps delivery (see p.306). With forceps, an episiotomy is likely but not obligatory.

- If your baby is in a breech position and there is a complication during delivery.

West. Episiotomies are used in order to avoid tears, which have ragged edges and are difficult to stitch together. Also, they can take longer to heal. But you can avoid tears if you stop pushing while your baby's head is being born, and allow your uterus to ease out the head gradually rather than suddenly. If your baby's head is delivered suddenly, you are likely to tear, so an episiotomy will be done if the perineum is under stress.

If an episiotomy is done too early, before your perineum has thinned out, muscle, skin, and blood vessels are damaged and there may be heavy bleeding. Tissues are crushed by the scissors as they are cut, and this can lead to bruising, swelling, slow healing, and a perineum that is stitched too tightly. This tightness can be very uncomfortable during the postnatal period, and may even leave a painful scar, which can prevent you from making love for months afterward. If you want to avoid an episiotomy, it's a good idea to make it clear in your notes and birth plan that you don't want it to be done unless entirely necessary. If you do have to have an episiotomy, you have the right to have a local anesthetic in the perineum before it's done, so insist on that.

Breech birth Research shows that normal vaginal delivery is riskier than a cesarean for a breech birth. Most breech babies are delivered by cesarean section, but usually with epidural anesthesia. Few midwives have experience of breech deliveries, so a breech baby will generally be delivered by a doctor.

Time What hospitals judge to be the normal length for labor differs from place to place. For example, the "right" length for the second stage can be two hours or 30 minutes, or somewhere in between, depending on the obstetrician or midwife. In fact, the length of labor varies from woman to woman, and from birth to birth, and it's the combination of what's normal for you with the hospital's policy that may cause problems.

In most cases, if the first stage is thought to have gone on too long, the membranes are ruptured (if this hasn't been done already), or an oxytocin drip is set up to increase the rate and strength of contractions. If the second stage is taking a long time, a doctor may suggest an episiotomy and forceps delivery. Many midwives, though, say it's usually obvious when labor is going well but is just taking some time, rather than being slow because something's wrong.

Being together It's rare for babies to be separated from their mothers after the birth unless they need special care or the mother asks for her baby to be taken away for a while. But your partner won't be able to stay with you in the hospital, as there just aren't suitable facilities in most places, and this can be difficult for him after all the excitement and emotion of the birth. Before you go into the hospital, ask how long your partner can stay with you after the birth. Many women say that they were too excited to sleep afterward and wished they had someone to talk to.

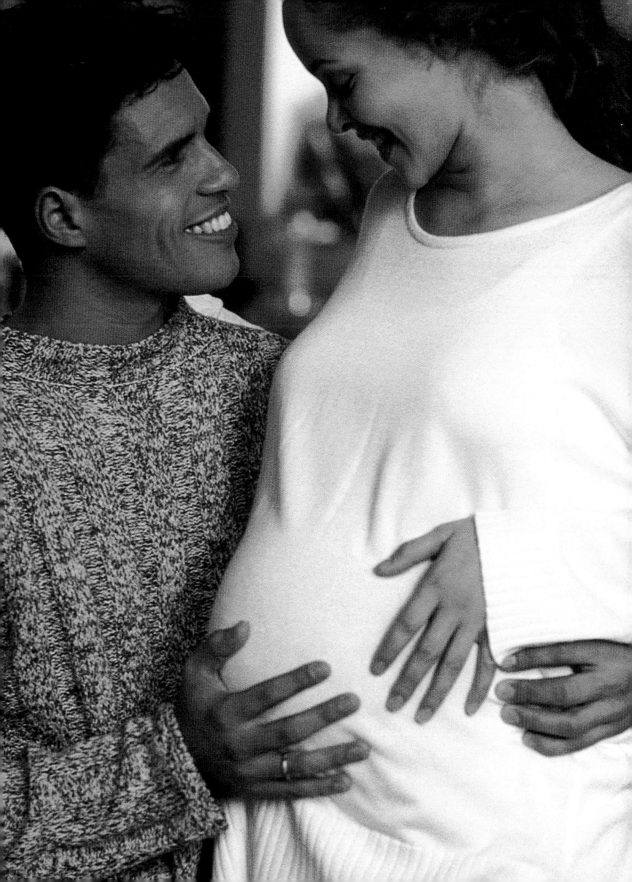

Childbirth philosophers

Over the last few decades, a number of people have influenced the way women and their caregivers approach childbirth. Their teaching and ideas have changed women's attitudes to prenatal and postnatal care and led to alterations in the atmosphere and procedures surrounding childbirth in the Western world. Most of these theories seek to help a woman to follow the lead of her body, in a loving and intimate environment.

DR. GRANTLEY DICK-READ

Dr. Dick-Read was the first obstetrician to realize that fear of giving birth was a main cause of pain in labor. He introduced the idea of natural childbirth, not only to the medical world but also to mothers. He recognized the need for proper education of mothers through prenatal classes and careful teaching, and also for emotional support, in the hope of eliminating fear and tension. His teaching was so basic that it's now taken for granted by all centers, and there's no method of childbirth that doesn't rely on his teaching, including breathing exercises, breathing control, and complete relaxation. Dick-Read's watchword was preparation—not only with information, but also by seeking help, reassurance, and sympathy.

FREDERICK LEBOYER

Leboyer was influenced by the psychiatrists Reich, Rank, and Janov, who shared the belief that later problems in life stem from the trauma of birth. His concerns are less with the mother and more to do with the baby's experience of labor and delivery, and how this affects that baby once grown up. The Leboyer method of delivery works best if seen as an attempt to help people understand what a newborn baby sees, hears, and feels.

In his book *Birth Without Violence*, Leboyer suggests that the birthing room should have soft lighting, and there should be as little noise and movement as possible to lessen birth's trauma. Leboyer also believes that immediate skin-to-skin contact is essential to calm the baby, and that she should be laid on her mother's stomach as soon as she's born. He also says that the newborn should then be bathed in warm water, since this is the closest she can get to the nurturing environment of the uterus.

Not all of this fits in with the physiology of what actually happens at birth. A baby needs to feel air on her face to stimulate her lungs to breathe for the first time: placing her in warm liquid may not be sufficiently stimulating for her to continue breathing. Many professionals say that there is no proof that Leboyer's

This birth preparation technique was developed by Dr. Robert Bradley. It's also known as husband-coached childbirth, and the involvement of a woman's partner is a key feature.

The Bradley method teaches women to accept the pain of labor, and to go with the flow under the guidance of her husband or partner, friend, or counselor. The coach attends childbirth classes with the mother, helps her with her exercise and breathing routine, and comforts, coaxes, and coaches her through labor and delivery.

The danger of this is that most women need to be distracted from the pain, to focus outside of themselves, so that they can cope. Going into the pain can be totally overwhelming.

Also, each labor is completely individual and may be unlike what you've practiced, and a woman often reacts to giving birth in a different way than she'd imagined. Some birth partners can become so enthusiastic about the coaching that they lose sight of the woman and her needs.

theories work. However, it's only right that every baby be welcomed into the world with reverence, so even if you don't agree with all of Leboyer's ideas, it's still interesting to read about his suggestions for a gentler birth.

DR. MICHEL ODENT

When he worked as a general surgeon, Dr. Odent was extremely shocked when he first saw women pushing their babies uphill against the force of gravity because their feet were held in stirrups. He realized this meant that stronger, and therefore more painful, contractions were needed; that labor was much slower and more exhausting; and there were more complications because mothers were in a position where the baby was held back from being delivered.

His initial shock led him to develop his own methods of childbirth, broadly based on traditional midwifery, at Pithiviers in France. Odent believes that, given the opportunity, women in labor return to a primitive biological state, where they function at a new level of animal awareness, lose their inhibitions, and enter a state of consciousness in which they will follow their basic instincts. He believes that the natural pain relievers released by the body, endorphins, are responsible for this.

Pithiviers has the lowest rate in France for episiotomies, forceps deliveries, and cesarean sections, and all medical interference is kept to a minimum. By no means all of the mothers giving birth there have been low-risk. Many were expecting complications (a breech baby, for example), but went on to have successful natural births at Pithiviers.

SHEILA KITZINGER

A very highly respected birth practitioner, who has enormous influence in the West, Kitzinger believes that birth is a very personal experience, and that a laboring mother should be an active "birth-giver," rather than a passive patient.

She likens the modern, managed birth in a modern, managed hospital to giving birth in captivity; in essence, to being in a zoo. She says that the zoo may be humanely and scientifically managed; the keepers may be kind and considerate, and pride themselves on a low mortality rate and the good condition of their charges; the visiting times may be frequent and the premises friendly and welcoming; there may be space to move around in the cage; those in charge may have tried to recreate the natural habitat, but the zoo still dictates the behavior of the captives.

She believes that the aim of maternity services should be first to allow parents a real choice, whether for a totally managed birth, a totally natural birth, or somewhere in between, and to respect their wishes about where and how their child is born. Second, she believes that birth is not an illness, and that a laboring mother and her partner should be treated not as patients, but as intelligent adults with a right to have the final say in decisions about the birth of their baby.

THE LAMAZE METHOD

This method of psychological counseling for childbirth was pioneered in Russia, and was then adopted in France by Dr. Lamaze.

More than 90 percent of women in Russia and 70 percent of French women are taught variations of the Lamaze method of childbirth. It's become equally popular in the United States, and is still the basis of the teaching of the National Childbirth Trust in Great Britain.

Lamaze believed that no matter how relaxed a woman was, she would almost certainly experience some pain during childbirth, and that she would have to cope with it.

Inspired by Ivan Pavlov's research into stimulus-response conditioning in dogs, Lamaze saw the value of conditioned learning in helping women to cope with the pain of childbirth.

The method has three main principles.

- Fear of labor is reduced or eliminated when you know and understand more about what's happening.

- You learn how to relax and become aware of your body and how to cope with pain.

- You consciously use rhythmic breathing patterns through each contraction to take your mind off the pain.

Birthing Centers

CHOOSING A BIRTHING CENTER

Choosing where to deliver your baby is a complicated decision that you'll want to make as early on in your pregnancy as possible. If you're thinking about having your baby at a birthing center, here are some important questions you'll want to ask:

- Is the birthing center approved by the Commission for the Accreditation of Birth Centers?

- Are the professionals on staff (such as midwives, doctors, and nurses) licensed healthcare providers?

- What are the procedures if complications arise and you need to be referred to an obstetrician or admitted to a hospital?

- Will your insurance plan pay for services at the birthing center or, if necessary, an emergency transfer to a hospital?

- What are the center's statistics for hospital transfers, episiotomies, and mortality?

- What procedures are followed after your baby's birth and how long is the typical postpartum stay at the center?

- How easy is it to get to the birthing center and does it offer prenatal education classes?

Birthing centers have become popular for many women because they provide a trio of advantages: midwife care, less medical intervention, and convenience. Many birthing centers are actually in or nearby a hospital with a doctor on call, making them an attractive choice for women whose pregnancies are considered low risk. Other advantages include the freedom to choose how mobile you want to be during labor, which birthing positions you'd like to try, and which comfort and labor aids – such as massage, relaxation techniques, a warm shower or a birthing pool – you want to use.

WHAT TO EXPECT

If you are thinking of having your baby at a birthing center you can expect a more family-centered and affordable birth experience than you would have in a hospital. Typically, a birth center is an independent facility, though some are housed inside hospitals. You can go there for prenatal care throughout your pregnancy, as well as for labor and childbirth when the time comes. Certified nurse-midwives provide most of the care in birth centers, although a physician is on call in case of an emergency. Not surprisingly, it's best to give birth at a birthing center only if you're as certain as you can be that you're at low risk for complications during childbirth.

THE ADVANTAGES

If you are a healthy woman at low risk for labor complications and want your healthcare provider to be a nurse-midwife, a birthing center may be the ideal choice for you, especially if you are commited to a more natural childbirth experience. Birthing centers offer a low-tech, personalized, and comfortable place for women to deliver their babies. There you can labor, deliver, and recover in the same room. And if a birth turns into a medical emergency, any accredited birth center will have a back-up arrangement with doctors at a nearby hospital.

Other advantages to laboring in a birthing center include comfortable, homelike rooms, where you can labor in the company of your partner, a close friend, and even your children, and have access to comforts such as a birthing pool. You also have the freedom to move around and wear what you like, as well as choose the position you'd like to be in for labor and delivery. Birthing centers are dedicated to natural childbirth, without medical interventions such as drugs or episiotomies. However, they do have IV's, oxygen, and infant resuscitation equipment. A handheld Doppler may also be used to monitor your baby's heartbeat, instead of an electronic fetal monitor, and analgesic drugs, such as Demerol, are also available if you want them, but epidurals are not. Pitocin is not used during labor to stimulate contractions, but may be used to control postpartum bleeding. All treatments and exams for both you and your baby are done with your supervision and consent and with a full explanation of what is happening. Birthing centers have no routine procedures that require you to be separated from your child. They also make it a priority to provide breastfeeding education and support during the prenatal period, in the first hour after birth, and later in the postpartum period. And because women who deliver in birthing centers usually stay for a shorter time and use fewer interventions, it costs about one-third less on average to deliver in a birthing center than it does in a hospital.

THE DISADVANTAGES

For women whose pregnancies are complicated, birthing centers are not the best option because they are not designed or equipped to handle complications that may arise either during your pregnancy or when you are in labor. Roughly 12 percent of women who begin their labor in birthing centers are transferred to hospitals for non-emergency reasons, such as when labor is not progressing and Pitocin is needed. Another drawback is the lack of access to pain medications. For example, if you plan on having an epidural (or want the option), you'll need to give birth in a hospital because an anesthesiologist is required to administer this form of pain relief.

Also, if you are transferred to your backup hospital, where your midwife may or may not have admitting privileges, there is a good possibility that your baby will be delivered by a doctor you've never met before. And being moved from place to place while you are laboring can be upsetting in itself.

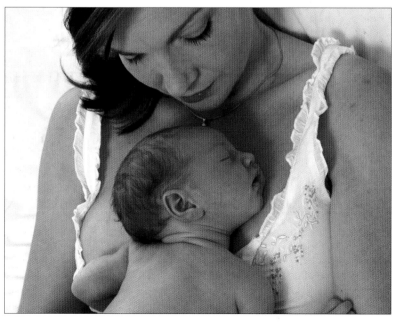

IS A BIRTHING CENTER RIGHT FOR YOU?

If you would like to have your baby in a birthing center but think that you might be in a high-risk category, talk to your doctor or midwife as early in your pregnancy as possible.

Your healthcare provider will take an extensive health history, perform a complete physical exam, and order the necessary lab work.

At each visit you'll be assessed to make sure that it's still appropriate for you to give birth at the birthing center. Here are some of the situations that might develop during your pregnancy that would put you into the high-risk category:

- Carrying twins (or more)
- Preeclampsia or other pregnancy-induced raised blood pressure
- Gestational diabetes
- Premature labor
- Baby in a breech or other abnormal position near due date
- Placenta previa
- Baby not growing normally
- Labor needs to be induced

A birthing center delivery
Natural childbirth, without technological interventions or a reliance on drugs, is the focus in birthing centers, and every measure is taken to keep the environment as homelike and comfortable as possible. An array of labor aids, the presence of committed, professional labor support, and your birth partner make the experience an intensely personal one.

Hospital birth

A hospital birth will vary depending on where you are and who cares for you (see p.120), but may include the following procedures. Discuss any issues with your doctor or midwife as soon as you can.

- You'll probably travel to the hospital while you're in labor.

- Your membranes may be ruptured and fetal monitoring equipment put in place (see p.275), at least for a short time.

- If labor slows down or stops, you'll probably be given oxytocin to stimulate uterine contractions.

- Pain-relieving drugs will be available, including an epidural.

- Your birth partner will be allowed to stay with you during labor and the birth unless there is an emergency that requires you to go to the operating room.

- You may be given an episiotomy if necessary to ease the delivery of your baby's head and prevent possible injuries to your perineal or vaginal tissues.

- You could be given oxytocin/pitocin (see p.291) to reduce the risk of bleeding after the placenta is delivered.

- You'll be given your baby to hold after birth, and encouraged to start breastfeeding.

- Pediatricians are available to assist with the newborn if there is a complication.

- If you are being cared for by a midwife in the hospital, a doctor will be available 24 hours a day in case of emergency or in case the midwife would like a second opinion.

Even though more and more women are choosing to deliver their babies in birthing centers, most babies are born in a hospital. The majority of women opt to give birth in a hospital, either because they are encouraged to do so by their medical advisers or because it's their preference. Most hospitals are now paying much more attention to the mother's wishes, so there's no reason why you shouldn't enjoy giving birth to your baby in a hospital setting.

WHAT TO EXPECT

The hospital surroundings will be unfamiliar, and this can make you feel anxious, but here are some tips to help you make yourself more comfortable. You'll probably have been told to leave all valuables at home, but when you get to the hospital, you may be asked to remove any remaining personal items such as jewelry. If this worries you, ask if you can keep your personal belongings with you in a bag. If you wear contact lenses, ask about the hospital's policy beforehand—they may prefer you to bring your glasses instead.

After admission When you arrive at the hospital, you'll need to go through brief hospital admission procedures. Your midwife or doctor will ask you about how your labor is going—how often you're having contractions and whether your water has broken, for example. Then she will examine your abdomen to confirm the situation, feel your baby's position, and check your baby's heart. Your blood pressure and temperature will be taken, and you'll be given an internal examination to see how far your cervix has dilated. They will probably ask you to wear a fetal monitor for about 20 minutes, but afterward you should be able to move around as much as you wish.

Giving birth If you've decided that you prefer to manage without drugs for as long as you can during labor, the midwives will usually be more than happy to help you cope using other methods of pain relief (see p.282). Bear in mind, though, that drug relief is available if you want it, and you can ask to start with smaller doses if you don't feel you need the full measure.

Once your baby is descending, you may be helped into a semi-reclining position. If you're in any danger of tearing, you may need to have an episiotomy (see p.109) when your baby's head is crowning. If forceps have to be used, an episiotomy (see p.306) is more likely. Your baby will be delivered onto your abdomen, and while you take your first look at each other, you'll be given an injection of Syntometrine into your thigh. This is to make sure that your uterus will contract firmly, reducing the chance of severe bleeding after the delivery of the placenta. Your baby will then be given the Apgar tests (see p.292) while you are cleaned up. If you need to have stitches, these are usually done at this point, either by the midwife or the doctor.

THE ADVANTAGES

For some mothers, a hospital birth gives the best chance of a successful and happy outcome. Having your baby in the hospital is the safest option if you suffer from a medical condition such as heart disease or diabetes, if you're expecting twins, if your baby is known to be breech, or if, as a first-time mother, your obstetrical history just presents too many unknown factors.

Should anything go wrong during the labor and birth, emergency medical assistance is on hand right away, and there's a wide range of pain-relief medication readily available should you want it. You may feel happier knowing that your baby can be given treatment in an intensive care unit if the need arises.

By staying in the hospital after the birth, you may get more rest than you would at home, especially if you have other children.

THE DISADVANTAGES

Once you're in the hospital, it's easy to feel overpowered by the atmosphere, although some are getting more relaxed about childbirth. Bear in mind that hospital staff have to follow rules and routines, and you're going to have to fit in with them. But that doesn't mean that you should have to do anything you aren't happy about. Your partner may feel a bit awkward and separate from the birth of his child, so try to include him in whatever way you can. It helps to find out as much as you can about the hospital procedures and setup beforehand so that you're more prepared once you go into labor.

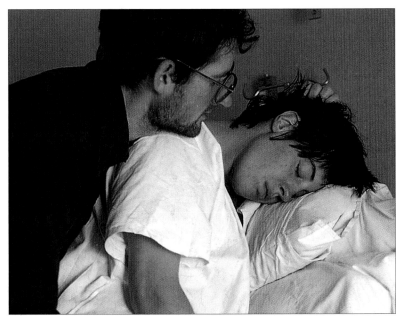

YOUR BABY'S EXPERIENCE

Your baby will be born surrounded by medical staff with the expertise to handle any problems that arise.

- An electrode to measure her heart rate may be attached to her scalp during labor.

- With the exception of epidural anesthesia, she'll experience any drugs that you are given, and this can mean that she feels drowsy or is slower to feed once she's born. Narcan can be given to quickly reverse these effects.

- She'll be handed to you to cuddle and get acquainted with for a few minutes right after the birth.

- Her umbilical cord will be clamped and cut as soon as she's been born.

- Her mouth and nose may be routinely suctioned to clear them of any mucus.

- She'll be weighed and examined (Apgar score) by the doctor or midwife (see p.292).

- She'll be returned to you, possibly cleaned and wrapped in blankets, to begin bonding and breastfeeding.

- Later on, she'll be more thoroughly examined by a doctor to check for any abnormalities.

Birth in the hospital
As far as possible, you should be allowed to assume positions that are comfortable for you, and to have your birth partner close at hand.

The care available

There are lots of things you'll need to think about or find out when you're choosing the hospital where you'd like to give birth. Here are some questions to ask yourself or others, before you decide.

- What kind of birth do I want?

- What birth facilities are there in my area?

- Am I prepared and am I able to travel for prenatal care? Can I be cared for by my doctor?

- What are the reputations of the hospitals in my area? Have I gotten as many different opinions, from as many different sources, as I possibly can?

- What are the staff at the different hospitals like? What are their views on labor and birth? Do I agree with them? You can sometimes find that there's a difference between a hospital's policies and the way the staff actually approach childbirth.

- Do I want immediate access to a neonatal intensive care unit?

- How long do I want to be in the hospital for, and what kind of accommodations are there?

- Do I want to feed my baby when and how I feel like it?

- Do I want my baby with me at night? All night?

- What are the visiting hours?

- Can my partner (and children) be with me whenever I want?

- Can my partner stay with me the first night after the birth?

You can ask your doctor, your midwife, or the leader of your prenatal class what she knows about the hospitals in your area. But the only way to really find out what a hospital can provide and whether it's right for you is to go and take a good look around and ask questions. There may, of course, be only one hospital in your area, but if you do have a choice, make sure you get satisfactory answers so that you can feel happy and confident about the hospital you choose.

TYPES OF HOSPITALS

There are different kinds of hospitals, most of which provide maternity care. Without question, teaching hospitals provide the most modern facilities. Here, doctors are always on duty, so if you run into any complications, there will be someone to attend you. And, as a rule, doctors at teaching hospitals are usually more experienced in dealing with complicated births. The smaller community hospitals are rare now, but they do tend to be more friendly and flexible, although midwives still have to follow the same guidelines as midwives in larger hospitals.

VISITING HOSPITALS

If you can, tour one or more hospitals with your partner before making your final choice. Most maternity hospitals give a formal tour, sometimes as part of general prenatal preparation classes, otherwise as part of the general welcome made to mothers signing up. Find out about when these tours take place and ask if you can join one before you make your decision.

GETTING TO KNOW YOUR HOSPITAL

Hospitals can be intimidating, but usually seem less so when you get to know them. Try to visit the hospital of your choice at least once, more if possible, so that you can meet some of the staff who'll be caring for you. You'll also have a chance to get the feel of the routine and look at the delivery room and other facilities. The more time you have to walk around, the more familiar you'll become with the surroundings so you're more relaxed when the big day comes. It's best if you and your partner do this together so that you both get to know the place and the people and will feel confident when you are actually there for the birth itself. Remember, though, that security considerations mean that maternity wards are now carefully monitored, so don't try to visit without an appointment. Any unannounced visitors are likely to be challenged.

It's a good idea for you and your partner to take a look around the outside of the hospital and find the emergency entrance. Many women go into labor at night, and having to search for the entrance in the dark is the last thing you need.

CHANGING YOUR HOSPITAL

If you do have problems and you find that your hospital is not meeting your expectations, you don't have to abandon the system altogether. A hospital is there to serve you; healthcare is a consumer issue and you do have the right to refuse certain procedures. If you're very unhappy with any aspect of the care at your hospital, you can arrange to be transferred to another one.

You could also try getting in touch with the head of the clinic or your obstetrician and explain your feelings and what you think is wrong with the clinic. If you find a sympathetic doctor who you get along with, you may change your mind about leaving, although it's unlikely that he or she will be there for your delivery. If you do feel you must change hospitals, your obstetrician will probably recommend another doctor at a center of your choice.

BIRTHING ROOMS

Most hospitals should have birthing rooms available. These are nonclinical and more like your own home, with comfortable chairs, low lighting, soft music, piles of cushions, and drinks and snacks on hand.

The whole aim of a birthing room is to help you relax, overcome fears, and relieve tension. A normal routine before the birth makes for a normal delivery, and once you're in a birthing room you won't be moved unless there's an emergency that needs immediate attention. There shouldn't be any sudden changes in movement, mood, and surroundings. You won't have to lie down to have your baby, and you don't need to be surrounded by intimidating equipment. In a birthing room, you can take up whatever position you want for the birth of your baby.

For many women, a birthing room provides the ideal compromise between home and hospital births. It provides surroundings and facilities as similar as possible to those at home, but with emergency expertise on hand and an epidural available if labor pains become overwhelming.

MATERNITY CARE CENTERS

Family-centered maternity care is available at some of the more progressive hospitals and larger medical centers. It's a philosophy aimed at caring for the whole family unit during labor, delivery, and after birth. A hospital that adopts this kind of maternity care respects the social, personal, and family importance of childbirth, and is likely to avoid some of the more controversial routine procedures and suggest alternatives.

Some aspects of hospital maternity care may appeal to you greatly, such as a Leboyer-type delivery, keeping parents and baby together, rooming in, early discharge, etc. These practices do vary from hospital to hospital and you'll need to visit to discuss your preferences with the staff. A hospital may say that it has family-centered care but you may find that it doesn't fulfill your expectations, so find out just what they are offering before committing yourself.

QUESTIONS TO ASK

When you're choosing a hospital, find out as much as you can by asking questions.

- Will I be able to wear my own clothes and personal effects (rings, contact lenses, glasses)?

- Can my partner or friend stay with me all the time? Will they ever be asked to leave?

- Will I be able to move around freely during labor, and give birth in any position I choose?

- Will I be able to have the same caregivers throughout labor?

- Can I bring in my own midwife to attend to me throughout labor?

- Are beanbags, birthing chairs, and stools provided?

- Does the hospital have birthing pools? If not, will I be able to use a rented one?

- What's the hospital policy on pain relief, electronic monitoring, and induction?

- What kind of pain relief is available, and is it available at all times?

- Will I be able to eat and drink if I want to?

- What's the hospital policy on episiotomies, cesareans, and the expulsion of the placenta?

- If I tear or have an episiotomy, are the midwives allowed to stitch me, or will I have to wait for a doctor?

YOUR ATTENDANTS

Medical professionals can have many different approaches to childbirth. Ask your obstetrician or midwife the following questions to get an idea of their views.

- What do you think about inducing labor and birth?

- When would you think it necessary to rupture the membranes?

- Do you think that electronic fetal monitoring is a valuable aid in every birth?

- Would you be worried if labor was slower than normal?

- What do you think about a mother moving around during labor, the use of water or a birth pool, and breathing techniques to help relieve pain? What drugs do you normally give to control pain?

- Would you mind if the lights were dimmed during labor?

- How often do you perform episiotomies?

- When would you think it necessary to do a cesarean section?

- Will we be able to have some time alone with our baby immediately after the birth?

Professional attendants

You do have some choice about who attends your labor—it's not simply a matter of opting for hospital expertise or a home midwife. Wherever you decide to have your baby, the system can usually be tailored to suit your individual needs. Most women like to have their partner or a friend with them during childbirth, and hospitals now welcome this. You may find it reassuring to have a birth coach, too— someone who's been through it before and knows what to do.

OBSTETRICIANS

An obstetrician is a doctor who specializes in pregnancy and childbirth. This doctor will provide your prenatal care, and the hospital you go to will depend upon his or her affiliation. Many doctors in a city will have privileges at more than one hospital, but doctors in the suburbs may practice at only one hospital. You may choose a doctor recommended by a friend or family member, or you could check your insurance company's list of providers in your area. You may decide you'd prefer a female doctor over a male one.

MIDWIVES

The modern, professional midwife is a specialist in childbirth. She can care for you throughout your pregnancy and during labor and delivery, and knows when to call for extra advice and assistance. Unlike the obstetrician, her focus is the normal, not the abnormal. She's interested in your general well-being, not just your uterus and how it may malfunction. Although midwifery is traditionally a female profession, there are now some male midwives as well.

Certified nurse-midwives (CNM) These midwives are registered nurses whose specialty is taking care of pregnant women and delivering babies. Like nurse-practitioners, they may also be able to diagnose and treat common illnesses in adults. In the US, they are graduates of programs that are accredited by the American College of Nurse-Midwives, they have passed a national certification exam, and they are licensed in all 50 states according to the relevant state laws. Certified nurse-midwives may work in a group practice with other midwives or with obstetricians, in a birthing center, or in a hospital. Rarely, they may deliver a child at home. Wherever midwives practice, they must have an obstetrician on call for assistance in case the pregnancy turns out to be high-risk or something goes wrong. Many insurance plans and HMOs are required by law to allow a woman to choose between an obstetrician and a nurse-midwife, but you should check your medical insurance carrier to make sure this is the case.

Certified midwives (CM) Some midwives do not obtain a general nursing degree before going into midwifery, although they do start with a degree in another health-related field. They go through the same educational and licensing system that was set up by the American College of Nurse-Midwives. This level of certification was started in 2000 and, therefore, is not yet common across the US.

Direct-entry midwives These midwives go directly into midwifery, obtaining their expertise through a combination of self-study, apprenticeship with other midwives, or a private midwifery program rather than going through the formal educational and licensing system set up by the American College of Nurse-Midwives. They are not legally recognized in 15 of the 50 states, and their fees are reimbursed by Medicaid in only ten of these.

NURSING STAFF

You may encounter a variety of nurses during your labor and delivery because each has a different role. Labor and delivery nurses help care for both mother and baby during delivery, postpartum nurses help the mother immediately after birth, and neonatal nurses take care of the new baby. Nurse-practitioners may provide additional support during your pregnancy because they are qualifed to diagnose and prescribe medicine.

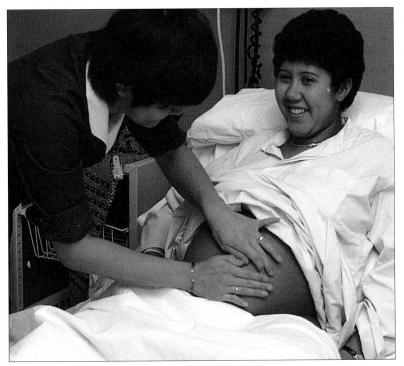

MIDWIVES AND OTHER BIRTH ATTENDANTS

This person will be your primary caregiver, so you'll want to form a good relationship. It may help to find out the following:

- What training and experience has she had?

- Does she work alone, or with other midwives? Will you have a chance to meet them?

- What are her views about managing labor?

- What's her backup system? Does she work closely with an obstetrician?

- What equipment, drugs, and resuscitation equipment for the baby does she carry?

- What prenatal care does she provide? Will she make home visits?

- Under what circumstances would she transfer you to a hospital?

Your birth attendant
The professional attendant who assists you to give birth should be someone you've met before and trust, and who'll give you the kind of support and encouragement you and your partner need. Ideally, your attendant helps to create an intimate atmosphere in which you feel happy working with your body to bring a new life into the world.

Birth plan

COVERING YOUR ALTERNATIVES

Your main birth plan will detail the kind of birth you'd prefer, your ideal, but it's a good idea to have an alternative version ready, just in case.

This alternative plan can set out the procedures that you'd prefer to be followed if complications should arise. On rare occasions, labor may become unexpectedly prolonged or difficult, or your baby may need special attention. If you think about all the possibilities beforehand, you'll make it easier for your birth attendants to take care of any situation as you wish.

Planning your labor
Make a note of all of the issues that are important to you and talk to your doctor about them.

Making your own plan for your baby's birth will help you make sure you have an active involvement in the way he's born and what happens immediately after the birth. Think about all the options and what you'd prefer, and talk everything over with your birth attendants and your partner. In this way, you'll build a bond of trust with everyone concerned and create a happier, more comfortable labor.

A CONSENSUS PLAN

Think about what's important to you and then find out as much as you can to see if what you want is feasible (see pp.118 & 120, and column, right). There's no point in making an unrealistic plan that can't be used once you are in labor.

Talk to your care provider about your birth plan early in your pregnancy. If you're having a hospital birth, ask your doctor to refer you to the hospital that's most in tune with your wishes if possible. It also helps to talk about what you want with your midwife, childbirth teacher, and other members of your prenatal team—they'll able to give you advice and tell you about the kinds of experiences other mothers have had in your local hospitals.

Hospital response Your hospital team will welcome the preparation you've done for the labor and will encourage you to get involved. Some mothers used to get bad reactions to birth plans from hospital staff because they might interfere with standard practices. That's unlikely now—in fact, there'll be space in your hospital notes for your preferences to be recorded.

Working together Cooperation is an important part of a birth plan. Working everything out in detail with all your attendants, including your partner, should ease anxieties and help you feel more in control of your baby's birth. Make sure staff are aware of any alternative plans you've made and stay friendly with your caregivers—they'll want to follow your wishes as far as they can, provided you and your baby are not at risk. Once you've talked about what's important to you, give a copy of the plan that's kept with your hospital notes to each of your birth partners or caregivers. This could be important if someone who doesn't know your wishes has to attend your labor. If you refuse any routine hospital procedures, you'll probably be asked to sign a refusal of treatment form. This protects the hospital from liability and give you more freedom of choice.

Special considerations Make a note on your birth plan of any particular needs you may have while you're in the hospital—for example, if you're a vegetarian or you need any other special diet.

PRESENTING YOUR BIRTH PLAN

These two birth plans give an idea of the different choices in childbirth, but there are many other variations. You can lay your plan out as a list, a letter, or a document like this example from a hospital.

Thanks for all the information you've provided in the prenatal classes and at the childbirth classes. I've thought carefully about how I'd like my labor and delivery to be.

My partner, John, will be my companion during labor. He's been to childbirth classes with me. If I have to have a cesarean section, I would like him to stay with me throughout the operation.

I understand that electronic fetal monitoring is routinely used and I'm happy to have this done.

If I need pain relief, I'd prefer to have an epidural, with as low a dose as possible so that I still have feeling in my legs and I'm aware of contractions. I would prefer for it to wear off for the second stage, since I'd like to push out the baby myself.

If everything goes well and I don't need pain relief, I would prefer to be able to walk around and give birth using a birthing stool, which I will provide myself.

I intend to breastfeed on demand and want my baby to sleep next to me if at all possible. I would also like my partner, John, to be able to stay with us for the first night.

I'm looking forward to coming into Central Hospital. I would like to put down a few points about the birth as the midwives have suggested. They are:

Support person	I will be accompanied by my sister, Sarah.
Monitoring	I would prefer to be monitored by a sonicaid or Pinnard stethoscope.
Positions	I will probably want to deliver the baby in a semi-upright position, since this is how I had my other two babies.
Pain relief	It's likely that I will need gas and air, as I did last time.
Episiotomy	I would prefer not to be cut if it can be avoided. I would welcome help in order to help prevent it.

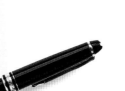

When?
Make sure you've talked to your caregivers about your plan by the eighth month.

IT'S YOUR CHOICE

Try to be open to all the possibilities that will help you feel confident about your labor. Don't feel the birth has to be totally managed or completely natural; it can be a blend of many things. Here are some alternatives:

- hospital/birthing center
- medical induction of labor if necessary/spontaneous start
- amniotomy if necessary/ spontaneous rupture of membranes
- fetus monitored electronically for a short time only/continuous fetal monitoring
- fasting only if high risk of cesarean/eat and drink as and when desired
- types of pain relief: Pethidine, epidural, gas and air, breathing exercises, TENS, diversion
- catheterization only with epidural/empty own bladder as necessary
- directed pushing/ spontaneous pushing
- deliberate breath-holding/no deliberate breath-holding
- elective episiotomy/episiotomy only if absolutely necessary
- mother not touching vaginal area/touching baby's head as it crowns, lifting baby out

Childbirth classes

It's a good idea to choose a childbirth teacher fairly early in your pregnancy; make plans to start classes in your seventh month or earlier.

The quality and approach of classes can vary—some are tightly structured with little question-and-answer time, others allow plenty of time to practice techniques. Some depend mainly on lectures, others on class participation. A good teacher is very often the key to whether a class is successful or not, so check with other couples you know who've attended classes before you make your final choice.

Select a teacher whose philosophy of birth fits in with the type of birth you'd like to have. It can be confusing and upsetting, if what you learn in class is not reflected in your later experience in the hospital or at a birthing center.

Find out how many couples are taught in each class. Half a dozen couples is ideal, since the teacher will have time to give all of you enough attention and you'll be able to get to know your classmates.

Childbirth teachers are generally very aware of and sensitive to the needs and problems of pregnancy. Yours will probably be more than happy to talk to you—even if you're not yet attending childbirth classes.

I'm an enthusiastic supporter of prepared childbirth, and I believe that everyone can benefit from going to childbirth classes. These classes are tremendously enjoyable. You'll make friends, and you may find that the other members of the group become a substitute for your extended family as you swap stories and experiences, so you don't feel alone and isolated. It's a great help to be able to share what you're going through with people who are in the same position, and it helps to relieve tension and anxiety. Many couples find they make strong, lasting friendships with the people they meet at classes.

PARENTING CLASSES

These are designed to give you information that will make you both feel more confident and are particularly useful for first-time parents. They cover three main areas:

First, the classes go through the processes of pregnancy and birth, including female anatomy and physiology, and the changes that are happening to you and the baby throughout your pregnancy. This will help you have a clearer understanding of what's involved and why things are happening. The teachers will also talk to you about the kinds of medical procedures that you can expect, and why these will be done. You'll be given plenty of opportunities to ask questions.

Second, you'll be taught relaxation, breathing, and exercise techniques. These will help you to control your own labor, reduce pain, and give you the confidence that only comes with being familiar with what's happening. It's bodies, not brains, that give birth, so be open to anything that helps you tune in to your body. Your partner will probably be taught how to give you a massage to help relieve your pain (see p.283).

Third, the teachers will talk you through the stages of labor and birth, and give tips on starting to breastfeed. They'll also give you practical advice on how to bathe and dress a baby, change diapers, and make up formula and bottle feed should you need it, all of which will help you feel more confident about caring for your newborn baby in the early days.

EXERCISE CLASSES

Strengthening the muscles used in childbirth can often mean you have an easier and more comfortable delivery. With this in mind, many hospitals hold prenatal classes that include some exercise and relaxation. There are also independent organizations that provide exercise classes for pregnant women—some are even for specific types of births. If you tell your instructor that you would like to have your baby while you are standing or squatting, you'll be given specific exercises to help strengthen your back, hips, pelvis, and thighs.

YOGA

Practicing yoga is an excellent way to prepare for childbirth because it emphasizes muscular control of the body, breathing, relaxation, and peace of mind. But yoga isn't something you can do casually—to be of any benefit, it must be done regularly, preferably starting long before you conceive. There are some special exercises for pregnancy, but it's best to have the guidance of a qualified teacher—particularly if you're pregnant.

TECHNIQUES OF CHILDBIRTH CLASSES

Many studies have shown that women who take childbirth classes have shorter labors. In one study, the average length of labor for women who'd been to classes was 13.56 hours, compared with an average 18.33 hours in another group of women who'd had no training. This is probably because knowing how to deal with pain means you have a more relaxed labor. Strategies for dealing with pain taught by childbirth classes include:

Cognitive control You dissociate your mind from the pain by visualizing a pleasant scenario for the pain. For example, you'll feel happier about contractions if, every time you have a pain, you imagine your baby moving farther down the birth canal, closer to being born. In this way, you'll concentrate on the joyous part of the sensation rather than the pain.

Distracting yourself can also help, although this works best in the early stages. Counting to 20, going through a list of possible names for your new baby, or concentrating on a beautiful picture or piece of music helps you to take your mind off the pain, and keeps it from completely filling your consciousness and over-whelming you.

Another way of taking your mind off the pain is to focus your attention on your breathing techniques. Think about each breath and become consciously aware of your breathing pattern.

Systematic relaxation You'll be taught exercises to relax all the various muscles of the body in turn to decrease your fear of pain and so increase your tolerance for it. This will help you to isolate pain in your contracting uterus, rather than allowing it to spread to other parts of your body.

Hawthorne effect This psychological research showed the importance of positive attention and motivation in any situation. If a mother receives extra, focused attention from a birth assistant, she's likely to cope better with labor.

Systematic desensitization You gradually become more tolerant of pain. An example used in many classes is your coach pinching your leg very hard to illustrate how painful a contraction will be. This pinching is repeated every time you go to a prenatal class, and by the end of the course you'll be able to tolerate harder squeezing for longer periods.

FATHER'S ROLE

Childbirth classes are an opportunity to show your partner just how central a role he is going to play.

Classes will help make a supportive man a more effective birth assistant as he gets more familiar with the processes of labor and delivery.

Some courses include father-only sessions when the men can talk freely about any problems or anxieties they have about the coming event. If a man is worried, he should get some support and advice from the teacher, as well as from other fathers-to-be.

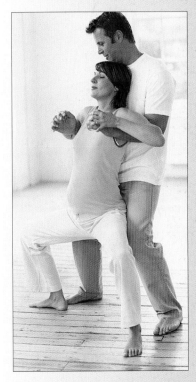

Team effort
Childbirth classes give a couple a unique opportunity to work together as a team toward a common goal—the birth of their baby. This teamwork often brings a special closeness.

CHAPTER 5

Food and eating in pregnancy

Eating healthily in pregnancy really means having a wide range of the right kind of foods—those rich in essential vitamins and minerals. If you make sure you eat plenty of fresh fruit and vegetables, whole grains, organically produced meat, and low-fat dairy products, you'll be doing the best for your baby.

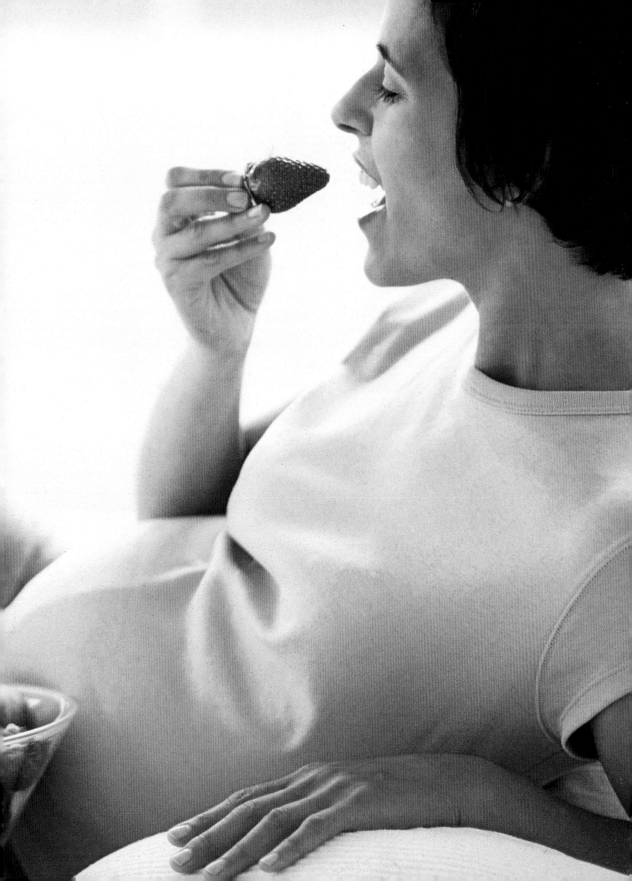

Food in pregnancy

EATING FOR YOURSELF

Your body works harder when you're carrying and giving birth to a baby than at any other time. It's important to eat well if you're to cope with the increased demands on your body, keep up your strength, and enjoy your pregnancy.

- Eat 200–300 more calories per day.

- Start to eat 5–6 small meals a day instead of 2–3 big ones.

- Make sure you eat enough protein and carbohydrates (see p.132). Protein supplies are essential nutrients for your developing baby. Carbohydrates fuel your energy needs.

- Eat foods containing vitamins, such as vitamin C, and minerals, particularly iron (see p.133). You'll need these for the healthy functioning of all your organs.

Gaining weight

Doctors generally recommend that a woman of average weight, who's having an average pregnancy, shouldn't gain more than 25–35 lb (11–16 kg) over the 40 weeks as shown in the chart on the right. About 6–8 lb (2.7–3.5 kg) of this is for the baby and the rest for the baby-support system (placenta, amniotic fluid, increased blood, fluid, fat, and breast tissue). Women carrying twins will gain 35–45 lb (16–20 kg) and should have 300 calories a day more than women carrying a single baby. Most women put on little or no weight during the first trimester, 1–2 lb (0.5–1 kg) a week between months four and eight, then very little, or none at all, in the last month. A slow, steady gain means that your body can adapt more easily to your increasing size, and your baby is provided with a continuous flow of nourishment.

When you're pregnant, you certainly don't want to bother with measuring portions and figuring out how many calories there are in what you're eating. And there's no need to do this as long as you follow some basic guidelines about healthy eating. One golden rule is that the closer food is to its natural state, the better it is for you. So fresh is best, frozen is next-best, and you should make canned foods your last choice. It's common sense.

EATING FOR TWO?

You'll probably feel hungrier than usual when you're expecting a baby—it's nature's way of making certain you eat enough for both of you. But you certainly don't need to "eat for two" as people used to believe. Most women only need to eat an extra 200–300 calories a day, far less than if you ate twice your normal amount of food. Much more important than the quantity of what you eat is the quality. Everything you eat should be good for you and your baby. Some mothers-to-be, such as those who previously ate an inadequate or unbalanced diet, may be nutritionally at risk and have special dietary needs—see also the column on p.138.

More problems develop if you eat too little rather than too much. Pregnancy is not the time for dieting. Research has shown

AVERAGE WEIGHT GAIN DURING PREGNANCY

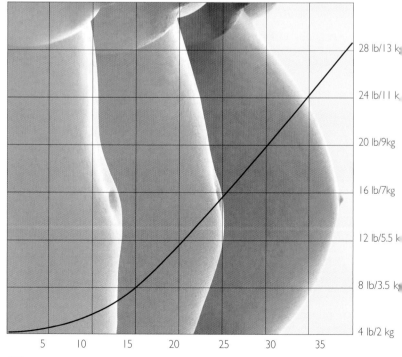

| | 28 lb/13 k |
| 24 lb/11 k |
| 20 lb/9kg |
| 16 lb/7kg |
| 12 lb/5.5 k |
| 8 lb/3.5 k |
| 4 lb/2 kg |

5   10   15   20   25   30   35

that when mothers-to-be eat poor diets, there's a higher incidence of spontaneous abortions, neonatal death, and low-birthweight babies than normal.

You owe it to yourself, as well as to your growing baby, to eat the diet that's best for both of you. Try to stick to the healthy eating guidelines on pages 134 and 135, but remember that you can balance your food intake over a 24- to 48-hour period rather than at each meal if you prefer. Just make sure you don't miss any meals—your baby grows all day, every day, and will suffer if you don't eat properly.

Junk foods such as chocolate bars and hamburgers and fries contain little more than fat and sugar. They don't do your baby any good, and your body converts these empty calories into fat, so don't eat them.

You'll put on some fat when you're pregnant, and your body needs this to convert to milk when you're breastfeeding. Although breastfeeding will help you lose the weight you put on during pregnancy, it's best to avoid really excessive weight gain; fat that's deposited at the tops of your arms and thighs is very difficult to get rid of after pregnancy.

Your baby's needs

While your baby is growing inside your womb, you are her only source of nourishment. Every calorie, vitamin, or gram of protein she needs must come from you. You're in sole charge of your unborn child's nutrition; you, and only you, can make sure the best-quality food reaches her.

You'll be doing your best for your baby if you eat lots of fresh fruit, vegetables, beans, peas, whole-grain cereals, fish, fowl, and low-fat dairy products. A Danish study showed that eating oily fish—such as salmon, mackerel, herring, and sardines—may help lessen the risk of premature birth. Make your diet as varied as possible, choosing from a wide range of foods.

Don't forget Mom

The other person to do your best for is yourself. Eating plenty of healthy foods throughout your pregnancy will mean that you have better reserves for coping with, and recovering from, the physical strains of pregnancy and the hard work of labor. Anemia and preeclampsia (see p.224) are much more common in mothers who have a poor diet, and some problems, including morning sickness and leg cramps, may be made worse by what you do or don't eat. Make sure you're eating plenty of fresh vegetables, grains, and fruits during pregnancy. They'll give you energy and may help prevent constipation.

A healthy diet will help to reduce excessive mood swings, fatigue, and many other common complaints of pregnancy (see pp.206–213). And if you cut out or restrict the amount of empty calories you eat, you'll have less excess fat to lose after your baby has been born.

EMPTY CALORIES

It's best to avoid the following foods when you're pregnant. They're full of sugar or sugar substitutes and refined flour, so they're no good for you or your baby.

- Any form of sweetener—this includes white and brown sugar, corn syrup, molasses, and artificial sweeteners such as saccharin and aspartame.
- Candy and chocolate bars.
- Soft drinks, such as cola and sweetened fruit juices.
- Commercially produced cookies, cakes, pastries, and pies, as well as jam and marmalade.
- Canned fruit in syrup.
- Nondairy creamer.
- Sweetened breakfast cereal.
- Ice cream or sherbet that contains added sugar. Freeze fruit juice or puréed fruit instead.
- Toppings or dressings that contain sugar, such as relish, pickles, salad dressing, spaghetti sauce, mayonnaise, peanut butter, and many others—read the labels.

SUPPLIES TO KEEP AT WORK

It's not always easy to stick to your healthy diet when you're at work. Planning ahead and keeping some supplies in the office will help.

In the office refrigerator:

- mineral water
- unsweetened fruit juice
- plain live-culture yogurt
- Dutch or Swiss cheese
- hard-boiled eggs
- fresh fruit
- "snack" vegetables—carrot and red pepper sticks, tomatoes
- whole-wheat bread
- jar of wheat germ.

In your desk drawer:

- whole-grain crackers, crispbread, or breadsticks, perhaps with seeds
- dried fruit
- nuts or seeds
- decaffeinated instant coffee and decaffeinated tea bags
- powdered skim milk for extra calcium in drinks.

In your bag:

- whole-grain crackers, crispbread, or breadsticks, perhaps with seeds
- dried fruit, nuts, and seeds
- fresh fruit or "snack" vegetables
- small thermos of unsweetened juice or milk
- glucose candy for emergencies.

Make sure everything is securely wrapped and sealed.

THE BEST FOOD TO EAT

Fresh food that's as close to its original state as possible is best for you and your baby. Eating good-quality food should be your goal throughout, as well as after, your pregnancy.

When you're out shopping, choose fresh produce; seasonal fruit and vegetables are always fresher and sometimes cheaper than imported, out-of-season items. Pick out firm fruit and vegetables and reject any that look tired or are going bad. Buy your meat and fish from stores you can trust—don't run the risk of getting a food-related illness (see p.139). If you can afford it, go for free-range or organic foods grown without pesticides and hormones (used particularly in beef and intensively farmed poultry); many organic foods carry a USDA organic label. Check the labeling of processed foods to see whether they include any genetically modified (GM) ingredients. Until the scientific research into the safety of these foods has been completed and fully debated, it's sensible to avoid GM foods during pregnancy.

Always keep some packs of frozen vegetables—they're good standbys when you can't get to the store. Avoid cans, except for whole tomatoes and fish such as sardines. Read the labels on any other packaged foods you buy, and remember that the closer an ingredient is to the top of the list, the more there is of that one ingredient. Sugar has many different names (see p.132) and can appear on a list more than once.

Foods that have been overrefined, such as white flour and white sugar, have had all of the natural goodness stripped out of them and fill you and your baby with nothing but excess calories. Choose whole-wheat bread and flour rather than "enriched" refined products; it's highly unlikely that the enrichment puts back in all that's been taken out. The two "waste" products of flour refining are bran (the fiber) and wheat germ (the heart of the wheat) and these contain most of the goodness. Bran is probably an unnecessary addition for the average pregnant woman (although it will help prevent constipation), but wheat germ contains lots of vitamins and minerals that are good for everyone. Wheat germ is crunchy and nutty and can be added to salads and sandwiches, as well as to cooked and baked dishes. You can buy wheat germ from health food stores and good supermarkets.

GOOD EATING HABITS

You'll probably need more than willpower if you're going to stick to your healthy regimen. The first step is to avoid eating food you know you shouldn't have because there's nothing else available. Keep some sugar-free fruit and nut bars and decaffeinated tea bags with you so you don't give in to temptations like cookies and coffee in the afternoon. If possible, prepare a batch of meals over the weekend that you can store and eat during the week. That will keep you from calling for a pizza delivery when you're too tired to cook. Banish junk food from your kitchen.

Think before you eat—a high-protein chicken and lettuce sandwich on whole-wheat bread that's rich in fiber and folic acid is much better for you than fat-rich bacon and mayonnaise on fiberless white! Invest in a healthy-eating cookbook and try out some dishes that are lower in fat and sugar but still taste delicious. Get in the habit of snacking on nutritious foods and eat little and often. Toward the end of your pregnancy, you'll probably find that eating larger amounts is difficult anyway.

VEGETARIAN MOTHERS

Many people prefer not to eat meat; many more limit their intake of meat, particularly red meat. This is fine, but when you're pregnant, you'll need to make sure you eat enough protein, vitamins, and iron to meet your own and your baby's needs (see also p.136). Plants contain proteins, too, but you need to eat them in the right combinations to provide you with most of the necessary amino acids that are found complete in animal forms of protein (see below).

You'll also need to make sure you're getting enough iron, since there's relatively little in plant foods, and certain substances interfere with how well iron is absorbed by your body (see p.133). If you eat no animal products at all, you'll have to work harder to make sure that you're not lacking in any nutrients—particularly calcium and vitamins B6, B12, and D, all of which are provided by dairy products. Although you don't need much B12, lack of it will eventually lead to pernicious anemia, so if your diet contains no animal products, it's best to take vitamin B12 supplements.

SHORTCUTS

When you're short of time, energy, or money, eating the right foods can like seem like too much trouble. Here are some ideas to help you eat well without too much effort:

- keep a range of frozen vegetables

- buy meat and fish in bulk, and freeze in meal-size portions

- cook meals ahead and freeze

- wash ready-made fresh salads, even if the label says "ready to eat"

- use a microwave oven—but don't stand next to or directly in front of it while it is in use

- keep meals simple—eat raw vegetables; steam, stir-fry, or broil for speed, or bake so you can leave food to cook on its own

- get help—grandparents-to-be will be glad to give you a hand.

COMPLEMENTARY PROTEINS

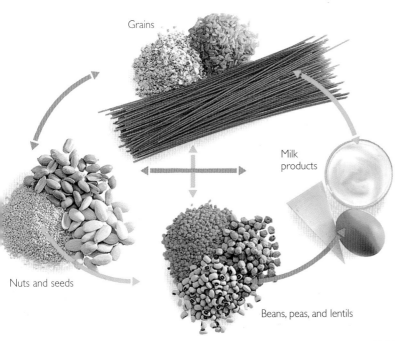

Grains

Milk products

Nuts and seeds

Beans, peas, and lentils

Combining proteins

All animal products provide first-class proteins—they contain all the essential amino acids the body needs in the right proportions.

Plant products contain second-class proteins—the amino acids that they provide are not in the right proportions. To make sure you get the necessary amino acids from plant foods, you need to eat the right combinations of foods. Peas, for instance, can be served with rice or corn; a handful of nuts can be added to rice and sweet corn salad.

◀▶ Generally complementary

◀▶ Sometimes complementary

CHOOSING PROTEINS

The needs of your growing baby mean that you'll have to eat 30 percent more protein than usual from the start of your pregnancy.

Your needs jump from 1¾–2¼ oz (45–60 g) to 3–4 oz (75–100 g) of protein daily, depending on how active you are.

Proteins are made up of amino acids, which are vital to individual body cells and tissues. We need a total of 20 different amino acids. Your body can make 12 of these, the nonessential amino acids, itself. The other eight, the essential acids, must be supplied by food you eat. These are contained in first-class proteins, found only in animal products such as meat, dairy foods, fish, poultry, and eggs. Buy organically reared produce if you can, especially poultry, eggs, and beef.

When you're choosing protein foods, think about what else they contain. Offal and meat are the richest sources of first-class proteins and contain vital B vitamins. But some meat, particularly red meat, can be very high in animal fat. It's best not to eat liver when you're pregnant, since it's high in vitamin A, which may be toxic to your baby.

Fish is a good choice of first-class protein for pregnant women. It's high in vitamins and nutritious fish oils, and is low in saturated fat.

Equivalent amounts of protein are one egg, one slice of hard cheese, two tablespoons of cottage cheese, or half a cup of beans.

Essential nutrition

What you eat when you're pregnant is even more important than you might think. Research shows that it not only affects your baby at birth, but also appears to have a long-term effect throughout your child's life—even into old age.

PROTEIN

Protein is probably the most essential food for your baby; the amino acids that make up protein are literally the building blocks of the body. The cells and tissues that make up muscles, bones, connective tissues, and many of your organ walls are formed from protein.

The type and quality of protein in food varies (see column, left). Meat, fish, and poultry are the best sources, but they can be expensive. Plant foods eaten together can be a cheaper way of supplying your body with enough protein. Whole-wheat bread or noodles with beans or cheese, or cornmeal or noodles with sesame seeds, nuts, and milk will keep your protein intake high. You need at least three servings of protein foods (see p.134) daily.

CARBOHYDRATES AND CALORIES

Carbohydrate foods should make up the bulk of your daily calorie intake, but make sure you eat the best, complex, carbohydrates and avoid empty calories (see p.129).

Simple carbohydrates are sugars in various forms. The most common types and sources are sucrose (cane sugar), glucose (honey), fructose (fruit), and maltose, lactose, and galactose (milk). These carbohydrates are absorbed quickly from the stomach and are a source of "instant energy," which can be useful when you're in dire need. Glucose candy may also be helpful when you feel nauseous.

Complex carbohydrates are the starches contained in grains, potatoes, lentils, beans, and peas. The body has to break them down into simple carbohydrates before it can use them, so they provide a steady supply of energy over a period of time. Complex unrefined carbohydrates (whole oats and brown rice) are also good sources of vitamins, minerals, and fiber.

VITAMINS

Vegetables and fruits are good sources of many vitamins and minerals. Some are rich in vitamin C; others contain vitamins A, B, E, minerals, and folic acid—all of which you need in your diet. Vitamins are quickly destroyed by exposure to light, air, and heat, and many can't be stored by the body, so you need to top off your supplies every day. Leafy green vegetables, yellow and red vegetables, and fruit supply vitamins A, E, B6, iron, zinc, and magnesium. Choose broccoli, spinach, watercress, carrots, tomatoes, bananas, apricots, and cherries.

Some vegetables, such as watercress, are rich in many vitamins and are an excellent choice for you and your baby. Others provide a selection of vitamins and minerals, as well as fiber.

Although we can get some B vitamins from vegetables and fruit, the bulk of our vitamin B intake comes from meat, fish, dairy products, grains, and nuts. Some of the B vitamins are only found in animal foods, so vegetarians must make sure they're getting enough in their diet. If you don't eat dairy products, you'll need to take vitamin B12 supplements—ask your doctor for a prescription.

Most women are advised to take prenatal vitamins, which are specially formulated for pregnant women, along with an iron supplement. Some mega-vitamin supplements contain excessive amounts of vitamin A and could be harmful to your baby.

Folic acid This is essential for making red blood cells and plays an important part in the growth of your baby, especially during the first 12 weeks. Folic acid is vital to the development of the nervous system, and research shows that folic acid supplements taken up to three months before conception and for the first 12 weeks of pregnancy significantly reduce the incidence of neural tube defects such as spina bifida. If you haven't started taking folic acid before conception, start as soon as you know you're pregnant. Folic acid is available in tablet form, and it's also in green leafy vegetables, cereals, and bread.

MINERALS

A varied, healthy diet should provide you with enough minerals and trace elements—essential chemicals that help the body function properly but cannot be made by it. High levels of iron and calcium, in particular, are needed for your baby's development.

Iron The body needs iron to make *hemoglobin* (the oxygen-carrying part of the red blood cells). When you're pregnant, your iron intake must be not only adequate (see column, right) but also continuous. You need to keep up supplies of extra iron to support the large increase in the amount of blood in your body during pregnancy because your baby's need for iron is constant. Iron can block the body's absorption of zinc, which is essential for the development of your baby's brain and nervous system, so you need to eat zinc-rich food, such as fish and wheat germ, separately from iron-rich food.

Calcium A baby's bones begin to form between four and six weeks, so you'll need plenty of calcium both before you conceive and while you're pregnant. Dairy products, leafy green vegetables, tofu, broccoli, and any fish containing bones (such as sardines) are rich in calcium. If you don't eat dairy products, you may need supplements. Vitamin D is needed for calcium absorption, so try to eat eggs or cheese every day.

DRINK PLENTY OF LIQUIDS

When you're pregnant you have nearly 50 percent more blood in your body than usual, so you need to keep up your fluid intake.

Water is best, though fruit juice is also good. Drinking plenty also helps to avoid the risk of urinary tract infections. Don't cut down on your fluid intake if your hands and feet swell—it won't make any difference to this type of fluid retention.

VITAMIN D

The action of light on the skin triggers the body to make Vitamin D.

- Most light-skinned people need about 40 minutes of daylight—it doesn't have to be sunny—every day to make enough vitamin D for their needs.

- Dark-skinned people living outside the tropics need progressively more sunlight depending on their skin tones.

KEEP UP YOUR IRON INTAKE

The amount of iron you need varies from woman to woman. Your doctor will keep track of your iron levels.

If you're lacking in iron when you become pregnant, or develop iron deficiency later, your doctor will prescribe an iron supplement or injections so you don't get anemia.

Nutritional values

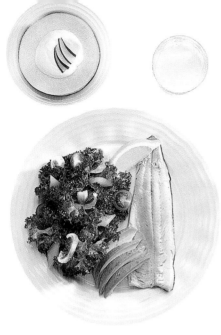

There's no need for you to spend lots of time measuring out portions and calculating your vitamin intake, but you might like some guidelines to help you make sure you're eating as well as possible. You can balance your intake of different nutrients over a couple of days, rather than at every meal.

DAILY NEEDS

So that you and your baby have the best possible diet, try to eat the following each day—each of the suggested sources represents a single portion. It's a good idea to vary the food you choose.

- First-class proteins—three servings
- Vitamin C foods—two servings
- Calcium foods—four servings in pregnancy, five when nursing
- Green leafy and yellow vegetables and fruits—three servings
- Other fruit and vegetables—one or two servings
- Whole grains and complex carbohydrates—four or five servings
- Iron-rich food—two servings
- Fluids—eight glasses a day, not coffee or alcohol. Water is best.

A balanced meal
This meal of trout and salad, melon with yogurt and nectarines, and a glass of milk is tasty and full of goodness.

What you need	Suggested sources	
Calcium foods	2 oz (50 g) hard cheese 4 oz (100 g) soft cheese 1½ cups cottage cheese 1 cup yogurt	1 cup milk, fresh or made up from powdered milk 3 oz (75 g) canned sardines, with bones
First-class protein foods	3 oz (75 g) hard cheese 4 oz (100 g) soft cheese 2 cups milk 1½ cups yogurt 3 large eggs	4 oz (100 g) fresh or canned fish 4 oz (100 g) shrimp 3 oz (75 g) beef, lamb, pork, poultry, offal (not liver), without the fat
Green leafy and yellow/red vegetables and fruit	½ cup broccoli florets 2 tbsp sliced carrots 1 cup peas, beans, spinach 3 tbsp diced bell pepper 1 cup sliced tomatoes	1 cup melon cubes 6 plums 1 mango, orange, grapefruit 2 apricots 4 peaches, apples, pears
Whole grains and complex carbohydrates	½ cup cooked barley, brown rice, millet, bulgur ¼ cup whole-wheat or soy flour 1 slice whole-wheat or soy bread 6 whole-wheat bread sticks	⅛ cup kidney beans, soybeans, chickpeas ½ cup lentils, peas 1 whole-grain pita bread or tortilla 6 whole-wheat cookies
Vitamin C foods	3 tbsp diced bell pepper 1 large tomato 1⅛ cups blackberries or raspberries ½ cup citrus juice	½ cup strawberries 1 large lemon or orange ½ medium grapefruit ¼ cup black currants

VITAMIN AND MINERAL SOURCES

Foods can provide all the vitamins and minerals we need, except for vitamin D. The chart below is a guide to the best sources of essential vitamins and minerals. They tend to be easily destroyed, so try to eat foods that are as fresh as possible. Some foods contain a range of vitamins and minerals.

Name	Food source
Vitamin A (retinol & carotene)	Whole milk, butter, cheese, egg yolk, oily fish, offal, green and yellow fruit and vegetables
Vitamin B1 (thiamine)	Whole grains, nuts, legumes, offal, pork, brewer's yeast, wheat germ
Vitamin B2 (riboflavin)	Brewer's yeast, wheat germ, whole grains, green vegetables, milk, cheese, eggs
Vitamin B3 (niacin)	Brewer's yeast, whole grains, wheat germ, offal, green vegetables, oily fish, eggs, milk
Vitamin B5 (pantothenic acid)	Offal, eggs, whole grains, cheese
Vitamin B6 (pyridoxine)	Brewer's yeast, whole grains, soy flour, offal, wheat germ, mushrooms, potatoes, avocados
Vitamin B12 (cyanocobalamin)	Meat, offal, fish, milk, eggs
Folic acid (part of B complex)	Raw leafy vegetables, peas, soy flour, oranges, bananas, walnuts
Vitamin C (ascorbic acid)	Rosehip syrup, bell peppers, citrus fruits, black currants, tomatoes
Vitamin D (calciferol)	Fortified milk, oily fish, eggs (particularly the yolks), butter
Vitamin E	Wheat germ, egg yolk, seeds, vegetable oils, broccoli
Calcium	Milk, cheese, small fish with bones, walnuts, sunflower seeds, tofu, yogurt, broccoli
Iron	Kidneys, fish, egg yolks, red meat, cereals, molasses, apricots, haricot or cannellini beans
Zinc	Wheat bran, eggs, nuts, onions, shellfish, sunflower seeds, wheat germ, whole wheat

PREPARING FOOD

Developing some good cooking habits will help you eat healthily.

- Trim fat off meat before cooking.

- Skim fat off the surface of casseroles and soups.

- Bake, steam, or broil instead of frying.

- Stir-fry food in a teaspoon of olive oil, plus a little water, or with a bouillon cube dissolved in a cup of water.

- Use nonstick pans and as little fat as possible when you make omelets or scrambled eggs.

- Use flavored vinegars, such as raspberry, basil, thyme, or garlic (homemade ones are better than store-bought), or yogurt for salad dressings, instead of mayonnaise or sour cream.

- Add dried skim milk to milky drinks, or when baking, for extra servings of calcium.

- Always choose low-fat, rather than full-fat, dairy products.

- Eat fruit and vegetables raw as often as you can.

The vegetarian mother

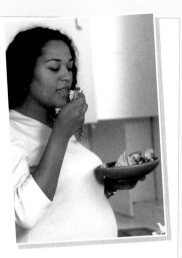

*Anne was anxious that her vegetarian diet
might not be able to support her baby's healthy
growth and development. We looked at her
various worries and, once we'd identified
possible protein and calcium deficiencies,
I suggested some ways of making sure her
diet contained enough of these nutrients.*

SPECIAL NEEDS FOR VEGETARIANS?

Having already had two babies, Anne knew that she
might need to make some changes to her diet, even
with her previous eating habits, but now that she was a
vegetarian, she wanted to check a few things.

For example, she'd heard that a vegetarian diet might
be short of vitamin B12; if so, would that harm her
baby? She'd also read something about folic acid and
spina bifida. Was her diet lacking in folic acid, and
should she take supplements? She knew that some
pregnant women take iron supplements; would she
need to?

Anne knew that the main change she had to make to
her diet would be to make sure she ate more protein,
but she wanted to know what kind of protein would be
best and which foods provide it. During pregnancy, the
body demands increased calcium intake. Would it be
best to take calcium tablets, or would she be able to get
enough by eating plenty of calcium-rich and calcium-
fortified foods?

EASY WAYS FOR ANNE TO MEET HER INCREASED NEEDS

Opinions on a vegetarian diet during pregnancy differ
widely. They range from those of vegans who believe
that women can carry a healthy baby to term without
eating any animal protein or even taking vitamin B12
supplements, to inflexible doctors who insist that meat
and fish are essential foods for a pregnant woman.
Both views are wrong.

In the case of vegans, if no animal products,
including dairy products, are eaten, vitamin B12
supplements are absolutely essential. B12 is vital to the
healthy growth and development of the fetus, as well as
that of a breastfed baby. Vegan mothers have to add
milk and eggs to their diet, or take synthetic B12,
during pregnancy and while they're breastfeeding.

A vegetarian diet that includes dairy products can
support a pregnancy, and later breastfeeding, perfectly
well, as long as you have more protein and calcium. All
pregnant women should increase their milk intake to a
pint a day (choose skim rather than whole milk). Anne
can also boost her protein and vitamin intake by
drinking vitamin-fortified soy milk and eating lots of
other soy and dairy products.

However, the simplest way for Anne to increase the
protein and vitamin content of her diet would be for
her to eat at least four eggs a week. Eggs will provide
iron, too, although not as much as red meat. While
some vegetarians claim that they can get the same

amount of iron that red meat provides by eating more green leafy vegetables, they'd have to eat almost five pounds of these vegetables per day to do so!

I advised Anne to accept her obstetrician's advice if he prescribed vitamin, iron, and calcium supplements, but reassured her that if he presses her on eating meat, she should contact the North American Vegetarian Society (see Addresses, p.370) for further information.

SUGGESTED DAILY VEGETARIAN MENU

Breakfast
Two slices of whole-wheat toast with yeast extract and peanut butter. Cup of decaffeinated tea with skim milk. One banana

Midmorning snack
Selection of raw vegetables with humus (chickpea dip) and whole-wheat pita bread

Lunch
Baked potato, topped with cottage cheese, red pepper, tomatoes, and watercress. Glass of tomato juice. Chopped nuts and dried fruit

Afternoon snack
Broccoli and cheese soup (preferably fresh) with chopped walnuts and low-fat sour cream. Two slices of rye bread

Dinner
Mushroom and tofu lasagna, spinach, steamed snow peas, and whole-wheat garlic bread. Fresh fruit with low-fat yogurt. Grapefruit juice

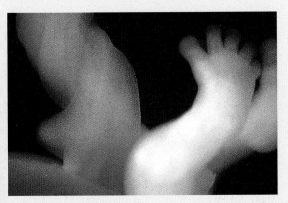

Your baby's lifeline
The umbilical cord links your baby with the placenta. All the nutrients necessary for healthy growth and development pass to your baby through the cord.

Bedtime snack
Boiled egg and whole-wheat toast with yeast extract. Glass of skim milk
This menu should take care of Anne's needs.

Anne's baby

Nature makes sure that a baby's nutritional needs are supplied by the body before the mother's. Anne's baby, therefore, could be better nourished than she is herself.

• **Iron** A baby needs plenty of iron for blood formation and organ growth. This can be supplied by eating iron-rich foods such as egg yolks, cereals, and molasses

• **Calcium** This mineral builds healthy bones and teeth. Anne needs a diet that is rich in calcium for her own needs as well for her baby's

• **Protein** Anne needs to eat a variety of protein-rich foods to nourish her baby's fast-growing muscles, bones, skin, and vital organs

• **Vitamin B12** The development of her baby's brain and nervous system depends on sufficient supplies of this vitamin. Anne, like every other mother, cannot afford to be deficient

• **Folic acid** The development of her baby's brain, spinal cord, and spine also depend on Anne's having sufficient levels of folic acid in her blood

• **Calories** The blood sugar of the baby is always lower than that of its mother because it's used so quickly. A constant supply is needed for healthy growth

**If any of the following points
apply to you, you could be
nutritionally vulnerable and
your baby may be at risk.
You'll need to get special
advice and help from your
doctor or clinic before and
during pregnancy.**

- If you've had a recent stillbirth
or miscarriage, or your children
are coming in quick succession
(at least 18 months between
babies is best for your health).

- If you smoke, or are a heavy
drinker.

- If you're allergic to certain foods,
such as cow's milk or wheat.

- If you suffer from a chronic
medical condition that means
you have to take regular long-
term medication.

- If you're under 18—your own
body is growing quickly and your
nutritional needs will be higher
than average when pregnant.

- If you're carrying more than
a single baby.

- If you've been under a lot of
stress or had a physical injury.

- If your job involves hard physical
work or is in a potentially dangerous environment (see p.168).

- If you were generally run-down
or underweight before
conception, or eating an
inadequate or unbalanced diet.

- If you are bulimic, anorexic, or
have a BMI (body mass index)
of less than 19.

Nutritional and food-related problems

It's very important to eat enough good food to satisfy your nutritional needs while you're pregnant; otherwise, you could put yourself and your developing baby at risk. Another danger can be eating food contaminated with bacteria that cause disease; examples are chicken or eggs contaminated with salmonella.

MALNUTRITION

You need to eat properly for your baby's sake. If you don't, there's a higher risk that you could miscarry or have a premature or low-birthweight baby, who will be more vulnerable at birth and later in life. (By the way, having a low birthweight baby does not mean labor will be easier.) Being poorly nourished yourself can also slow the growth of the placenta, and low placental weight is related to a higher infant mortality rate. Your baby's brain develops most rapidly in the last trimester of pregnancy (and in the first month of life after birth) so if you're undernourished, it can affect your baby's brain function.

A poor diet during pregnancy can continue to affect a child throughout his life, and may mean he's more likely to suffer such middle-age diseases as high blood pressure, coronary artery disease, and obesity. If there's not enough nutrition getting through to your womb, the baby diverts what's available to those cells that are immediately important, and away from those cells that will not be important until later in life—in effect, your unborn baby trades a long life for short-term survival.

On the other hand, if you have enough good food and give birth to a good-sized baby, such a baby will be easier to care for, more vigorous, active, mentally alert, and less likely to suffer from colic, diarrhea, anemia, and infections.

Fresh foods are best, and if you can't afford them, the United States Department of Agricultue Food and Nutrition Service can help with subsidized food stamps. Avoid processed foods and those containing lots of additives, flavorings, and colorings.

Processed foods Many of these foods contain chemicals to improve flavor, nutritional value, and shelf life. As a general rule, it's best to avoid these, especially when you're pregnant—in particular, processed cheese and meats, cheese spreads, and sausages. Check the lists of ingredients on labels for additives, including food colorings and preservatives. Always make sure that you eat any packaged food well before its expiration date, and don't buy any foods that don't list their ingredients. It's also a good idea to avoid highly salted foods, particularly those containing monosodium glutamate (MSG), which can cause dehydration and headaches.

Preserved food   Smoked fish, meat and cheese, pickled food, and sausages often contain nitrates. These can react with the hemoglobin in your blood and reduce its oxygen-carrying power, so they are best avoided.

Drinks   Caffeine (in tea, coffee, and hot chocolate) is a stimulant, so try to cut back on them when you're pregnant. The tannin in tea interferes with iron absorption, so drink organic herbal teas instead. Soft drinks always contain sugar or sweeteners, so limit your intake of them. Mineral water is fine.

FOOD HAZARDS

Some foods can be contaminated with large enough numbers of bacteria to cause illness, particularly in vulnerable people—such as pregnant women and babies.

Listeriosis   Foods that can contain large numbers of listeria bacteria include soft cheese, unpasteurized milk, prepackaged coleslaw, cooked chilled foods, pâtés, and meat that hasn't been properly cooked. Listeria bacteria is normally destroyed at pasteurizing temperatures, but if infected food is then refrigerated, the bacteria may continue to multiply. For this reason, you shouldn't eat chilled food after its expiration date. Listeriosis can spread through direct contact with infected live animals, such as sheep. Symptoms are flulike: a high temperature and aches and pains, and also sore throat and eyes, diarrhea, and stomach pain. An unborn child affected through his mother's blood may be stillborn, and listeriosis may be a cause of recurrent miscarriage.

Salmonella   Infection with salmonella is often traced back to contaminated eggs and chicken meat, so avoid foods that contain raw eggs. Cook eggs and chicken well, and choose free-range eggs and fowl. Symptoms, including headache, nausea, abdominal pain, diarrhea, shivering, and fever, develop suddenly from 12–48 hours after infection and last two or three days. If the infection spreads into your bloodstream, you'll need to take antibiotics.

Toxoplasmosis   This common infection can be picked up by eating raw or undercooked pork or steak, or by coming into contact with the feces of infected cats and dogs. Don't dispose of your cat's and dog's feces unless you wear gloves and wash your hands in disinfectant immediately afterward. (see p.169).

Dysentery   This disease is carried in the feces of an affected person. It causes dehydration, severe diarrhea, and abdominal pain, and is dangerous for pregnant women. Amoebic dysentery is rare outside tropical areas, but bacterial dysentery is more common. It's usually passed on when an infected person fails to wash his or her hands properly after going to the bathroom and then handles food.

FOOD SAFETY

Never take unnecessary risks when handling and storing food; bacteria can multiply very rapidly.

- Always use clean utensils between jobs, or tastings.
- Always wash hands after going to the bathroom and before touching food, and make sure you cover any infections or cuts.
- Defrost and cook food thoroughly, especially poultry.
- Never let raw meat or eggs come in contact with other foods.
- Avoid dented and rusty cans and any food that looks or smells spoiled.
- Make sure dairy products have been well pasteurized.
- Don't refreeze food that has already been defrosted.
- Reheat food thoroughly and only once. Throw away leftovers.

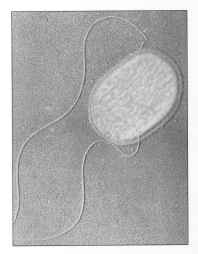

Salmonella bacteria
The highly magnified picture above shows one of the many hundreds of different strains of the potentially hazardous salmonella bacteria.

The diabetic mother

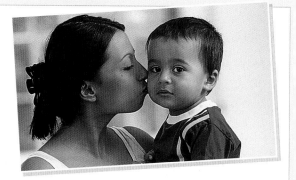

third pregnancy should be fine, but she's well aware of the importance of frequent prenatal checks. She knows that uncontrolled diabetes would lead to complications for her and to far more serious ones for her baby.

There's no need for women who have or develop diabetes during pregnancy to worry that they'll have a difficult pregnancy or have problems producing a normal, healthy baby. As long as diabetes is carefully managed, with the obstetrician and diabetic physician in close cooperation, the outcome should be good.

PREGNANCY AND DIABETES

As well as being 50 percent more likely than men to become diabetic, women have a tendency to develop the disease during pregnancy. Certain women are recognized as potential diabetics. They've usually had at least one heavy baby or have a family history of diabetes in parents or siblings. Other women can develop diabetes during pregnancy. Some may remain diabetic after pregnancy, but others go back to normal.

Pregnancy can complicate established diabetes, causing the kidneys to function less effectively as well as causing eye changes. While most sufferers will have been treated with insulin, some women with diabetes may have been treated with diet alone or with diet and blood-sugar-lowering (hypoglycemic) tablets. The extra demands of pregnancy will require that insulin be prescribed, so any diabetic who plans to get pregnant should change to insulin before conceiving.

Having been an insulin-dependent diabetic for two years, Jill was meticulous about her prepregnancy

preparations. She planned this present baby and made sure her diabetes was fully assessed well before she became pregnant. In particular, she was concerned about controlling her blood sugar levels, the functioning of her kidneys, and the health of her eyes. In the months before conceiving, she kept careful control of her diabetes. She took folic acid supplements in the period before conceiving.

KEEPING CONTROL DURING PREGNANCY

Jill knows that diabetes can mean a greater risk that her baby will have cardiac and skeletal problems, but that good control of her diabetes during preconception and the first trimester should greatly reduce this risk (see Health considerations, p.18). She came to ask my advice very early in the pregnancy.

I explained to Jill that now she's pregnant, she may need less insulin for the first three months. Then her body will start to produce hormones with an anti-insulin effect, so she'll need more insulin than before.

CHECKING BLOOD SUGAR

In order to keep control of her diabetes, Jill will need to test her blood sugar several times a day and adjust her dosage of insulin accordingly. Jill knows that regulating her sugar levels carefully brings the best results for herself and her baby, but that this may sometimes be difficult. It's rare nowadays, though, for a pregnant woman with diabetes to be admitted to the hospital to improve blood sugar control, since the food there is usually very different from her diet at home and she would need different levels of insulin.

POSSIBLE PRENATAL COMPLICATIONS

Pregnant women with diabetes usually go to a special prenatal clinic so they can be seen by an obstetrician and a specialist in diabetes. There may also be a dietician, a specialist nurse, and a midwife. Diabetic women usually have extra scans at 28, 32, and 36 weeks to check their baby's growth but may have them more often if there are any causes for concern.

As an established diabetic, Jill may have a number of disorders while she's pregnant because of fluctuations in her blood-sugar levels. She may suffer urinary tract infections, thrush (see p.212), high blood pressure, preeclampsia (see p.224) and *polyhydramnios* (an excess of amniotic fluid, present in one out of five diabetic pregnancies). She could also go into premature labor.

PROBLEMS FOR HER BABY

Jill's baby, too, may have problems if her diabetes gets out of control. If a mother's blood sugar levels get high, sugar crosses the placenta and is converted into fat, muscle, and enlarged organs. The baby then becomes overweight and may be difficult to deliver vaginally. The baby produces large quantities of insulin to cope with the high sugar levels. At birth, when he's suddenly cut off from the source of sugar, the baby experiences a sudden, severe drop in blood sugar, while his insulin production remains high. If left untreated, this causes profound *hypoglycemia* (shortage of blood sugar), which can ultimately result in coma and death. This situation, however, will never arise with good prenatal care.

A preterm baby of a diabetic mother can be prone to respiratory distress syndrome, since the diabetes prevents the baby's lungs from producing the surfactant they need to aid breathing.

A GOOD OUTLOOK

The good news for Jill is that her careful control of her diabetes will make a big difference. Diabetic women never used to be warned of the risks of having babies at all. Now they are helped to control their condition, with help from their obstetrician and their diabetic physician, so that they can have a healthy baby. Unless there are complications, such as high blood pressure or pelvic disproportion, and as long as her diabetes stays under control, Jill should have a normal delivery.

Jill will probably be advised to have an induction at 39 weeks if her baby isn't born by then, so he doesn't grow too big. I advised her to have a glucose and insulin intravenous drip to control the diabetes during labor, and continuous fetal heart monitoring and fetal blood sampling to detect any fetal distress. After her baby's been checked in a neonatal intensive unit in case he needs any immediate treatment, he'll be given to Jill so he can be breastfed.

Jill's baby

As long as Jill remains under constant care, the risks to her baby won't be too great. Her doctor will be aware of the following:

• Jill's baby may be very large, so he may have to be delivered with forceps or by cesarean section

• He may suffer from mild *hypoxia* (low oxygen supply to the tissues) shortly before birth, and this can lead to neonatal jaundice (see p.342), a condition that can be treated after birth

• He'll be carefully checked after birth for any complications. In some hospitals, all babies of diabetic mothers are taken to intensive care so their blood sugar levels can be closely checked.

• Jill should breastfeed her baby as soon as possible in order to counteract any hypoglycemia (shortage of blood sugar) he may have after birth

• Some diabetic mothers have bigger and bigger babies that are very heavy at birth—perhaps 10–11 lb (4.5–5 kg). While such a large baby may be delivered easily, some obstetricians prefer to induce before term (at 36 weeks, say) after amniocentesis to check pulmonary development. Or they may opt for a cesarean before the baby has reached its full size.

CHAPTER 6

A healthy pregnancy

Keeping both your body and your mind in shape during pregnancy is very important. Exercising will help you do both. Everyone gets stressed and anxious sometimes, and you may even be faced with some potentially dangerous situations and substances. If you find ways of coping with and avoiding any problems that come up, you'll have a truly healthy pregnancy.

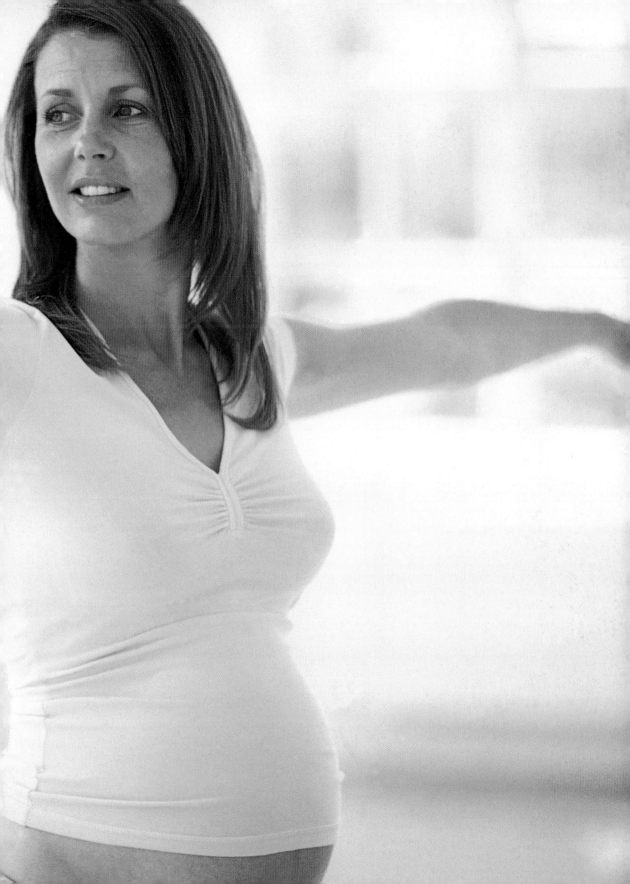

GOOD FOR YOU

Getting some regular exercise helps you feel happier as well keeping you in shape. It's an enjoyable way of getting ready for the months of change ahead.

- Hormones called endorphins, which your body releases when you exercise, will lift your spirits.

- You'll feel more contented and relaxed as your body releases tranquilizing hormones after you exercise.

- Your self-awareness will improve as you learn how to use your body in new ways.

- Regular exercise helps ease back-aches, leg cramps, constipation, and breathlessness.

- You'll find you have more energy.

- You'll be better prepared for the work of labor.

- After delivery, you'll get your figure back more quickly.

- You'll meet other moms at prenatal exercise classes, so you'll make more friends.

- Share your exercise routine with your partner or other members of your family and they'll shape up, too.

- You'll find you have less leg and ankle edema because you were able to "mobilize" the fluid while exercising.

Exercise for a healthy pregnancy

Regular exercise will build up your stamina and improve your suppleness and strength. This will help you cope with the extra demands made on your body as it adapts to pregnancy and childbirth. By exercising you can also develop a better understanding of what your body can do and learn different ways of relaxing.

Exercising helps you feel positive, so you're less likely to think of yourself as clumsy, fat, or ungainly, particularly in the last three months. Your circulation will improve, and that can help to ease tension. Labor may be easier and more comfortable if your muscle tone is good, and many of the exercises you learn in prenatal classes, combined with relaxation and breathing techniques, will help you trust your body during labor. And if you stay in good shape during pregnancy, you'll get your figure back more quickly after your baby's birth.

YOUR EXERCISE ROUTINE

You might think it's impossible to fit exercise into your schedule every day. But many of the best exercises for pregnancy, as shown on the following pages, can be done while you're doing something else: you can do pelvic floor exercises while you're brushing your teeth; foot and ankle exercises while sitting at your desk; and tailor-sitting when watching television.

Start your routine gently and gradually build up to what feels right for you. Before each exercise, take a few deep breaths. This gets the blood flowing around your body and gives all your muscles a good supply of oxygen. If you feel any pain, cramping, or shortness of breath, stop exercising, and when you start again, make sure you go more slowly. If you're out of breath, your baby won't be getting enough oxygen either. Getting oxygen to your baby is your body's priority, so you may feel short of breath doing activities you had no problem with before pregnancy.

Doing a little exercise several times a day is better than a lotall at once, and then none at all. Normally a woman can restore her energy by lying down for half an hour, but when you're pregnant, it can take half a day to recover from fatigue. So be kind to yourself and choose exercise that you enjoy and find relaxing.

GOOD WAYS TO EXERCISE

Most sports are fine, as long you've been doing that sport regularly before your pregnancy and you keep it up consistently once you're pregnant so that you stay in shape. Check the list for some of the best activities and those to avoid.

Swimming This is an excellent way to exercise when you're pregnant. Swimming tones most of your muscles and is a good way to build up your stamina. Your body weight is supported by the water, so you're unlikely to strain or injure any of your muscles and joints. Some gyms offer special swimming classes for pregnant women.

Yoga This helps increase your suppleness and reduces tension. It also teaches you to control your breathing and concentration, which are useful skills during labor.

Walking Even if you're not usually very active, you'll be able to manage some regular walks of a mile or more. Walking is good for your digestion, your circulation, and your figure. Try to walk tall, with your buttocks tucked under your spine, your shoulders back, and your head held up, not hanging down. Toward the end of pregnancy, though, you may find that the cartilage in your pelvic joints has softened so much that you get a backache if you walk more than a short distance. Always wear well-cushioned flat shoes when you go out for a walk.

Dancing As long as you're not too energetic, it's fine to dance as often as you like throughout pregnancy.

GO CAREFULLY

It's safest not to continue cycling, skiing, and horseback riding once you get big, because your balance is thrown off by the extra weight out in front. Other activities, including those listed below, are best avoided because they put your body under unnecessary stress that could harm both you and your baby.

Jogging This is very hard on your breasts and jarring for your back, spine, pelvis, hips, and knees. Don't jog when pregnant.

Backpacking Weight-bearing activities like this are not good because they put a severe strain on the ligaments in your back. Remember that when you're pregnant, progesterone relaxes your ligaments, and unlike muscles, which can go back to their old shapes, ligaments remain stretched.

Sit-ups Avoid any exercise that pulls on your abdominal muscles. The longitudinal muscles of the abdomen are designed to separate in the middle to allow room for your enlarging uterus—sitting straight up from a lying position forces them to part even farther. If you strain these muscles, it may take longer for you to get back your abdominal tone after the birth. Never exercise flat on your back after your fourth month. By that time your uterus is heavy enough to compress the veins taking blood to your heart, reducing blood flow to your head, making you feel dizzy and faint. To sit up from a lying position, always roll over on to your side and use your arms to push you up sideways.

GOOD FOR YOUR BABY

Every time you exercise within your limits, your baby gets a surge of oxygen into her blood that sets her metabolism alight and gives her a real high. All her tissues, especially her brain, function at their peak.

- The hormones that your body releases when you exercise pass across the placenta and reach your baby. So when you start to exercise, your baby receives an emotional lift from your adrenaline.

- While you're exercising, your baby also feels the positive effect of endorphins. These are our own natural morphinelike substances, released while exercising, that make us feel extremely good and happy.

- After exercise, endorphins have a profound tranquilizing effect that can last up to eight hours, and your baby experiences this, too.

- The movements you make when you exercise are very soothing and good for your baby. She feels comforted by the rocking movements.

- As you exercise, your abdominal muscles exert a kind of massage on your baby that's comforting and soothing.

- During exercise, your blood flow is at its highest and so your baby's growth and development benefit.

Stretching

WHY WARM UP?

A gentle warm-up routine gets your body ready for more demanding exercises and is easy to fit into your daily life.

Warming up helps to relieve tension. It gently warms up your muscles and joints and prevents muscles from overstretching, reducing the risk of injury. You may suffer from stiffness and cramps if you don't warm up.

Before beginning any exercise routine, always warm up gently (see left) with these stretching exercises. They'll stimulate your blood circulation, giving you and your baby a good supply of oxygen. Repeat each exercise five to ten times. Make sure you're comfortable while you stretch and that your posture is good.

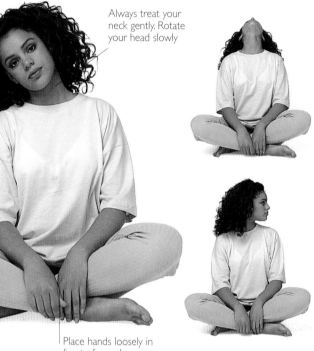

Always treat your neck gently. Rotate your head slowly

Head and neck
Gently tilt your head over to one side, then lift your chin and rotate your head gently over to the other side and down. Repeat, starting from the other side. Keeping your head straight, turn it slowly to the right, back to the front, and then back to the left. Return to face the front.

Place hands loosely in front of your legs

Keep your neck and back straight

Waist
Sitting comfortably with your legs crossed, straighten your back and gently stretch your neck upward. Breathe out and turn your upper body to the right, placing your right hand behind you. Place your left hand on your right knee and use this hand as a lever to twist your body a little farther, gently stretching the muscles of your waist. Repeat in the other direction.

Place your hand on your knee to help control the stretch

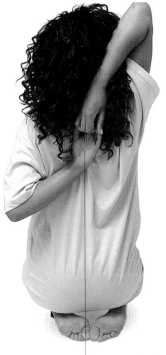

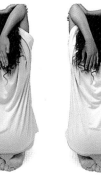

TAKE CARE

- Work on a firm surface

- Always keep your back straight. Support your back against a wall or with pillows if you need to

- Start your routine slowly and gently

- If you feel pain, discomfort, or fatigue, stop immediately

- Always remember to breathe normally—otherwise, you'll reduce the flow of blood to your baby

- Never point your toes— always flex your foot to prevent cramps

Arms and shoulders

Sitting with your legs tucked underneath you, lift your right arm up and slowly stretch it to the ceiling. Bend it at the elbow and drop your hand down behind your back. Put your left hand on your right elbow, pushing it farther down your back. Put your left arm down behind your back and reach up to grasp the right hand. Stretch for 20 seconds, then relax. Repeat with other arm.

Clasp your hands together lightly if you can; if you can't reach, don't worry

Legs and feet

Sit with your back straight and your legs stretched out in front of you. Place your hands on the floor next to your hips to support your weight. Bend your knee slowly and then straighten. Repeat with other leg. This will tone the muscles in your calf and thigh and helps to ease cramps.

Keep your back straight and your weight central

Improving circulation

Raise your foot off the floor and flex it outward. Then draw large circles in the air by moving only your ankles.

Bend your foot toward you to make the muscles work harder; be careful not to strain

YOUR PELVIC FLOOR

Your pelvic floor muscles form a funnel that supports your uterus, bowel, and bladder, and closes the entrances to your vagina, rectum, and urethra.

The pelvic floor muscles lie in two main groups, making a figure eight around your urethra, vagina, and anus. Muscle fibers come from back and front, high up on your lower back and pubic bones. The layers of muscle overlap and are thickest at the perineum.

When you're pregnant, the extra progesterone in your body softens and relaxes your muscles, and pressure from your enlarging uterus can stretch and weaken your pelvic floor. Half of all women who've had babies find they have a weakness in their pelvic floor. As a result they may feel uncomfortable or suffer so-called "stress incontinence"— leaking a little urine when laughing, coughing, or sneezing.

To counter this, physiotherapists have developed exercises you can do to keep your pelvic floor toned.

Pull in and tense the muscles around your vagina and anus. Hold as long as you can without straining. Relax. Repeat 25 times or more each day.

Start doing this exercise again as soon as you can after your baby is born to lessen the risk of a prolapse. Early exercise will tone up your vagina for sexual intercourse, too. Try to make the exercise part of your daily routine.

Body exercises

If you do some exercises for your whole body, you'll relieve the strain caused by your extra weight and strengthen important muscles. Also, if you learn to move your pelvis easily during pregnancy, you'll find it's easier to get into a comfortable position during labor. Janet Balaskas, who firmly believes in active birth, specializes in prenatal exercises based on yoga positions. Some of her suggestions are shown here.

Make sure your back is straight

Forward bend

1. Place your feet 12 in (30 cm) apart, keeping them parallel. Clasp your hands behind your back. Bend slowly forward from your hips, keeping your back straight. Breathe deeply for a few breaths, then rise slowly.

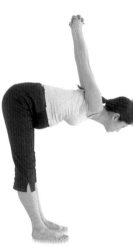

2. You should only do this step if you are able to do Step 1 comfortably. After bending forward, slowly raise your hands until they're as far above your head as possible.

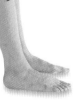

Pelvic tuck-in

Kneel down on all fours with your knees about 12 in (30 cm) apart. Clench your buttock muscles and tuck in your pelvis so that your back arches upward into a hump. Hold for a few seconds, and then release, making sure you don't let your back sink downward. Repeat several times.

Make the same movements and gently rock your pelvis up and down

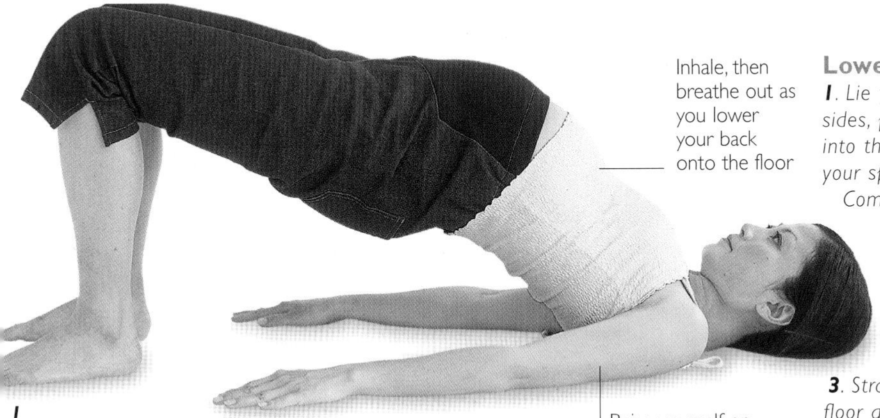

Inhale, then breathe out as you lower your back onto the floor

Lower back release

1. Lie flat with your arms by your sides, palms down. Press your feet into the floor. Lift your pelvis so that your spine rises as high as your neck. Come down one vertebra at a time.

2. Keeping your lower back in contact with the floor, gently hug your knees. Hold for a few minutes, breathing deeply.

3. Straighten your right leg on the floor and gently hug your left knee. Repeat with other leg.

4. Bend both knees and cross your feet at the ankles. Then rotate your hips clockwise, making tiny circles with your lower back on the floor. Repeat the movement in the other direction.

Raise yourself on supported arms to strengthen thighs and lower back

I

2

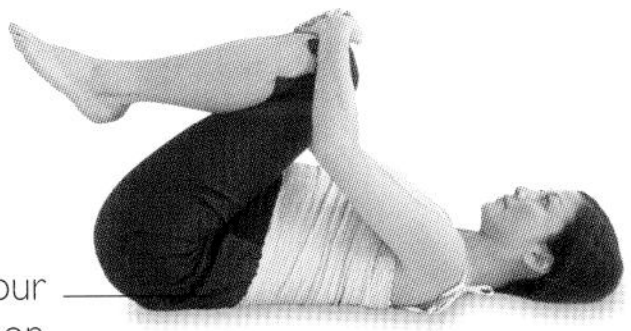

Keep your lower spine on the floor

Hold your knee for a few moments, breathing deeply

3

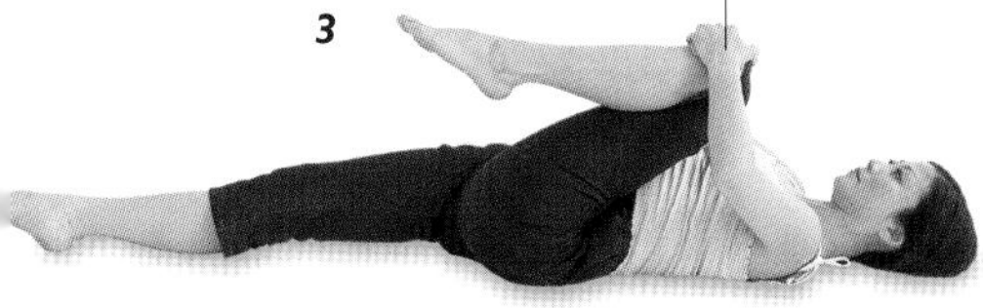

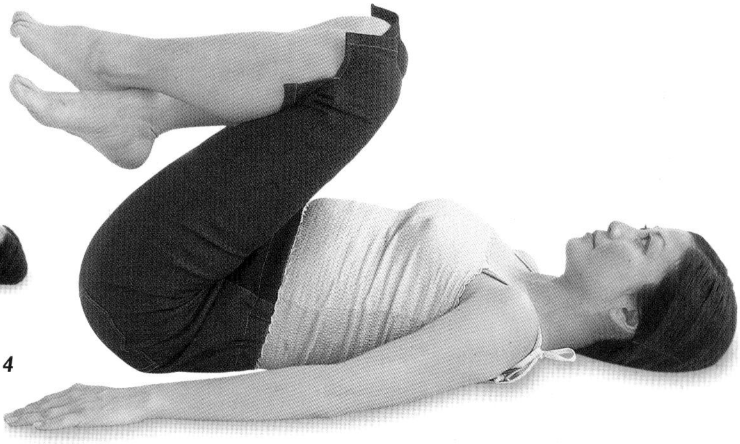

4

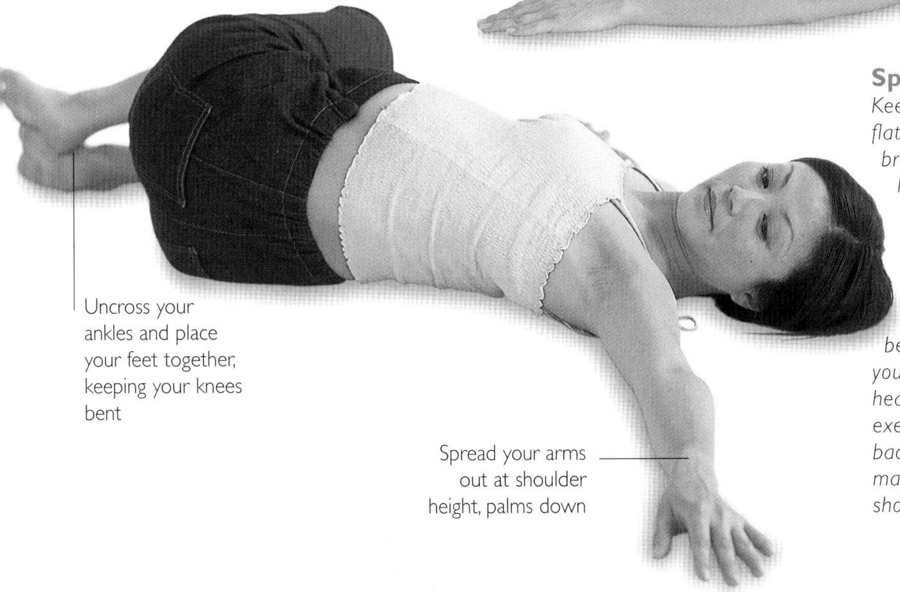

Spinal twist

Keep your shoulders and arms flat on the ground and, as you breathe out, slowly turn your knees over to the right and your head over to the left. This gently twists the spine. Hold this position for a few seconds. Come back to the center, keeping your knees bent, and then relax. Then roll your knees to the left and your head to the right. Repeat the exercise. Avoid lying flat on your back for prolonged periods. You may need pillows to prop up your shoulders so you don't get dizzy.

Uncross your ankles and place your feet together, keeping your knees bent

Spread your arms out at shoulder height, palms down

Shaping up for labor

If you prepare your mind and body beforehand, you're more likely to have a comfortable labor. You'll find the following exercises very useful during pregnancy. You may want to give birth while squatting, and tailor-sitting will strengthen your thigh muscles and increase circulation to your pelvis, making your joints more supple. This exercise also helps to stretch your pelvis and relax the tissues of your perineum.

After exercising, spend 20–30 minutes relaxing, and, if possible, arrange a regular break during your day. You don't have to sleep—five or ten minutes with your eyes closed and your feet up is enough to refresh you. Learning relaxation techniques will be a great help during labor, when tension can make the pain worse. If you're able to concentrate on the rhythm of your breathing, you'll feel less anxious and save your energy.

If you find it hard to pull your feet close to your groin, you can start with them about 12 in (30 cm) away from your body and gradually bring them closer. With practice, your muscles will loosen

Tailor-sitting

Sit on the floor, and stretch your legs out in front. Make sure your back is straight. Bend your knees and bring the soles of your feet together, then pull them as close as you can to your groin. Open out your thighs and lower your knees toward the floor. Relax your shoulders and the back of your neck. Breathe deeply. Concentrate on breathing down toward your pelvis resting on the floor, relaxing as you breathe out. As you breathe in, lift up and stretch your spine while keeping your pelvis on the ground.

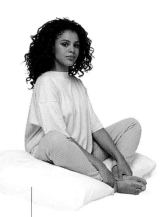

Support your thighs with some pillows or blankets, or sit against a wall at first if you find it easier

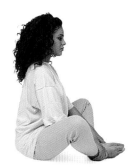

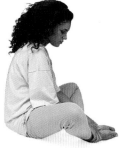

Correct   Incorrect

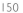

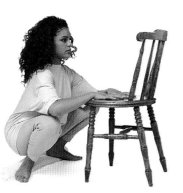

Safe balance

If you need to, hold on to something steady, such as a chair, low stool, or window sill, to support your back as you squat, and place a towel underneath your heels. You can also lean against a wall.

Squat to make your pelvis more flexible, stretch and strengthen your thigh and back muscles, and relieve back pain

Squatting

Stand with your back lengthened and straight, and your feet 18 in (45 cm) apart. Squat down as low as you can. Linking your hands, spread and hold your knees apart with your elbows. Try to get your heels on the ground with your weight evenly distributed between heels and toes; don't worry if you have to raise your heels. Hold the squat for a few minutes, or for as long as you're comfortable. Then come forward to kneel or stand up. Squatting can become a natural part of your daily life—for example, when you're lifting something low.

RELAXATION

It's comfortable to lie with your legs up on a chair or a bed, but as you get bigger, try to avoid lying flat on your back. You may find it helpful to support your shoulders with pillows so you don't feel dizzy. You can relax like this while your other children play nearby.

Lie with your feet up to relieve swollen ankles and feet

Clear your mind and breathe in deeply. Hold for a count of five and breathe out. Relax all parts of your body

Lying this way eases pressure on your major blood vessels and your abdomen

Lying down

Lie on your side with a pillow under your head. Bend your upper arm and leg upward and place a pillow under this knee; keep your lower leg straightened. Close your eyes and concentrate just on your breathing.

Massage for relaxation

MASSAGE EXTRAS

A few extras can make your massage even more luxurious. Have everything ready before you start so you don't have to break the rhythm.

Scented oils will help hands glide over your skin, and leave it soft and smooth. The fragrance of the oil will add to the atmosphere, making each occasion special.

Try rubbing feathers, fabric, and other soft-textured materials against the skin to leave it tingling.

Cover any exposed skin with some warm, fluffy towels so you don't get cold.

Use spinal rolls for firm, smooth counter-pressure (see p.296).

Gently brushing your hair with light strokes of a soft bristle hairbrush can be very relaxing.

Getting a massage from your partner, or giving yourself one, is a wonderful way to relax and unwind. Massage stimulates the nerve endings in your skin, improves your circulation, and soothes tired muscles, giving you a sense of peace and well-being.

SOOTHING TOUCH

Use some good-quality massage oil (one with a vegetable oil base) to smooth your skin and make your massage more pleasurable. To create a comfortable, relaxing atmosphere: dim the lights, put on some soft music, and put some pillows or cushions around and underneath you. Later on in your pregnancy, you may find it's more comfortable to lie on your side supported by pillows, or to sit astride a chair.

You can massage most parts of your body, apart from your back, quite effectively yourself. Using the palms and fingers of one hand, work clockwise around each breast, stroking from the base

SELF MASSAGE

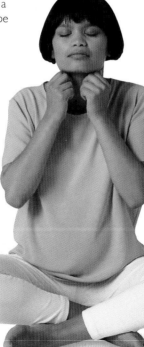

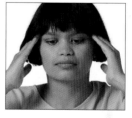

Soothe your forehead
Cover your face with your hands. Place your fingertips on your forehead and rest the heels of your hands on your chin. After a few seconds, draw your hands toward your ears.

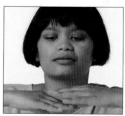

Tone your chin
Stimulate the blood circulation under your chin with brisk movements. Using the backs of both hands, gently slap upward with one after the other.

Firm your neck
Make gentle pinching movements around your jawbone. Softly squeeze the skin between your thumb and the knuckles of your index finger. Be careful not to drag your skin.

toward your nipple; gently knead your nipples between your fingers and thumb. Massage your abdomen, hips, and thighs, with the palms of your hands, using smooth, circular movements.

If anyone else is giving you a massage, make sure that their hands are warm before starting and that they've taken off any rings, bracelets, or watches. When you're both comfortable, take a few deep breaths to help you relax. It's best for the masseur to begin massaging you gently. The pressure can gradually be increased if it's comfortable for you, but always keep the movements slow and gentle.

Circling Using the palms of both hands at once, make circling strokes in the same direction away from the spine. Lighten the pressure when massaging over the abdomen and breasts.

Effleurage Make light, feathery, circular movements with the fingertips as though tickling the skin. This can be done all over the abdomen during pregnancy.

Gliding Place the palms of both hands on either side of the lower back, with the fingers pointing to your head. Push the hands up to the shoulders, without exerting body weight on to the hands. Slowly glide the hands down the sides of the body back to the starting point.

ESSENTIAL OILS

Using aromatic oils in your massage can help you feel relaxed and refreshed. Their scents also help conjure up wonderful images.

These oils are distilled from flowers, trees, and herbs, and are said to have healing qualities. For example, lavender oil relieves headaches and insomnia. There are some essential oils that shouldn't be used in pregnancy, so always check with an experienced aromatherapist before using anything. Blend the oil with a carrier oil such as almond or olive before applying it to your skin.

MASSAGE BY A PARTNER

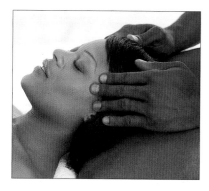

Forehead massage
Using your fingertips, make tiny circular movements all over her forehead, working from one side to the other and then back again.

Back massage
The extra weight your partner is carrying in front can cause strain. Gently massaging her lower back can help to ease any discomfort.

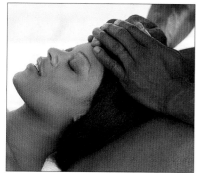

Tension soother
Soothe tension with this gentle movement. Place your hands on her forehead so that your fingertips just meet in the middle and hold lightly. Press gently, then release and hold lightly again before lifting your hands away.

Ease strain by gently pressing her lower back

Emotional changes

WILL MY MOODS AFFECT MY BABY?

You may worry that your changing moods will somehow affect your baby.

Your baby does react to your moods and she may start kicking when you're angry or upset, but your different emotions don't appear to have any harmful effect on your baby (see A mother's influence, p.192).

Dreams and nightmares can be very vivid, and you may find that you wake up suddenly, feeling hot, drenched in sweat, and with your heart racing. Don't worry—this won't harm your baby.

On the other hand, your baby enjoys your good moods, when you're excited and happy. When you feel good, your baby feels good. When you're relaxed, your baby also feels tranquil.

If there's something that makes you feel content and happy, such as listening to music, dancing gently, or painting, do as much of it as you can and share the good feelings with your baby.

It's not only your body that alters during pregnancy; your emotions will change rapidly, too, and you'll experience feelings you've never had before. It'll help if you accept that you will feel upset from time to time—all pregnant women do—and that there are things you can do to help you cope with your mood swings.

Changes in your hormone levels cause your moods to make sudden swings from elation to depression. Your changing body shape can disturb your self-image. And we all occasionally feel anxious about how good we're going to be as parents. Emotionally, pregnancy can be very difficult.

HORMONAL CHANGES

There are enormous changes in your body during pregnancy, and because of this, your mood is likely to change often. You might find yourself being hypercritical and irritable, you might have exaggerated reactions to minor events, you may feel unsure of yourself and panicky sometimes, and you may have bouts of depression and crying.

It's normal to go through all of these things because you're less in control of your feelings than usual. The swinging levels of hormones have taken over and are controlling your moods the way a conductor controls an orchestra. So don't feel guilty or ashamed if you show your irritation, anger, or frustration. If you explain what's happening, most people will understand. At work, you may have to struggle to keep up an appearance of calm. This effort will definitely pay off, especially if you plan to go back to your job after the birth of your baby.

CHANGING BODY SHAPE

Normally, you have a while to get used to a change in the way you look, such as losing or gaining weight or growing your hair. But when you're pregnant, you don't have time to adjust to your changing shape, and you may feel strange, even unrelated to the body in which you find yourself. You might worry that you're putting on too much weight and that you'll look fat and unattractive during or after pregnancy.

Thinking of pregnant women as fat, and therefore ugly, is essentially an Anglo-Saxon attitude: many other cultures see pregnant women as sensuous and beautiful. Don't look at your increasing curves with despair; think of them as a reaffirmation of life. See your roundness as ripeness, and glory in your body's fertility. Feel confident and proud of your shape.

CONFLICTING FEELINGS

However positive you are about your pregnancy, it's normal to have conflicting feelings sometimes. One moment you're thrilled at the prospect of your new baby, the next you're feeling terrified of your new responsibilities. Becoming a parent is a time of reassessment and change, of worries and fears.

The first and most important thing you have to do is to accept your pregnancy. This may sound obvious, but there are some women who blithely sail through the early months of pregnancy giving it as little thought as possible, which is especially easy until the baby begins to show.

You and the baby's father have to come to terms with the pregnancy and begin to think about the reality. Until now, your thoughts about a baby and parenthood may always have been in soft focus, a pastel picture of a loving threesome.

Conflicting feelings are sure to surface once you begin to accept the realities to come. Don't worry—it's good to have conflicting feelings. It's normal to feel this way, so don't feel bad about it. It means that you're genuinely coming to terms with the situation. You won't have the shock that some people get because they wait to face all this when they bring their baby home.

FEARS

Perhaps you worry about labor—whether you'll be able to cope with the pain, whether you'll scream, lose control of your bowels, or need an episiotomy or an emergency cesarean. Most of us do get anxious about these things, but there's no need. Labor is usually straightforward, and it doesn't really matter how you behave. You may be surprised at how calm you are, or you may not be calm at all, and both are okay. Just remember that your birth attendants have seen it all before, so there's nothing for you to feel embarrassed about.

You may worry about how good a parent you'll be, whether you'll hurt or harm your baby, or not care for her properly. These are normal feelings and represent very reasonable fears. Many people don't know much about baby care and worry about doing a good job. The answer is to get some hands-on experience—handle and care for a newborn baby if you can. Perhaps you could babysit for a friend's baby, or spend some time with her. If you change and cuddle someone else's baby, it'll give you some confidence. Try to get your fears into perspective—you probably had similar worries about starting a job.

DREAMS

You may find that your dreams become more frequent, and even frightening, in the last trimester. Many pregnant women report common themes, and all express deep feelings and concerns that are entirely natural—everybody worries at one time or another that something will be wrong or go wrong with their baby. You may have dreams about losing your baby; and this is usually an expression of fear about miscarrying or having a stillborn baby.

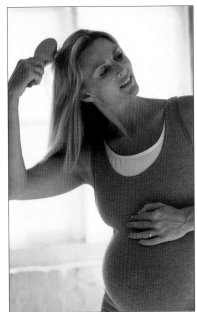

Your changing shape
The more positive you are about the way you look while you're pregnant, the better you'll feel.

KEEPING A DIARY

Keeping a diary at any time of your life can give you information and insights about yourself that you might not have the time to recognize.

Your diary is a place where you can let go of thoughts and feelings that you may not want to share, and it'll also help you to focus on yourself. Later, your child may enjoy reading your diary herself—especially when she's about to start her own family.

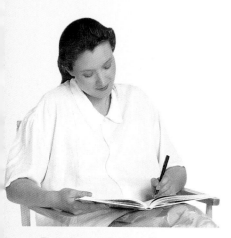

Pregnancy journal
If you can take the time to keep a pregnancy journal, you'll have a cherished record of this special time in your life.

Dreams like these may be the brain's way of preparing for an unwanted outcome and also help to bring these feelings to the surface. Dreams can act as a release for your anxieties.

Dreams, nightmares, and thoughts in general may also be a way of expressing hostility to your unborn child—she's going to overtake your life, disrupting your privacy and comfortable routine. They may express feelings you may not be able to cope with or even be consciously aware of. Again, don't make the mistake of taking dreams literally and then feeling guilty or afraid.

SUPERSTITIONS

You may find you're more superstitious than usual. In the past, superstition and old wives' tales were ways of explaining an inexplicable world. But with the excellent medical care available today, your chances of having a damaged child are very low. Something you see as a bad omen certainly doesn't mean that anything will go wrong with your baby.

COPING WITH EMOTIONAL CHANGES

If you can, look on the emotional turmoil you're going through as a positive force as you adjust to being pregnant and becoming a mother. Don't imagine that having second thoughts or fears means you've made a mistake. You're just tossing this around in your head the way one wrestles with any big life decision. Yet social conditioning can make us feel guilty if we don't walk around with a madonna-like expression and saintly attitude to everything. That's absurd. Being pregnant isn't all fun. Accepting the reality is the best thing you can do for yourself and your child.

Spend time daydreaming Imagining and thinking about your baby helps you to build your relationship with her even before she's born, so don't feel silly if you find yourself spending a couple of hours doing nothing but thinking about your baby. Making that connection with the tiny person growing inside you is the first step in accepting your child.

Many mothers find they have an undisguised preference for a girl or a boy in their daydreams. Although it isn't usually a problem if your newborn turns out to be the opposite sex from the one you wanted, it can mean have to readjust, so try not to get too carried away with your plans!

Consider your parents Your parents are about to become grandparents, perhaps for the first time. They may be delighted, they may be upset, or they may feel a combination of both reactions. In other words, they might be feeling as confused about their new role as you are about yours. Some people see becoming grandparents as meaning that they're getting old, and this can be unsettling for someone who perhaps feels only just middle-aged. Try to be understanding and loving with your parents. Include them in your pregnancy, talk to them about what's happening, and share your feelings with them.

Confront your isolation A pregnant woman can feel isolated. Many women postpone having children, and some decide against it altogether. You may find that you're the first in your social circle to start a family, and that you don't know any other pregnant women or full-fledged mothers. It can be lonely. There's so much that you want to know and talk about. You may have little niggles and worries that you feel are too irrelevant or silly to talk about at your prenatal clinic, and you may wish you knew someone who was going through the same thing or who already had a child. If you feel like this, find someone you can talk to—join parent groups, make friends with other pregnant women in your childbirth classes, and ask your friends or family if they know any pregnant women, or parents with young children, whom you could get to know. You may find these relationships go on long after your baby is born. And don't forget your partner—if you're feeling isolated, he probably is, too, so talk to him, include him, and expand your social circle together.

Communicate Wanting to talk through and share what you're feeling and thinking during your pregnancy is natural. Your partner is an obvious first choice, and he'll probably be anxious to talk to you. There are bound to be things that he'd like to talk about: worries, things that he may have not wanted to discuss with you because he thought that he might upset you, or you might think it was silly, or because you were too busy, or too tired. Keep talking. You need each other more now than ever before. Denying or ignoring your fears and feelings won't make them go away. Suppressed feelings have a very nasty way of festering and then surfacing when you're least able to deal with them, turning into full-blown problems. If you bring these problems out in the open when they first come up, you'll be able to deal with them and get on with your lives.

COPING WITH MATERIAL CHANGES

Everyday difficulties that you'd normally deal with quite calmly can turn into dramas during pregnancy. Keep a level head, and try not to overreact if you can help it.

Finances Financial problems are always one of the main causes of problems between a couple, and they can become especially troubling during pregnancy. You may find it difficult to cope with a reduction in income, even if you plan to return to work, but remember that you're in this together. Work out before the birth how you'll manage on your income once your baby has arrived.

Housing Moving or expanding your home may be something that you have to think about—perhaps you need extra space, or there may be a lack of facilities in your area. All this can be stressful, and tends to be worse when you're pregnant. If you must move—and it's not really the best idea from a physical point of view—do it before your pregnancy is too advanced.

GRANDPARENTS

A new baby means a new role not only for you but maybe for your parents, too.

Once your baby's born, they're bound to revel in their roles as doting grandparents, but they may feel they're still too young when you first tell them the good news.

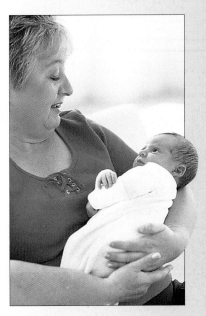

A source of help
Your parents can be invaluable sources of information, expertise, and reassurance when you have a new baby to care for.

Body care

Pregnancy hormones can affect almost every part of your body, including your breasts, skin, hair, teeth, and gums. To keep your body in good shape, you'll probably need to make some changes in your daily routine. Your growing abdomen may affect your posture, too, so check the way you stand and move (see p.160).

Skin

Your skin will probably "bloom" during pregnancy. All the extra hormones encourage the skin to hold moisture that plumps it out, making it more supple, less oily, and less prone to pimples. The extra blood circulating around your body also makes your skin glow. But there can be problems, too. Red patches may get bigger, acne may worsen, areas may become dry and scaly, and you may notice deeper pigmentation across your face.

Skin care Here are a few general tips for looking after your skin during pregnancy. Soap removes natural oils from the skin, so use it as little as possible. Try using baby lotion, or glycerine-based soap and body wash. Always add some oils to your bath to lessen the dehydrating effects of hard water, and don't lie in the tub for too long, since this dehydrates the skin. Aromatherapy oils have a particularly wonderful effect and leave a film of protective oil on your skin that keeps it supple, and prevents dehydration and damage due to water loss. Makeup can help cheer you up, and it helps moisturize the skin as it prevents water loss.

Deeper pigmentation This happens to nearly every woman, especially on areas of the body that have pigmentation already, such as freckles, moles, and the areolae of the breasts. Your genitalia, the skin on the inside of your thighs, underneath your eyes, and in your armpits may become darker, too. A dark line, called the linea nigra, often appears down the center of your stomach. It marks the division of your abdominal muscles, which separate slightly to make room for your expanding uterus. Even after you've had your baby, the linea nigra and the areolae usually remain darker for a while, but will gradually fade.

Sunlight intensifies areas of skin that are already pigmented, and many women find that they tan more easily when they're pregnant. Since ultraviolet A (UVA) rays can lead to skin cancer, and the effect they have on the unborn baby is unknown, it's important to avoid sunburn. If you're out in the sun, use a sun block, especially on pigmented areas such as your nipples. Keep your skin covered up in hot sun, and don't use sunbeds.

Chloasma This is a special form of pigmentation, also called the mask of pregnancy, which appears as brown patches on the bridge

MAKEUP TIPS

The tone and color of your skin can alter when you're pregnant, so you may want to make some changes to your usual makeup routine.

Fine lines or wrinkles If your skin gets drier than usual, any lines will look more obvious. Stop using products such as shiny or glittery eyeshadows, heavy foundations, and colored powders—they draw attention to lines and wrinkles.

Extra-greasy skin To combat this, use an astringent lotion, oil-free foundation, and finish your makeup with a dust of translucent powder.

Extra-dry skin This is very rare in pregnancy, but if your skin becomes so dry that it flakes, it's best to stop wearing makeup. Keep moisturizing your skin well. Otherwise, use an oil-based film of foundation and some powder to help to slow water loss. Thick, creamy moisturizers will also act as a barrier to water loss on dry patches.

High color and spider veins Stipple a thin, light coat of matt foundation onto your cheeks—use a beige color that's free of any pink. When it's dry, cover with your regular foundation and some translucent powder.

Dark circles Put on a thin layer of foundation, then stipple on an undereye coverup cream and leave to dry. Cover with another thin layer of foundation and blend carefully. Finish with a dusting of translucent powder.

of the nose, cheeks, and neck. The only way to handle chloasma is to make it less noticeable with a blemish stick or the coverup cosmetics used for birthmarks. Never try to bleach out the pigment; the patches will begin to fade within three months of labor. Conversely, some black women develop patches of paler skin on their faces and necks. These will probably disappear after delivery and can be camouflaged during pregnancy.

Spider veins When you're pregnant, all your blood vessels become sensitive—they rapidly dilate when you're hot, and constrict quickly when you're cold. As a result, tiny broken blood vessels called spider veins may appear on your face, particularly on your cheeks. Don't worry; they'll fade soon after delivery, and will probably have disappeared altogether within three months.

Pimples If you've always had a tendency to get pimples before periods, you may get them now. This is particularly likely in the first trimester, when the pregnancy hormones stimulating the sebaceous glands in the skin haven't yet reached a balanced level. Keep your skin as clean as you can, and use a cleanser two or three times a day to prevent breakouts. If a pimple does appear, apply a tiny smear of antiseptic cream. Never squeeze your pimples—this only spreads the infection into the deeper layers of the skin.

Stretch marks About 90 percent of pregnant women get stretch marks. These usually appear across the abdomen, although they can also affect the thighs, hips, breasts, and the upper arms. Nothing you put on your skin (including oil) and nothing you can eat will prevent stretch marks because they're caused by the breakdown of protein in the skin by the high levels of pregnancy hormones. If you gain weight gradually, that should allow the skin to stretch without tearing, although some women are blessed with more elastic skin than others. While the reddish streaks may look prominent while you're pregnant, during the weeks after delivery they'll become paler, and shrink until they're nothing more than faint silvery streaks that you'll barely notice.

TEETH

During pregnancy, you're more likely than usual to suffer gum problems because of your increased blood supply and the high level of progesterone, which softens all of your body's tissues. The increased blood volume also puts pressure on the tiny capillaries around your gum margin, which often bleed easily. A balanced diet helps prevent tooth and gum problems. Eating plenty of calcium-rich foods and high-quality protein, along with a good supply of vitamins B, C, and D, helps to protect you. It's important to see your dentist at least once during your pregnancy and have your teeth cleaned professionally to reduce the risk of gum infections. Be sure to tell your dentist that you're pregnant, since it's safest to avoid X-rays.

YOUR HAIR

During pregnancy, many women find that their hair changes in quality, quantity, and manageability.

The high levels of hormones stop your usual cycle of hair growth and loss. Usually some hair grows and some is lost every day. When you're pregnant, your hair is arrested in the growth phase.

After delivery, the cycle passes into a resting phase and you might lose lots of hair. Hair loss can go on for up to two years and may be alarming, but don't worry, it will stop—pregnancy never causes baldness. The hair you lose once your baby is born is simply the hair you would normally have lost throughout the whole of the nine months of pregnancy.

If your hair becomes more difficult to manage, think about changing to a simpler hair style that's easier to care for. Choose the mildest shampoo you can find. When you wash your hair, use only one application of shampoo, massage gently to a lather, leave for 30 seconds, and rinse off.

Body and facial hair may increase in quantity and even get darker in color.

CHECK YOUR POSTURE

Making sure your posture is good should help you suffer less of the backache and fatigue that can happen as your pregnancy advances.

Bad posture, caused by the increasing weight of your baby, is a common problem in pregnancy. Your growing abdomen thrusts your center of gravity forward, and to balance this you may tend to arch your back. This puts your back muscles under constant strain and can cause backaches.

When you're standing, sitting, or walking, check that your posture is correct—your neck and back should be in a straight line.

Avoiding problems

Pregnancy hormones stretch and soften your ligaments, particularly those in the lower back, so they tend to strain more easily. If you're careful, though, you can avoid the unnecessary back problems and tiredness that many women suffer during their pregnancy.

Don't bend down
When you're doing jobs at home or working in the yard and you need to work on something at floor level, sit or kneel down so it's in easy reach. Whenever you can, avoid bending or stooping.

Always keep your back straight, and lift by straightening your legs

Sit back on your heels, but don't let your legs fall asleep

Hold whatever you're lifting with both hands

Lifting and carrying
When you want to lift something from the floor, reach down to it by bending your knees, keeping your back as straight as you can. When you pick it up, hold it close to your body and lift it by straightening your legs, so that you use the strength of your leg and thigh muscles to do the actual lifting. Never struggle to lift objects that are too heavy—get someone to help you. Don't try lifting heavy things to or from high shelves or upward. If you're carrying heavy bags, try to divide the weight equally between both your hands.

Getting up

When you want to get up after lying down on the floor—after exercising, for instance—take it in easy stages. First, turn on to your side (see below), then use your hands to support yourself as you move yourself into a kneeling position (see top right). From there, keeping your back straight and using the strength of your thigh muscles, push yourself up into a sitting position (see bottom right). From here, you can stand up without straining your abdomen.

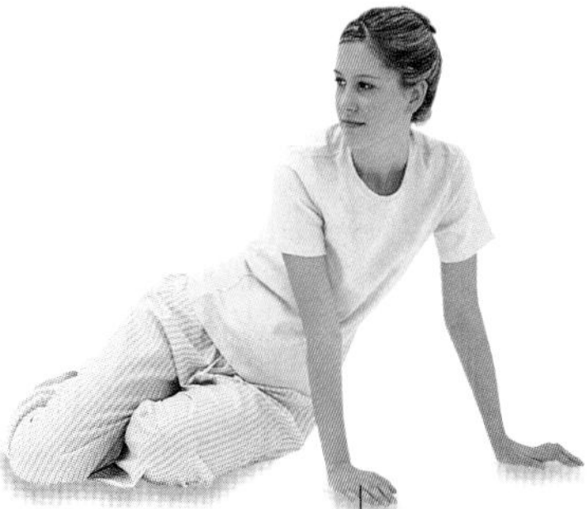

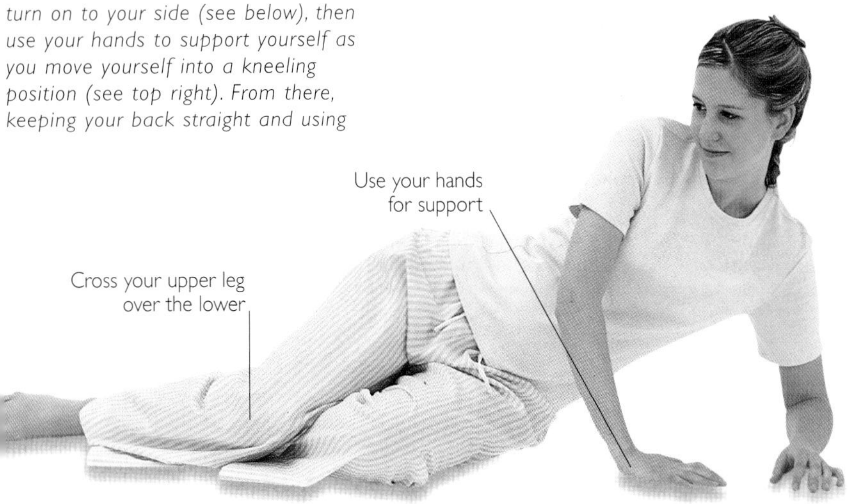

Cross your upper leg over the lower

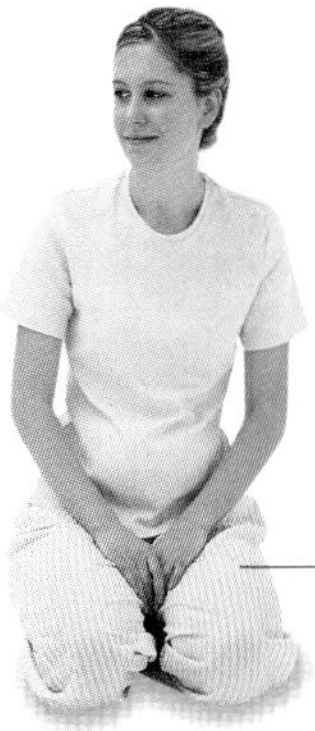

Use your hands for support

Use your hands to support yourself

Push up with your thighs

Nail and skin problems

POSSIBLE PROBLEM	WHAT TO DO
Itching or chafed skin The skin of your extended abdomen may become quite itchy when you're pregnant, and the area between your thighs may become chafed.	Massage your skin with baby lotion to stimulate the blood supply and soothe irritation. Keep the skin on your thighs dry, dust with powder, and wear cotton underwear.
Rashes A rash in your groin and under your breasts can be caused by excess weight gain and the sweat that gathers in the folds of your skin. Not bathing often enough increases the risk.	Keep your groin area and the skin under your breasts clean, and apply calamine or other drying lotion. Wear a good bra that supports your breasts properly.
Pigmentation Many women find that their skin pigmentation changes when they're pregnant; this particularly affects areas that already darker, such as moles and the areolae of the breasts.	Use a sun block to protect your skin from the ultraviolet rays in sunlight. The extra pigmentation will disappear after the birth.
Nails Your fingernails grow faster than usual when you're pregnant. They may also become brittle and split, or break more easily than they did before your pregnancy.	Keep your nails short and well trimmed. Wear gloves when you're washing dishes or working in the garden.

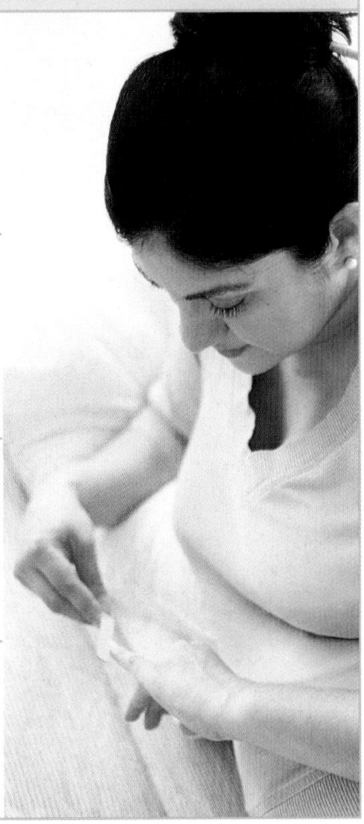

What to wear

Comfort is the top priority where clothes are concerned when you're pregnant. As you get bigger, try to stay one step ahead—there's nothing worse than feeling constricted in clothes that are too small for you. You'll probably feel warmer than usual during pregnancy because your blood is circulating around your body at a faster rate. Your feet and legs may tend to swell, particularly toward the end of the day, so choose your shoes and hosiery with extra care.

CLOTHES

You don't need to buy lots of expensive maternity clothes. If you have a few specially bought basics, such as a pair of maternity jeans with an expandable front panel, a selection of properly fitted maternity bras, some maternity cotton or wool tights and leggings with expandable gussets, and one or two maternity dresses for special occasions, you can add a few inexpensive items, such as ethnic dresses, drawstring cotton pants, and comfortable tops and sweaters—some of which you can wear after your pregnancy. Lots of pregnant women no longer want to wear tentlike clothes, preferring to show off their new shape.

Before you splurge on any special outfits, find out if any of your friends or neighbors have maternity clothes that you could borrow. In some areas you'll find shops that specialize in nearly-new maternity clothes, where you can buy clothes at bargain prices. It's best to avoid synthetic fabrics if you can—natural fabrics will be far more comfortable. Polyester, for example, tends to trap moisture and is uncomfortable in hot weather.

Work clothes If you work in a relaxed environment, you may be able to wear "business casual" clothes, such as leggings with a pretty top or a cool cotton skirt and T-shirt. But if your workplace is more formal, you may have to invest in some larger jackets, pants, and skirts than you'd normally wear, or some special maternity outfits.

If you wear a uniform to work, let your employers know that you're pregnant in plenty of time so they can provide you with new clothes when you need them or give you some financial help to get a new uniform for yourself. If you normally wear heels to work, change to flat shoes.

SHOES

The bigger you get, the more unstable you become, so it's best to wear flat or low-heeled, comfortable, easy-fitting shoes. Make sure they support your foot well, are roomy enough, and preferably have a nonslip sole for safety. Tennis shoes or sneakers are ideal; choose a pair with a Velcro fastening, because later in your pregnancy you might find it hard to bend down to tie laces. You'll

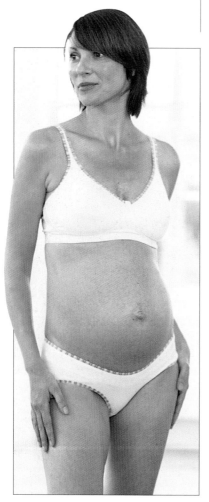

Maternity underwear
A well-fitting bra that gives you good support is vital for your comfort during pregnancy—and for your figure afterward.

find that there are plenty of attractive flat shoes that are versatile and hard-wearing. Your feet will swell during pregnancy, so choose a size bigger than normal, and avoid anything with a heel. Best of all, go barefoot whenever you can.

UNDERWEAR

Bra A good bra is essential when you're pregnant. Your breasts will get bigger, particularly during the first three months, and if you don't support them, they're likely to sag later. This is because the sling of fibrous tissue to which they are attached never gets its shape back once it's stretched. A well-fitting bra will help to prevent stretching in the first place.

When you buy a bra, it's best to have it properly fitted. A large department store or a shop specializing in maternity clothes or lingerie will have specially trained staff to help you. Look for a bra that gives you good support with a deep band underneath the cups and wide shoulder straps that don't cut deep into your skin. Back-fastening bras may be better than front-fastening. Only buy a couple of bras to begin with, since your breasts will continue to get bigger, and you'll have to get a larger size later in pregnancy. If your breasts become very big, it helps to wear a light bra in bed at night to give them extra support.

Just before your due date, buy two or three front-opening feeding bras so that you can breastfeed your baby easily. You can buy feeding bras at any maternity shop or department store.

Girdles Some women find wearing a light maternity girdle helpful, especially in the second and third trimester. The best have a front panel that grows with you and gives light support for your tummy, which can relieve your back of strain and help prevent backaches.

Socks Choose cotton socks that are loose-fitting. Synthetic materials don't have any give and can cut really deeply into swollen feet. Also, they don't let you sweat, so the skin may become waterlogged and soft. It's best to avoid knee-high socks—they can form a restricting band around the top of your calf, and encourage varicose veins (see p.212).

Pantyhose Even sheer maternity pantyhose will give you a lot of support. You'll find lots of different types in plenty of colors in maternity shops and most department stores.

Stockings If you have a tendency to suffer from thrush (see p.212), you might prefer to wear stockings and a garter belt instead of pantyhose. You'll probably find that support stockings, or ones containing a high percentage of Lycra, are the most comfortable, although they don't give you as much support as maternity pantyhose. Garter belts that fit on your hips under your abdomen will be most comfortable, so find a belt that's big enough and shorten the straps if you need to.

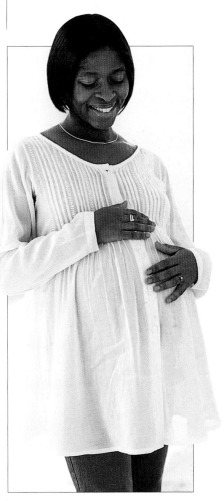

Maternity outerwear
Choose clothes that are comfortable and practical to wear during your pregnancy. Bear in mind that the seasons change as you grow bigger.

TIPS FOR YOUR DAY

A few little changes to your normal working lifestyle can make your day more comfortable.

Put your feet up Sit down as much as possible, and put your feet up whenever you can. Use something such as an overturned wastebasket or an open drawer as a footstool.

Relaxation exercises Do some simple neck, shoulder, pelvic, and foot exercises when you're traveling to work and when at work. These help to release tension and improve your circulation.

Practice squatting Use the squatting position whenever you have to bend down, or if you're tired of standing and there's no chair handy. This'll help to strengthen your thighs, and prepare you to use this position at the delivery.

Eat well Keep some healthy snacks handy (see p.130). Although you may still have feelings of nausea, you may want something to eat at inconvenient moments. A whole-wheat cookie or cracker and a glass of skim milk will fill you up and help you feel better if you're nauseous.

Take it easy Try to take things more slowly. Stop whenever you feel tired, and take a rest.

A working pregnancy

There's no reason why you can't continue working well into your pregnancy if you want to, unless your working environment could be dangerous for your baby. Harmful materials or fumes, or heavy physical work, for example, can be damaging. If you do want to go on working during your pregnancy and return to your job after your baby is born, make sure you have all the information you need to protect both your health and your job.

When you're pregnant, your body does change and you may be uncomfortable at times, but working can help you feel more normal. By continuing to work, you can keep up this important and stable aspect of your life at a time when you may be feeling disoriented in other ways because of the physical and emotional changes of pregnancy.

Exercising your rights

Most employers will be eager to help you continue working during your pregnancy and after your maternity leave, but it's up to you to tell them what you want to do. You need to let them know when you plan to stop work before your baby's born and when you'll be coming back afterward.

Protect your job Talk to your employer or your trade union representative about what maternity leave and pay you're entitled to (see p.64). You're allowed time off with pay for prenatal care, and this includes time to go to relaxation classes.

Protect your health If there's a chance that some aspect of your work will harm your baby—for example, exposure to X-rays, doing heavy lifting, or handling harmful chemicals—your employer should find you another job while you're pregnant, or, if this isn't possible, suspend you on full pay. This is your right, under the Occupational Safety and Health Act, no matter how many hours you work or how long you've been employed.

Adapting your routine

Working long hours may leave you feeling very tired, and bouts of morning sickness can make the situation even more difficult. Overtiredness can make feelings of nausea worse, and you might also find yourself losing concentration and falling asleep. Added to this, traveling to work, especially if you use public transportation, can be absolutely exhausting, particularly in the later stages of your pregnancy.

Making changes If there's anything about your job that worries you, find out if you can make changes until your baby is born. You may be able to start and finish work at a different time to avoid traveling during rush hour, for example. If your job involves a lot of standing or walking, find out if there's something you can do that allows you to spend more time sitting.

Take it easy Don't push yourself too hard. Be more relaxed about household tasks—your health and that of your baby are far more important. Relaxation is vital, and it's important to make time to take care of your body with an exercise routine and massage.

Ask for help If your partner doesn't already share the cooking and cleaning, ask him to do so. Maybe you could leave most of the household jobs until the weekend and do them together. If you let colleagues know you're pregnant from early on, they're more likely to understand your emotional and physical changes, such as mood swings, lack of energy, and need for comfort.

DECIDING WHEN TO STOP

Some women happily continue working until they near labor. In the US women are allowed and encouraged to work until term, as long as the pregnancy is uncomplicated and the baby is growing well. However, the Pregnancy Discrimination Act (PDA) protects the right of women who do have complications at some point during their pregnancy to receive the same disability leave and pay that is given to employees with any other disability.

DECIDING WHEN TO RETURN

Think carefully about when you'll want to go back to work after your baby is born, and what you'll do when you return. You may want to go back under different working conditions, and you'll need to talk to your employer about this. For example, you might want to try working part-time or try a job share, flexi-work, or some freelance activity that allows you to work from home. Bear in mind that both you and your partner are entitled to take a year's extra parental leave (unpaid) during your child's first five years, provided you've worked for your employer for at least a year (see p.64).

SHARING RESPONSIBILITIES

If you've agreed between you that one of you will go back to work and the other partner will care for the baby at home, the carer will need a lot of support, especially in the early days. Try to share the responsibilities; don't assume your partner will always fix problems or be the one to cope when, say, your baby is ill. If you're both working, share the household jobs and the daily routine, including picking up your baby from daycare or getting home first to take over from the nanny. Far from being a chore, these precious moments alone with your baby will be something you'll come to cherish.

YOUR BABY'S SAFETY

Watch out for any chemicals in your workplace that could damage your baby. If you're worried, talk to your doctor and employer about the risks and take steps to avoid any dangers.

Many pregnant women working in offices are worried about the dangers of exposure to radiation from photocopiers and computers. However, research shows that these very low levels of radiation won't harm your baby.

Very few workplaces allow smoking at all, and those that do keep it to certain areas. Do your best to avoid places where people smoke because passive smoking (inhaling cigarette smoke in the atmosphere) is just as bad for you and your baby as smoking cigarettes yourself.

Choosing single parenthood

Case study

Name Rosemary Hutchinson
Age 38 years
Past medical history Appendix removed at age 15
Obstetric history One abortion at 11 weeks ten years ago. She is now 14 weeks pregnant

Ros never saw motherhood as the most pleasurable aspect of being a woman. She always found work fulfilling and felt that a career was more satisfying for her. Even as a small girl, Ros was determined not to "dwindle" into marriage or adopt the role of housewife. She always takes responsibility for contraception and believes that she has the right to decide whether or not to have a baby. Ros made the decision to abort an 11-week pregnancy when she was 28 years old because she didn't want to interrupt her career.

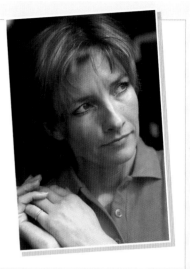

Ros is a lawyer. She studied politics, philosophy, and economics in college and went on to earn a law degree, which included a period of practical training. She now works as a highly respected lawyer, specializing in family law.

THE CHILD'S FATHER

Ros has had two long-term relationships but didn't feel she could settle down with either man. She didn't want to make any form of long-term commitment that meant giving up her independence.

This independence has had its price. As she got older, Ros began to fear that her fertility was diminishing and time was running out. She began to yearn for a baby, but still didn't want to commit herself to any man.

During a recent passionate and rather whirlwind affair with a younger man, Ros decided that she'd be more than happy if her lover, Timothy, was to become the father of her baby. She couldn't see the relationship lasting, though, and didn't particularly want it to.

She talked the idea over with Timothy, who agreed that he didn't want to make any long-term commitment to Ros either, although he was happy to father her baby. The affair has now ended, but they've remained firm friends, and Ros has just begun the second trimester of her pregnancy.

A HEALTHY BABY

This will be Ros's only child, and she wants to do everything she can to make sure her baby will be healthy. She went to a genetic counselor before getting pregnant because a cousin on her father's side suffers from hemophilia (see p.25). Since her father hadn't suffered from the disease, the counselor reassured Ros that she wasn't carrying the gene.

After she'd talked to Timothy about the possibility of his fathering her child, Ros asked him about his family background. Happily, everything seemed to be normal.

Prenatal care

On her first visit, Ros found out that her lifestyle was more important than her age in determining the smoothness of her pregnancy and her delivery. She's being very careful about her diet (see p.128) and exercise (see p.144), and she's not smoking, drinking, or taking any medication.

All of her medical tests have proved normal, and she knows that she shouldn't put on too much weight, that her blood pressure will be carefully checked, and that she must be on the lookout for signs of water retention (tight rings, swollen ankles) since this could be a warning sign of preeclampsia (see p.224). At her last prenatal checkup, Ros had a scan to check for any obvious abnormalities in the baby, among other things. Everything was normal. Although ultrasound scanning revealed no abnormality, Ros is eager to have the added check for genetic or chromosomal diseases provided by amniocentesis (see p.185). She'll also have a specimen of blood checked for her alpha-fetoprotein (AFP) levels.

PREGNANCY AND LABOR

Ros hopes that by cutting down her workload and working flexible hours, she'll be able to work right up until labor. Although Ros's law firm has approved her request for 12 weeks of maternity leave—while she receives her full salary—Ros plans to return to work a few weeks earlier. Given her tough working schedule, Ros knows how important it is to rest. Already she puts her feet up for 20 minutes at lunchtime and tries to snatch a nap in her office or in the car during the afternoon. She's rigorous about getting enough sleep, has stopped socializing except on weekends, and is in bed by 9:30 p.m. I advised her to learn deep muscle and mental relaxation and to keep doing her yoga.

Ros is determined to have the very best medical care available during labor and has chosen to have her baby at a large teaching hospital that's at the forefront of technology. She wants to have an active birth, and she's pleased that she'll be attended by an obstetrician she trusts— she won't have a birth partner and so will depend on her medical team for support during labor. She's made a birth plan (see p.122), which has been added to her hospital notes.

AFTER THE BIRTH

Ros can afford to hire a full-time nanny who will live in with her and the baby as soon as she returns from her hospital delivery. She's glad she's taken the time now, rather than after the birth, to interview nannies and hire someone she likes and trusts. The nanny will be on night duty after a few weeks so that Ros can return to work feeling rested.

Ros wants to breastfeed her baby for as long as she can, and she's prepared to express her milk and store or freeze it so that her baby has the benefits of breast milk even when Ros herself is at work.

I warned Ros that one of the hardest things about being a single parent is that she won't have anyone to share great moments with—when her baby first smiles or says her first words, for example. I also warned her that although her baby won't suffer from having only one parent, it does mean that the demands on Ros herself will be very high.

Ros's work will continue to give her great satisfaction, but I encouraged her to have as active a social life as she can, too. It's all too easy to become isolated when you're caring for a small child by yourself. I suggested that she investigate organizations such as Single Parents By Choice, where she can meet other parents who are raising children without partners. Organizations such as this one also offer invaluable emotional support, networking opportunities, and practical advice.

Ros's baby

Ros's baby will have only one parent right from the start, so her experience of life will e somewhat different from a child who has two parents caring for her.

• **Feeding** She'll have the advantage of being breastfed, even though Ros is going back to work. However, this does mean that she'll have to get used to being bottlefed by her nanny and breastfed by her mother.

• **Care** Ros will be able to give her baby just as much care as two parents would. Her baby will also become very attached to her nanny, who'll be a very important person in her life, but there's nothing wrong with this.

• **Time** Ros's baby won't see her mother all the time, but when she is with her, it will be special time.

• **Relationships** Ros and her child will tend to be everything to each other, which may lead to a rather intense one-to-one relationship. Babies do need and thrive on having plenty of contact with people other than their parents, so it's important that Ros's baby has a chance to interact with a wide range of people—both children and adults. She'll gain a great deal from having this broad network of support and loving care.

DRUGS AND YOUR BABY

Check with a doctor before taking any drug—prescription or nonprescription. Obviously, you must always tell any doctor you see that you're pregnant.

It's best not to take anything while you're pregnant unless your doctor confirms that the benefit to you outweighs any risk to your baby. The long-term effects of some drugs on the unborn child are still unknown. Other drugs are known to be dangerous to the fetus and should be completely avoided (see below).

Avoiding hazards

Many activities that are normally harmless may pose risks when you're pregnant. Cleaning out the cat's litter box, coming in contact with harmful chemicals at work, passive smoking while socializing, or having vaccinations for traveling all may affect the development of your unborn baby, and it's wise to take precautions.

AT HOME
Although few of us can move to a perfect environment while pregnant, you can do your best to avoid some risks, such as handling raw meat, touching other people's pets and cleaning litter boxes, breathing in exhaust gases from cars, and working with pesticides in the yard. Avoid alcohol, coffee, and teas containing caffeine as far as possible. Herbal teas are generally safe (but don't drink raspberry-leaf tea, which is said to trigger contractions). Avoid pesticides by choosing organic herbal teas.

Drug	Use	Possible side effects for your baby
Amphetamines	Stimulant	May cause heart defects and blood diseases
Anabolic steroids	Body-building	Can have a masculinizing effect on a female fetus
Tetracycline	Treats acne	Can color both first and permanent teeth yellow
Streptomycin	Treats tuberculosis	Can cause deafness in infants
Antihistamines	Allergies/travel sickness	Some cause malformations; check with doctor
Anti-nausea drugs	Combats nausea	May cause malformations, but can be used safely to treat morning sickness; check with doctor
Aspirin	Painkiller	Can cause problems with blood clotting
Diuretics	Rid body of excess fluid	Can cause fetal blood disorders
Narcotics (morphine, etc.)	Painkillers	Addictive; baby may become addicted to morphine and suffer withdrawal symptoms
Acetaminophen	Reduces fever	Safe in small doses
LSD, marijuana	Recreational	Risk of chromosomal damage, and miscarriage
Sulfonamides	Treat infections	Can cause jaundice in the baby at birth
Anti-inflammatories (ibuprofen, etc.)	Relieve pain and inflammation	Can cause premature closing of an important valve in baby's circulatory system

Harmful chemicals Try not to use aerosol spray products at home—you can get alternatives. Although modern aerosols contain halogenated hydrocarbons (rather than CFCs), which have not been shown to harm fetus or mother, my feeling is that we're all exposed to so many invisible sources of potentially harmful chemicals, and it's wise to take every possible precaution during pregnancy.

Avoid substances that give off vapors, such as glue and gasoline. These may be toxic and should never be inhaled, whether you're pregnant or not. Read the label of any material you use, and don't handle any that could be harmful. Some common examples are cleaning fluids, contact cement, creosote, volatile paint, lacquers, thinners, some glues, and oven cleaner. Coloring or perming your hair is probably safe, but I'd suggest waiting until after the first three months, when the most crucial organs in your baby's body have formed.

Hot baths It seems that saunas and hot whirlpools can be involved in fetal abnormalities, particularly those of the baby's nervous system, in exactly the same way as fever. When your body is subjected to extreme heat over a lengthy period, you can become overheated, which may affect your baby. Don't use saunas and whirlpools, especially in the first trimester, and take warm, rather than hot, baths.

Television rays Rays have not been shown to form ionizing radiation. It won't do you any harm to sit within several feet of the screen, but do make sure you're sitting comfortably.

Immunizations Because your entire immune system is changing under the influence of your pregnancy and may be weakened, you can have unpredictable responses to immunizations. If you've been exposed to infectious diseases or if you have to travel somewhere that requires immunizations, talk to your doctor. In general, vaccinations that are prepared using live viruses—including measles, rubella (German measles), mumps, and yellow fever vaccinations—are not given. All pregnant women should receive the flu vaccine.

AT WORK

When you find out that you're pregnant, you may have worries about your job: How safe is my workplace? Will the demands of my job put my pregnancy at risk? How long can I go on working? If your job is strenuous, involving a lot of standing, walking, lifting, or climbing, it may be hard for you to get enough rest during your pregnancy, and you may get very tired. Your doctor may suggest that you reduce your working hours, transfer to less strenuous work, or stop working several weeks before your EDD. In all circumstances, pregnant women must avoid doing anything that exposes them to physical danger, including some police work, motorcycle racing, and so on.

TOXOPLASMOSIS AND YOUR BABY

This parasite normally produces only mild flulike symptoms in an adult, but it can seriously damage an unborn child.

It can cause brain damage and blindness in a baby, and can even be fatal. It's most dangerous during the third trimester.

Toxoplasma is carried in the feces of infected animals, particularly cats, but most people get it from eating undercooked meat, particularly poultry. About 80 percent of the population has had it and has developed antibodies, but the younger you are, the less likely you are to be immune. You can ask your doctor to do a blood test.

Guidelines to follow:

- don't eat raw or undercooked meat, especially pork, rare steak, or steak tartare

- don't feed raw meat to your cat or dog. Keep their food bowls away from everything else

- do wear gloves when gardening, and don't garden in soil used by cats

- don't empty your cat's litter box or use your dog's poop-scoop. If you have to, wear gloves and wash your hands in disinfectant immediately afterward

- do wash your hands after gardening, or petting your animals

- do cook meat to an internal temperature of at least 129°F/54°C in order to kill bacteria. Use a meat thermometer to be sure

- if your cat hunts, treat it regularly for worms and parasites.

YOUR RISK OF INFECTION

In the first 12 weeks of pregnancy, try your best to avoid contact with anyone, especially a young child, who has a high fever, even if the fever is not thought to be caused by German measles (see p.19).

If you get mumps when you're pregnant, it'll run the same course as if you weren't pregnant. There's a slightly higher risk of miscarriage if you get the disease in the first 12 weeks.

You won't be vaccinated against mumps during pregnancy because it's a live vaccine which could affect your baby.

Chickenpox is rare among adults, so it's uncommon in pregnancy. There's some evidence that the disease can cause fetal malformations.

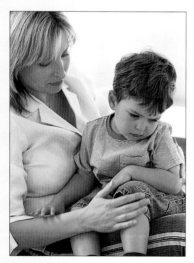

Infection
If you have young children, there's not much you can do to keep away from them if they're sick. If you're a schoolteacher, be fairly strict about sending home any feverish child.

Your doctor may also suggest that it's safest for you to stop working if you have certain diseases, such as a heart condition; if you have a history of more than one premature baby or miscarriage; or if you're expecting more than one baby. Women who are suffering from preeclampsia or placenta previa will be also be advised to stop work.

At work, watch out for anything that could be potentially harmful and make sure your employer transfers you to a hazard-free working place or job. Especially avoid:

• Chemicals used in manufacturing and other industries—for example, lead, mercury, vinyl chloride, dry-cleaning fluids, paint fumes, and solvents

• Animals, which present a risk of toxoplasmosis

• Exposure to infectious diseases, especially childhood rashes

• Exposure to toxic wastes of any kind

• Exposure to cigarette smoke (passive smoking), which can happen in public places and offices that don't have smoking restrictions

• Unacceptable levels of ionizing radiation. It's generally accepted that day-to-day exposure to ultraviolet or infrared radiation given off by equipment such as printers, photocopiers, and computer screens is not dangerous to you or your baby. But just to be extra-careful, if you make photocopies every day, it's a good idea to keep the top of the photocopier closed when the machine is copying.

Otherwise, if you're a healthy woman, with a normal pregnancy and working in a job with no hazards greater than those you meet in everyday life, you can usually work until close to your expected delivery date.

SOCIALIZING

Infections are caught from people we come in contact with in our daily life. Although you don't want to become a hermit when you're pregnant, or wear a surgical mask when talking to people, it does pay to be cautious—especially around children (see column, left) or adults who are running a temperature.

Colds and flu won't harm your baby, but do your best to avoid fevers. If your temperature is very high, ask your doctor what medications are safe to take—aspirin is not usually recommended in pregnancy except for certain conditions. You can also try using a damp sponge and a fan to cool your skin down. Don't take cold or flu medicines that contain antihistamines unless your doctor says it's okay. There's some evidence that particularly virulent flu viruses can cause miscarriage.

TRAVELING

There's no evidence that travel brings on labor or leads to miscarriage or any other complication of pregnancy. It is wise, though, to be extra-careful about travel if you've miscarried before or have a history of premature labor. Ask your doctor for the name of an obstetrician in the area you're visiting and, in the last trimester, limit yourself to trips within easy reach of home.

Trains Reserve a seat in advance if possible, and on longer trips, make sure you don't sit next to the dining car, since the smell may make you feel nauseous. Eat lightly to lessen the risk of travel sickness. Don't lean on, or stand close to, train doors, since they have been known to fly open (this obviously applies even when you're not pregnant).

Cars Traveling by car can be exhausting, so limit your trips. Stop at regular intervals so you can take a short walk to keep your circulation going. Always fasten your seat belt, but buckle it low, across your pelvis, and use the shoulder harness. Keep driving as long as you're comfortable behind the wheel, but you must stop as soon as you begin to feel at all cramped. This may seem obvious, but don't drive yourself to the hospital if you're in labor!

Air travel Traveling by plane isn't a good idea after your seventh month, because of pressure changes in the cabin. If you must fly at this time, ask the airline if they'll need to see a doctor's letter before letting you on the plane. If you sit over the wings or toward the front of the plane, you'll feel less of the plane's motion. Don't fly in small private planes with unpressurized cabins.

While flying, eat lightly because pregnancy makes you more prone to motion sickness. Make sure you empty your bladder before you board in case there's a delay in taking off, or the seat-belt sign stays on for a long time. When fastening your seat belt, make sure you buckle it low on your hips. It's best to avoid having any carbonated drinks, which can cause gas. To keep your legs from developing edema (accumulation of fluid), take frequent walks around the plane.

Foreign travel Always follow the guidelines I've given to protect against listeria and other food-related diseases (see p.139). Drink bottled water when in doubt.

Ask your doctor about immunizations you may need for travel to some destinations (typhoid fever vaccinations, for example, could harm your baby). Even if you've been exposed or are in a typhoid epidemic, the bad effects of the live vaccine will have to be weighed against the risk to your baby. You should refuse to have a yellow fever vaccination unless you've had direct exposure. You may need rabies and tetanus vaccinations, particularly if you've had any risk of exposure. Chloroquine may be used for malaria, but only if you're going to an endemic area. The polio vaccine may be given during pregnancy if you are not already immune.

GOOD TRAVELING

A little extra care will make traveling when you're pregnant a more comfortable experience.

- Leave more than enough time for your trip.

- Aim to leave more time than you normally would for any connections you have to make so you don't have to rush.

- Travel in short bursts rather than a long stretch.

- Travel safely (see main text).

- Carry a drink, such as milk or fruit juice, in a bottle or Thermos.

- Take some easy-to-carry food with you, such as whole-wheat crackers, cold hard-boiled eggs, raw fruit or vegetables, and nibbles like dried fruit, nuts, and seeds.

- Have some glucose candy or raisins to help prevent nausea caused by low blood sugar.

- Wear an eye mask and some ear plugs so that you can get some sleep when traveling by train or plane.

CHAPTER 7

Your prenatal care

Excellent prenatal care should be rewarded with healthy mothers and babies. The routine tests you'll have usually pick up any problems as soon as they arise, and there are special tests for mothers and babies with particular needs. At your prenatal clinic you'll also have the chance to ask questions about your pregnancy and to meet other women going through the same experiences as you are.

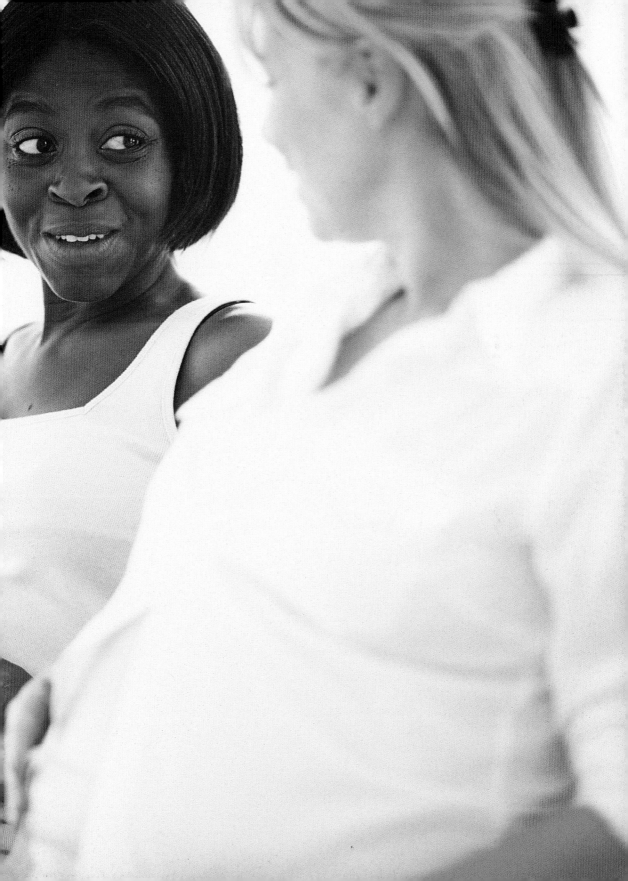

Prenatal care

YOUR FIRST VISIT

When you make your first visit to the prenatal clinic, you may be asked about the following:

- your personal details and circumstances

- childhood illnesses or any serious illnesses you've had

- illnesses that run in your family, or in your partner's family

- if there are twins in your family

- your menstrual history—when your periods started, how long your average cycle is, how many days you bleed, and the date of your last period (see p.62)

- what symptoms of pregnancy you have, and your general health

- details of previous births, pregnancies, or problems in conceiving

- if you take a prescription medicine or suffer from any allergies.

You'll have consultations, checkups, and tests throughout your pregnancy to make sure you and your baby are doing fine. Most pregnancies are perfectly normal, but it's vital to have these checkups to make sure all is well and to spot possible problems early, before any harm is done.

THE PRENATAL CLINIC

Your prenatal checkups may be at your doctor's office, your local clinic, or the hospital. You'll probably have a "check-in" appointment at 11 or 12 weeks or so, and you can expect about 10 further visits if it's your first pregnancy and about seven if it's not. The exact number and timing of prenatal checkups varies from area to area. If you have any complications, such as a multiple birth, a medical condition you had before you became pregnant, or you're at risk for some other reason, you'll have checkups more frequently.

Most prenatal care is now handled locally, so appointments are much less stressful than when most women had to go to hospital clinics. There's a more relaxed atmosphere, and if you do need to a hospital clinic, you'll probably find it less crowded than it used to be.

There'll be times, though, when you have to wait around, especially if you're having an ultrasound scan or a blood test. Take something to read or to do while you're there, and take some food and something to drink with you in case you have a long wait but don't want to risk going out for a snack and missing your appointment. Ask your partner to go with you if he can. If you have other children, it's best to ask someone to take care of them if possible, rather than take them with you.

The clinic can be a good place to start making friends with other expectant mothers, so chat with whoever's there.

TALKING TO YOUR CAREGIVERS

Midwives at a hospital-based prenatal clinic may find it hard to find time to talk to you as much as you'd like. Community clinics should be more relaxed, and you'll be able to find out what alternatives are open to you, talk about your preferences, and get reassurance about any worries and fears. If you feel that you're being hurried through your appointment, ask your midwife for some more time. Don't let yourself be intimidated, but do bear in mind that many women feel very emotional and weepy when pregnant, so you may cry much more easily than usual in any stressful situation. If you have strong preferences, but worry that you won't be able to stand up for yourself, take your partner along for moral support. It'll help to make a list of points you want to talk about beforehand and go over them together.

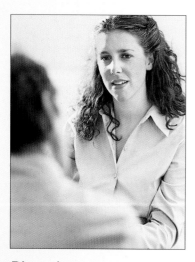

Discussing your pregnancy
Don't hesitate to ask for more time if you have questions you want answered.

UNDERSTANDING YOUR RECORDS

When you go to your first prenatal visit, you will be given a card with your due date, prenatal labs, and a visit summary (vital signs, weight, urine dipstick). Bring the card to all your visits so that your doctor or midwife can update it. Be sure to carry the card with you at all times, in case of an emergency. Your medical records will be copied by your doctor and sent directly to the hospital or birthing center so they are there when you arrive.

Your records may be difficult to understand because many of the medical terms are abbreviated. Compare the abbreviations on your records with those listed below. If your records still don't make sense, ask your midwife or doctor to explain.

Carry your records at all times, and remember to take them with you to the hospital when you go into labor.

Abbreviations and terms on your records

NAD No acute distress

Alb Albumin in urine (a name for one of the proteins found in the urine sample)

BP Blood pressure

FHH/NH Fetal heart heard or not heard

FH Fetal heart

FMF Fetal movements felt

Ceph Cephalic, baby is lying head down

Vx Vertex, baby is lying head down

Br Breech, baby is bottom down

LMP Last menstrual period

EDD/EDC Estimated date of delivery/confinement

Hb Hemoglobin levels to check for anemia

Eng/E Engaged The baby's head has dropped down into the pelvis ready for birth

NE Not engaged

Para 0 Woman has had no other children

Para 1 (etc.) Woman has had one or more children

Fe Iron has been prescribed

Height of fundus The height of the top of the uterus. The baby pushes this up as it grows and often the height is used to work out how many weeks you are. Some clinics measure the height of the fundus (from the top of the pubic bone to the top of the uterus) with a tape measure in centimeters

Relation of PP to brim This is the brim of your pelvis. The presenting part (PP) of the baby to the brim later in your pregnancy will be the part in the cervix ready to be born

PET Preeclamptic toxemia

Long L Longitudinal lie; the baby is lying parallel to your spine in your uterus

RSA Right sacrum anterior—the most common breech presentation

AFP Alpha-fetoprotein

CS Cesarean section

H/T Hypertension (high blood pressure)

MSU Midstream urine sample

Primigravida First pregnancy

Multigravida More than one pregnancy

VE Vaginal examination

BABY'S POSITION

Terms used to describe how your baby is lying appear as abbreviations on your chart. They refer to where the back of the baby's head (occiput) is in relation to your body, so ROA means the back of his head is to the front on your right.

Key to abbreviations: L: left side (or lateral, meaning the woman's side); R: right side; A: anterior (to the front); P: posterior (to the back); O: occiput (back of the baby's head)

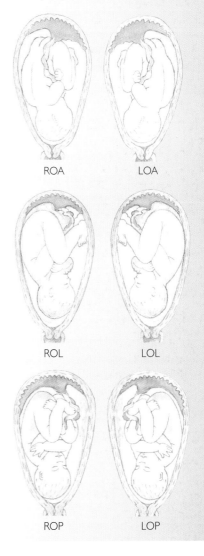

ROA   LOA

ROL   LOL

ROP   LOP

Routine checks

While you're pregnant, you'll have some routine checks to make sure both you and your baby are doing well. Some may be done at every visit, or at different times during your pregnancy. Other tests only need to be carried out once. If the tests show that there is, or may be, a problem, you'll be monitored closely and prompt action will be taken if necessary.

HEIGHT

Your height will be measured at your first visit. If you are petite, your midwife may suspect that you have a small pelvic inlet and outlet. The chances are, though, that your baby will match your particular physical build.

WEIGHT

Women are weighed at every visit. If you lose weight in the first trimester, it's usually because of nausea and vomiting due to morning sickness and nothing to worry about. Maternal weight gain used to be taken as a reliable indicator of the growth of the baby. Recent research, however, shows that external examination, blood and urinary tests, and especially ultrasound scans are much more accurate in measuring fetal growth. A sudden weight gain could mean you have fluid retention, a sign of preeclampsia (see p.224).

Checking your legs
Your doctor or midwife will examine your legs and ankles for any signs of varicose veins, swelling, or puffiness.

LEGS AND HANDS

At every visit your legs will be checked for varicose veins, and your ankles and hands will be examined for signs of swelling and puffiness (edema). A little swelling in the final weeks of pregnancy is normal, particularly in the evening, but excessive puffiness may give an early warning of preeclampsia (see p.224).

BREASTS

Your breasts will be checked for lumps and the condition of your nipples at your first visit. They won't usually be checked again, but if you're worried about anything, ask your midwife.

URINE

When you go for your first visit, you'll be asked for a sample of midstream urine to test for any underlying bladder or kidney infection. To collect a midstream sample, you'll be given a sterile pad to clean your vulva and a sterile container. You pass the first few drops of urine into the toilet bowl and collect some midstream urine in the container. You then finish urinating into the toilet.

You'll be asked to bring a morning sample of urine with you on other visits. This will be tested for urinary infection; for sugar, to make sure you're not developing diabetes; and for *ketones*, which are the classic sign that diabetes is established and needs urgent treatment (see p. 140). A rare cause of *ketonuria* (raised levels of ketones) is very severe vomiting in pregnancy, called *hyperemesis gravidarum*, which means you have to go to the hospital right away. If you do have diabetes, it may disappear once your baby is born but come back in future pregnancies. A trace of protein in your urine in late pregnancy is a strong warning of preeclampsia. This will be looked into at once because of the risks of miscarriage, a small-for-dates baby, and premature delivery (see p.298).

Blood tests

Also at your first prenatal visit, you'll be asked for a blood sample, usually from a vein in your arm. This is used to check your basic blood group (A,B,O), and also your Rhesus (Rh) blood group (positive or negative), in case a blood transfusion becomes necessary. If you are Rh-negative, you'll be tested for Rhesus incompatibility with your baby (see p.202).

HIV AND HEPATITIS B

Hepatitis B
All pregnant women should have a blood test for Hepatitis B. Infected women can be given treatment to avoid passing the disease on to the baby.

HIV
HIV screening is now recommended for all pregnant women. Treatment is available for women who test positive to lessen the risk that the disease will be passed on to the baby. It's important to diagnose HIV early, since this improves the likelihood of having a healthy baby.

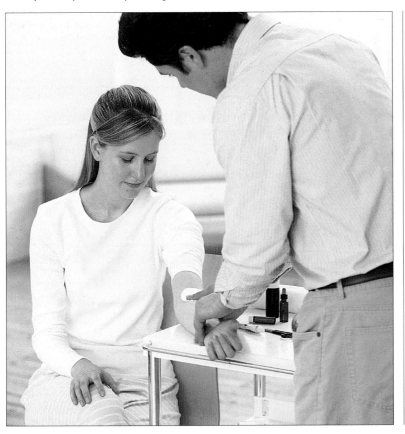

Taking a blood sample
Blood tests are important for finding out if you have, or are likely to have, any problems.

BABY'S HEARTBEAT

Your baby's heartbeat will be monitored at every visit from week 14. Your baby's heart beats almost twice as fast as yours (about 140 beats per minute compared with 72 beats per minute), and sounds just like a tiny galloping horse.

Pinnard stethoscope The doctor or midwife may listen to your baby's heartbeat using a traditional device known as a Pinnard stethoscope, although these are now rapidly falling out of use.

Doppler It's more likely that a Doppler scanner will be used. This is a small portable instrument (about the size of a telephone). It's placed on your stomach and uses ultrasound (see also p.180) to listen to the baby's heartbeat. The scanner magnifies the sound of your baby's heartbeat, so you can hear it, too.

Electronic monitor There are two kinds of electronic monitors. One, an external monitor, is strapped around your abdomen and sensors record the baby's heartbeat. The other, an internal monitor, has a tiny electrode that is clipped to the baby's scalp and records the heartbeat more accurately. These monitors are used only during labor. The latest monitors use radio waves so you can still walk around while being monitored.

Your hemoglobin level will also be checked. This is a measure of the oxygen-carrying power of your red blood cells. The normal level is between 12 and 14 grams; if yours falls below 10 grams, you may be given treatment for anemia. Iron and folic acid raise the oxygen-carrying power of your blood, so it's essential to eat a healthy diet with plenty of vitamins and minerals (see p.128).

The blood test will also show whether or not you've had German measles (rubella) (see p.19)—if you have, you're immune. Also, any sexually transmitted diseases, such as syphilis, will be revealed, and some genetic disorders, such as sickle cell anemia and thalassemia (see pp.24 & 25), are detectable in blood. You may also have a special screening blood test to help rule out certain types of fetal abnormalities.

You can also ask to have your blood tested for toxoplasmosis infection (see p.169). *Toxoplasma* is a parasite that can be picked up from cat feces and also from eating poorly cooked lamb or pork. Toxoplasmosis is harmless to adults, but it can cross the placenta and cause blindness, epilepsy, and developmental delay in the baby.

Pregnant women aren't routinely screened for toxoplasmosis. The results can be hard to interpret, which means it's difficult to predict if the baby is affected, and this can cause extra stress for the mother. Ideally, you should be tested before getting pregnant. You won't necessarily be given this test unless you're thought to be at risk, so if you're worried—particularly if you have pets that hunt outside—ask for the test.

EXTERNAL EXAMINATION

At every visit your caregiver or obstetrician will gently feel your abdomen and the top of your uterus (fundus) to check the size of your growing baby. This gives a good idea of whether your baby is about the right size for your dates. After 26–28 weeks the doctor or midwife will also feel for your baby's "poles" (head and rump) so they can assess what position your baby is lying in (see p.175). Your belly will be palpated to check your baby's size and growth.

BLOOD PRESSURE

You'll have this taken at every visit. As always, it measures the pressure at which your heart is pumping blood through your body. The reading is made up of two numbers: the upper one is the *systolic* pressure—when the heart contracts it pushes out blood and "beats." This is measured when the arm band is tight. As the pressure is released, the lower, or *diastolic*, reading is made. This is the resting pressure between beats.

The statistically average blood pressure reading in pregnancy is 120 over 70, although blood pressure differs with age, and there is a range of blood pressures that are considered normal. A higher reading than normal during pregnancy may be a sign of preeclampsia (see p.224) and you'll probably be advised to go into the hospital for evaluation. Constant checks are made so that changes are quickly noted.

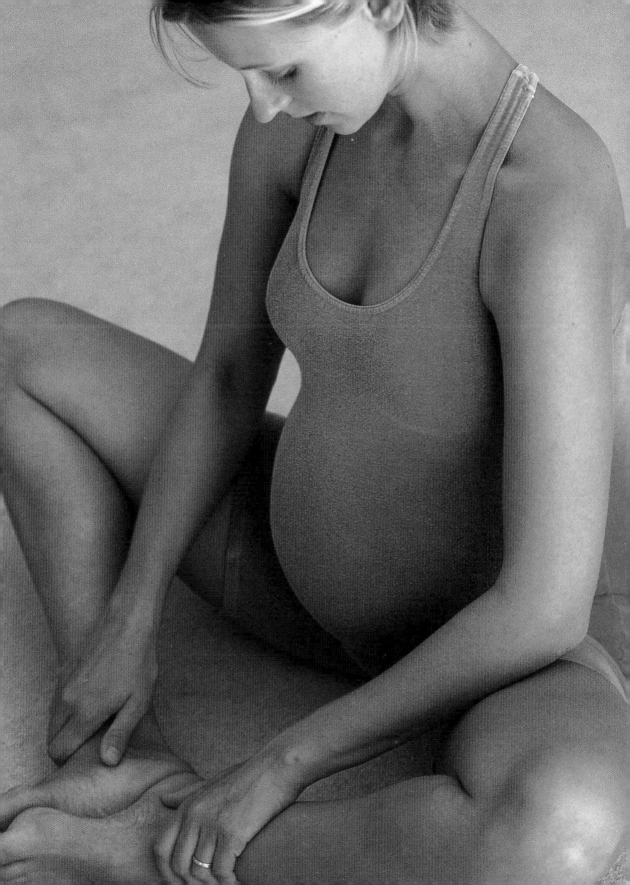

Ultrasound scan

WHY YOU HAVE SCANS

An ultrasound scan is done during your pregnancy to make sure your baby is developing normally. Sometimes you may need extra scans. Main reasons for these are:

- as part of infertility assessment
- to identify abdominal problems such as an ectopic pregnancy
- if the doctors suspect an imminent miscarriage
- to check for a multiple pregnancy
- for an anatomic survey.

One of the most helpful of medical technologies, ultrasound is now a routine part of prenatal care. Ultrasound scans are used to check your baby's general well-being and position, and guide doctors when they're carrying out any special tests and operations. You'll be given two scans—the first at around 12–13 weeks, to confirm dates and check whether you're expecting more than one baby. If your first visit to your midwife or doctor is after 13 weeks, you'll have a scan then. Between 18 and 20 weeks you'll have another scan to make sure your baby is growing well and there are no abnormalities. If all looks fine, you won't have any more scans.

HOW IT WORKS

The process is based on a sonar device that reveals objects in fluid, which was first used by the US Navy to detect submarines during World War II. A crystal, inside a device called a *transducer*, converts an electrical current into high-frequency sound waves, which the human ear can't detect. The sound waves form a beam that penetrates the abdomen as the transducer is moved back and forth. The beam reflects off material in its path, and the

HAVING A SCAN

Having an ultrasound scan usually takes about 15 minutes and doesn't hurt. You'll probably be asked to drink about a pint of water, and not empty your bladder before arriving at the clinic. This may be a little uncomfortable but it's worth it—a full bladder provides a clearer picture of your baby on the screen. At the clinic you'll be asked to lie down on a bed and lift up your top to expose your abdomen. An oil or gel, which acts as a conductor of the sound waves, is rubbed on your abdomen, and the transducer is passed over this area in different directions. You can just lie back and enjoy your first view of your baby as the image appears on the screen.

The operator will explain the image on the screen and point out different parts of your baby's body

Sound wave echoes from your baby are shown as an image on the ultrasound screen

Ultrasound machine

Oil rubbed on your stomach prevents air from blocking the transmission of sound waves

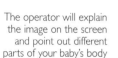

transducer records these echoes. The echoes are converted into electrical signals, which produce an image that can be displayed on a screen. The beam can only penetrate fluids and soft tissue such as the *amniotic sac*, kidneys, and liver. It cannot pass through bone, or register gas. An ultrasound scan is increasingly used to assess the threat of miscarriage, make sure you're not having an ectopic pregnancy, and assist in infertility treatments, such as IVF, and fetal surgery (see p.200).

YOUR SCAN

Your ultrasound scan can be a thrilling moment for you and your partner—a chance to see your baby for the very first time. Scanning equipment has been improved and refined over the years, and the technique is not intrusive.

You should be able to hear your baby's heartbeat, and to see the gentle movement of her hands and feet, waving and kicking, as she floats in the amniotic fluid. Ask the ultrasound operator to explain the image on the screen to you, since some details may be difficult to make out. Some clinics will offer you a print of the image of your baby as a memento to cherish, although they may charge you for this.

IS IT SAFE?

There are no known risks to your baby from an ultrasound scan. There have been some worries about long-term effects, such as hearing impairment caused by the impact of sound waves, but recent research suggests that ultrasound is not harmful to mother or baby. The waves are of a very low intensity, and so it's safe for the scan to be performed repeatedly.

WHY YOU MIGHT HAVE A SCAN

An ultrasound scan shows if your baby is healthy. It may also be used for the following reasons:

- to check your baby's location and development of the placenta

- to check on your baby's growth rate, particularly if you're not sure about the date of conception

- to find out whether your baby is ready to be born if overdue

- to confirm that your baby is in the usual head-down position, and not bottom-down, after week 38

- to detect certain fetal abnormalities, such as spina bifida

- to monitor the baby throughout special tests such as amniocentesis and fetoscopy

- to assist in operations performed on a baby in the uterus.

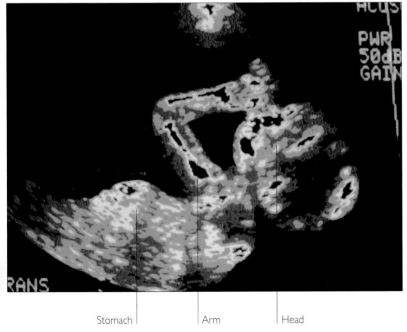

Ultrasound scan
A scan of your baby will show that she's healthy, how she's lying—and whether you're expecting more than one. This scan shows a baby in its mother's uterus. The baby floats in the amniotic sac, moving around all the time and doing things such as sucking its thumb, yawning, blinking, and urinating.

| Stomach | Arm | Head |

181

Twins

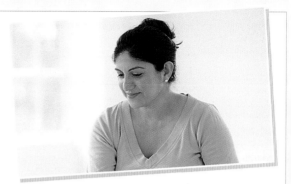

Karen was told she was expecting twins when she had an ultrasound scan at 14 weeks. She knew from the beginning that there was something different about this pregnancy. For one thing, she was constantly sick in the first couple of months, which she hadn't been previously. She also looked huge—at three months, she looked about five! Consequently, it wasn't a total surprise when her scan showed that she was carrying twins.

Once they'd got over the initial shock of finding out that they were expecting twins, Karen and Joe were delighted, if a little bit apprehensive. Their first concerns were for the well-being of Karen and the twins throughout the pregnancy, and then how they would manage to cope with the extra responsibilities that having two babies would bring.

SUSPECTING A MULTIPLE PREGNANCY

Many women guess early on that there's something different about their pregnancies when they're carrying twins. Size is often a clue, as well as the shape—twins tend to push the abdomen out sideways as well as forward. Twins can be diagnosed by week eight of the pregnancy by an ultrasound scan.

KAREN'S SPECIAL NEEDS

Some women sail through a twin pregnancy with very few or no side effects. Some don't. The extra stress of carrying two babies can increase feelings of tiredness and sickness as your body adjusts. Also, twin pregnancies need to be watched carefully for raised blood pressure, anemia, edema, and preeclampsia (see p.224). Like all expectant mothers of twins, Karen will go to her prenatal clinic more often than a woman expecting one baby. Her doctor will watch for edema, and may admit her to the hospital if she seems likely to develop preeclampsia. She must have a good, high-protein diet.

Sheer size can be a problem in later pregnancy, and it can be hard to get comfortable. I suggested to Karen that she might find that being in water helps, since it supports her weight. Gentle swimming would be fine as long as her doctor agrees. She might also like to rent a birthing pool (see Addresses, p.370) as an extra-large bathtub in which she can relax. Making love is not usually prohibited, although Karen should follow her doctor's advice and check with her right away if she has any discharge or bleeding or if she has contractions.

Among women expecting twins, those who don't get enough rest are much more likely to go into premature labor than those who've had complete rest from the fifth month. Whatever work you do during a twin pregnancy, including caring for young children, make sure it isn't too strenuous. I advised Karen to try to arrange some extra help with her older children, and have at least three hours of bed rest each day.

LABOR AND TWINS

A twin labor is always managed in the hospital because of the risks. Doctors and midwives are highly sensitive to the difficulties that can arise, but as long as the second twin's heart rate is normal, the doctor will wait to deliver the baby. The second twin may be monitored by ultrasound or Doppler until it is delivered.

WILL THEY BE IDENTICAL OR FRATERNAL?

One-third of all twins are identical. They are always the same sex and usually share the placenta, although this depends on how late the egg splits. Half of fraternal twins are boy–girl pairs and half are same sex. Their placentas are separate, but may be fused together. The incidence of identical twins appears to be completely random, while fraternal twins often run in families, inherited through the mother's side. There's no history of twins in Karen's family. The likelihood of having non-inherited, fraternal twins rises until a woman is in her mid-thirties, then drops again. It also seems to be higher if she's tall, well-built, and conceives easily. The chances of having fraternal twins also appear to increase with each subsequent child.

Twins shown by ultrasound

Ultrasound scans can show if you're carrying two babies. Sometimes,,though, one may be behind the other and not easily seen. If twins are still suspected despite only one being seen on the ultrasound, you'll probably have another scan in 5–6 weeks.

IDENTICAL TWINS

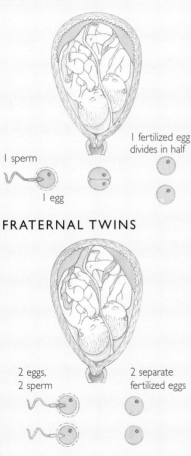

1 sperm

1 egg

1 fertilized egg divides in half

FRATERNAL TWINS

2 eggs, 2 sperm

2 separate fertilized eggs

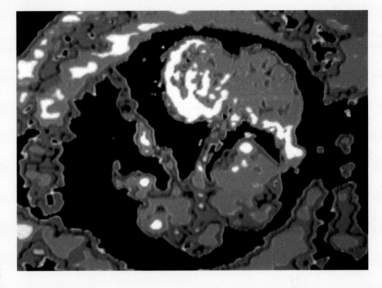

Karen's babies

A twin pregnancy and birth is different in several important ways.

• Twins have a shorter gestation period than single babies—they're normally born at 37 weeks rather than 40 weeks. This is mostly because there's just not enough space in the mother's womb, although other external factors are also important.

• Because they have a shorter gestation period, twins weigh less than single babies.

• There are extra risks for the second-born because once the uterus contracts down and the first twin is delivered, there is a risk that the second twin's placenta will separate. If this happens, an emergency cesarean section is performed for the delivery of the twin.

Special tests

During your prenatal care you can have a number of special screening, and diagnostic tests to check for various complications or defects affecting the baby. These tests can be reassuring if they rule out something you're worrying about, such as a genetic defect like cystic fibrosis, but they may also reveal a problem that makes you question whether you want to go on with your pregnancy. Situations like this put an enormous emotional strain for parents-to-be, so it's important to talk in detail to your doctor beforehand about the risks of having the tests and the implications of their results.

SCREENING TESTS

Most maternity clinics now have a number of tests available to screen mothers for a variety of possible fetal abnormalities. These screening tests don't tell you for certain whether anything is wrong, but if a test shows that there may be a problem, you may have some more diagnostic tests to confirm or rule it out.

Nuchal Translucency (NT) Scan The risk of having a baby with Down syndrome or some other chromosomal defect can be assessed around 11–14 weeks using a special ultrasound scan called a nuchal translucency scan. The ultrasound measures the thickness of the skin at the back of the fetus's neck—it's thicker in babies with Down syndrome. On the same day as the scan, you'll have a finger prick blood test for levels of pregnancy-associated plasma protein-A (PAPP-A) and human chorionic gonadotropin (hCG).

Combining a blood test with the nuchal scan raises the sensitivity of the screen to about 91 percent. Based on the results of blood tests, nuchal translucency measurement, and your age, a physician is able calculate your baby's risk of Down syndrome. A positive test does not mean that your baby has Down syndrome, however—only that your risk is greater.

Triple serum screen This test was developed by St. Bartholomew's Hospital in London. A sample of the pregnant mother's blood is taken between 14 and 20 weeks to measure the levels of three substances—*estriol, human chorionic gonadotrophin,* and *alpha-fetoprotein.* The results are assessed in relation to the mother's age to predict the chance of her baby's suffering from Down syndrome. If the chances seem high (more than one in 250), doctors will suggest you have amniocentesis. If you're not offered a triple serum screen, you can ask to have it.

AFP test Alpha-fetoprotein is found in varying amounts in your blood throughout pregnancy. Between 16 and 18 weeks the levels are usually low. If a blood test is done at this time and the levels are 2–3 times higher than the average of a sample group, it may show that there's a neurological problem. Some neural tube defects are too small to detect with ultrasound alone. If the AFP test is abnormal, you'll have a "targeted" scan of the spine, abdomen, and placenta; and perhaps an amniocentesis. Although nuchal translucency measurement has replaced AFP testing in many clinics as a screening test for Down syndrome (see opposite), it cannot replace screening for neural tube defects.

DIAGNOSTIC TESTS

These tests are used to confirm abnormalities in the fetus, and are generally only used after screening tests or ultrasound scans have shown that you may be at a high risk. The main diagnostic tests are amniocentesis and chorionic villus sampling (CVS). Amniocentesis is the most common diagnostic test; CVS is not available in all clinics, and it carries a higher risk of miscarriage, but it does give an early diagnosis.

You and your partner will need to think very carefully about the implications of having these tests and talk them through together and with your doctor. Ask for special counseling if you think you may need it.

AMNIOCENTESIS

Amniotic fluid contains cells from the baby's skin and other organs that can be used to diagnose his condition. Amniocentesis is the name given to the procedure that withdraws this fluid from the uterus.

Why it's done You'll probably want to have amniocentesis if you are over the age of 35, as the risk of chromosomal abnormalities (such as Down syndrome) increases with age (see column, right). It may also be suggested after serum screening, or if a nuchal scan shows a risk of Down syndrome (see opposite). Amniocentesis can also reveal other important information that may be sometimes helpful in determining the care and progress of your pregnancy.

Amniocentesis can be used to check for metabolic disorders, but it is preferable to have them diagnosed earlier in pregnancy by CVS (chorionic villus sampling—see p.186). At one time amniocentesis was also used to check the *bilirubin* content of the fluid to help work out if a Rhesus-positive baby needed a blood transfusion while still in the mother's uterus, but this is now done by a *Doppler* scan to check for fetal anemia (see p.187).

What it can reveal Where there is cause for concern, an amniocentesis test may show the following:

• The sex of the baby: cells sloughed off by the fetus accumulate in the amniotic fluid. Under the microscope, male cells can be distinguished from female cells and the baby's sex determined. In gender-linked genetically linked disorders such as hemophilia, a male child will have a 50 percent chance of being affected.

OLDER MOTHERS

Your age is just one of several factors that can affect the outcome of your pregnancy. Your diet is much more important.

If your general health is good, you shouldn't be treated any differently from younger women during your pregnancy. Age is a factor, though, in certain fetal abnormalities, and an older mother may have a higher risk of maternal diabetes and placental insufficiency. You may be screened for these more frequently.

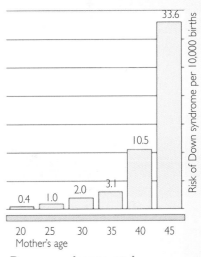

Down syndrome and your age
Maternal age seems to be an important factor in Down syndrome. As you can see from the graph, the risk of having a baby with this condition rises as you get older, but isn't really significant until after 35 years of age. But since most babies are born to women under 35 who don't have screening for Down syndrome, there are more Down babies in the pre-35 age group than in the post-35 age group.

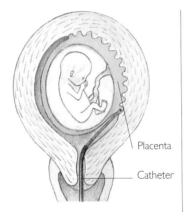

Chorionic sampling
Using ultrasound guidance, a small amount of chorion (placental tissue) is taken from the uterus through the cervix with the aid of a catheter.

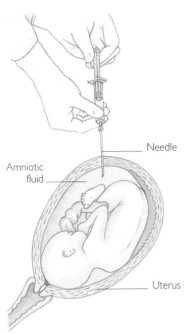

Amniocentesis
Amniotic fluid is extracted only after an ultrasound scan has determined the position of the fetus and the placenta. Using ultrasound as a guide, the doctor passes a needle through the abdominal wall and of amniotic fluid is withdrawn.

• The chemical composition of the fluid: this can reveal metabolic disorders caused by missing or defective enzymes

• The chromosome count: determined by examining discarded cells. Any deviation from the normal chromosomal structure usually means that the baby may have a disability.

How is it done? Amniocentesis is usually carried out at 16–18 weeks. Guided by ultrasound, the doctor inserts a hollow needle into the amniotic sac through the front of the abdominal wall. About 20cc (a few tablespoons) of amniotic fluid is usually withdrawn, and this is then spun in a centrifuge to separate the cells shed by the baby from the rest of the liquid. The cells then have to be cultured, and it takes about three weeks for the results to come through—a very stressful period for couples. Many women talk about putting their pregnancies "on hold" during this time, until the results confirm that the baby is unaffected.

Amniocentesis is only undertaken with ultrasound monitoring to guide the needle into the amniotic sac, so that neither the placenta nor the fetus is harmed. The risk that the procedure will induce a miscarriage in early pregnancy is small—about one in 200. There's also a very small risk (less than one percent) of your waters breaking, and your baby could develop respiratory difficulties after birth.

Chorionic villus sampling (CVS)

Chorionic villi, fingerlike outgrowths on the edge of the chorion, are genetically identical to the fetus. They develop earlier than amniotic fluid, so examining a sample of chorionic villi provides valuable information about your baby's genes and chromosomes before it's possible to carry out amniocentesis between 10-11weeks.

What it can reveal The most important group of mothers needing CVS are those at risk of having a Down syndrome baby. An abnormality of hemoglobin, such as sickle-cell disease or thalassemia, can also be diagnosed with CVS. Inborn errors of metabolism are, fortunately, rare, but if a family is afflicted, the incidence may be as high as one in four. The basic defect is an enzyme deficiency, and direct enzyme analysis on the chorionic tissue gives a diagnosis within two days. Single gene disorders, such as cystic fibrosis, hemophilia, Huntington's chorea, and muscular dystrophy, can be detected with the use of CVS.

How is it done? CVS is also carried out under ultrasound control, usually between 10 and 12 weeks, before the amniotic sac completely fills the uterine cavity. Two routes are used, the transcervical route and the transabdominal route. For the first, the cervix is first examined using a speculum. A plastic or metal catheter is then introduced through the cervical canal, across the uterine cavity, and then into the outside edge of the placenta. A small amount of chorionic villi tissue is then removed for analysis.

The second procedure follows that of amniocentesis, but with a sample being taken of the placental tissue rather than of the amniotic fluid. The risk of miscarriage following CVS is about one percent higher than the spontaneous miscarriage rate (see p.218). The advantage of CVS is that it gives an initial result within 24–48 hours, with full results in about a week. This is helpful if the risks are high and you don't want to have to wait until your pregnancy is at a more advanced stage for the results of amniocentesis.

UMBILICAL VEIN SAMPLING (CORDOCENTESIS)

Also known as Percutaneous Umbilical Cord Blood Sampling (PUBS), this procedure is used to check the makeup of fetal blood and, in cases of fetal anemia, for intrauterine blood transfusion. It's also used to check for infections and to assess your baby's levels of hemoglobin. Umbilical vein sampling is no longer used in cases of suspected slow growth. Instead, Doppler scans provide the necessary information and these are available in most clinics.

Infection detection Rubella, toxoplasmosis, and the herpes virus may be detected by performing a specific radio analysis of certain proteins that are present in a baby's blood.

Rhesus isoimmunization In cases of Rhesus incompatibility (see p.202), assessing the baby's hemoglobin is the best way to determine the severity of blood-cell destruction and whether a blood transfusion for the baby in the womb (also done through the umbilical vein) needs to be carried out.

How is it done? Under ultrasonic control, a hollow needle is passed through the front wall of the mother's abdomen and uterus into a blood vessel in the umbilical cord, about half an inch (1 cm) from where it emerges from the placenta. A small quantity of blood can then be removed for testing. The risk to the fetus appears to be about 1–2 percent. Umbilical vein sampling can replace any investigation currently undertaken on a blood sample.

DOPPLER SCAN

The Doppler scan uses black-and-white or color images to look at the blood flow between the placenta and your baby through the umbilical cord. It uses a slightly different type of sound wave from a normal ultrasound scan, which bounces off moving red blood cells and shows how fast they're moving through the fetus's blood vessels. Doppler is used to check when a baby is small for dates or seems not to be growing as fast as it should.

Doppler can be used to assess whether the developing fetus has anemia, although the only way to tell for certain is by the PUBS test. Doppler is also used to find out whether a Rhesus-positive baby needs a blood transfusion in the womb.

Testing for abnormalities

Case study

Name Daniella Stamp
Age 26 years
Past medical history Nothing abnormal
Family history Nothing of note
Obstetric history Dysmenorrhea (very painful periods)

Daniella and her partner Will had decided to try for a baby after he'd secured a good promotion at work, which meant they could afford to move into a bigger house. Daniella was particularly eager to have her babies while she was young and fit. After Daniella had missed two periods and a home pregnancy test proved positive, she and Will visited their family doctor, who referred them to the prenatal clinic at the local city hospital. They both found this visit impersonal and intimidating.

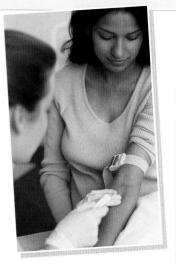

Modern technology allows doctors to investigate the health of the fetus before birth at earlier and earlier stages. Like Daniella, most pregnant women are now offered routine screening tests. These sometimes lead to much more invasive diagnostic tests for confirmation, with little discussion of the implications.

WHEN SCREENING IS OFFERED

At the clinic Daniella and Will were given a list of routine screening tests that would be carried out during Daniella's pregnancy. There was no explanation or discussion about these tests. As a young, healthy first-time mother, Daniella hadn't expected to be screened for fetal abnormalities. They both found the idea frightening, and it started them thinking about the implications of screening tests. They're both eager to have a natural birth and resistant to the technological approach they met at the hospital. Daniella wants a minimum of medical interference at her labor. They would have chosen a birthing center, but their doctor advised a hospital delivery as this was her first baby.

ROUTINE SCREENING TESTS

They were told that Daniella could start having tests to screen for abnormalities in her baby at 11–12 weeks with the first ultrasound scan. Then at 14-plus weeks, a blood test (known as the triple serum screen, see p.184) would be taken to look for Down syndrome, spina bifida, and gastrointestinal or genitourinary anomalies. At 16–20 weeks, she'd have an ultrasound scan, possibly followed by amniocentesis (a diagnostic test) if either screening test suggested a risk of abnormality in her baby.

Daniella is completely confused. She doesn't understand the difference between a screening test and a diagnostic test, and she doesn't really understand why they are necessary.

SCREENING AND PROBABILITY

I explained to Daniella that a screening test is by definition a blunt instrument. It doesn't give any precise information. It can do no more than pick up a tendency for something to happen. The way doctors express this tendency is in terms of probability.

So if a blood test gives a one in 150 chance of the baby's having Down syndrome, it means that if Daniella had 150 babies, one of them would have Down. This is a very small risk, but for Daniella, any risk of Down syndrome is a big risk; she wants the test to come back entirely negative. As I pointed out, on the scale of probability, one in 150 is exceedingly low. But these days any result higher than one in 250 means that Daniella will be offered more tests. The next step would be a precise diagnostic test to detect a specific abnormality. This is normally only done if a screening test is positive.

DIAGNOSTIC TESTS

Such tests are precise enough to give the answer "yes" or "no"; "present" or "absent"; "normal" or "abnormal." Unfortunately, they're quite invasive, and the most widely used, amniocentesis (see p.185), involves drawing a specimen of amniotic fluid containing cells from the baby out of the uterus—a delicate operation requiring skilled guidance with ultrasound. The cells are then examined for chromosomal or genetic damage in a specialist laboratory. I told Daniella that amniocentesis itself also carries a risk of miscarriage of about one in 200 (0.5 percent).

At this point Daniella asked the right question: "How long before I get the result?" In most clinics, even the best, it's a three-week wait. Daniella was upset. She said she'd be wracked with fear in half that time. I can only agree. It's brutal and inhumane to make a pregnant mother wait three weeks to find out if she's carrying a normal baby, especially as she may be feeling her baby move by the time the result comes through. "And what if the amniocentesis confirms Down syndrome?", Daniella asked. The blunt answer is: "You'd be counseled about whether to terminate the pregnancy."

OTHER TYPES OF TESTS

Daniella is feeling more and more upset. She'd never thought about the possibility of termination. Her dilemma might be eased with a nuchal scan, which could be done as early as 11 weeks and would alert her and Will to the possibility of a chromosome defect in her baby. This could be followed immediately with a diagnostic test, such as chorionic villus sampling or CVS (see p.186). This can be done much earlier in pregnancy and results can be obtained in as little as three days. Like amniocentesis, CVS carries a small risk of miscarriage. However, I could see Daniella was getting confused, so I gave her the checklist below to help.

WHAT IF SOMETHING IS FOUND?

The thought of terminating their pregnancy is an enormous shock. Will and Daniella feel the very idea of aborting their baby is unthinkable, whether or not tests show that their baby is normal. They are certain they'll go on with the pregnancy whatever the test results. They are unshakable in their desire to love and nurture their baby, whether or not he or she has a disability.

Their determination makes them wonder whether they should have any screening tests at all, in that the results wouldn't change anything. They also need to weigh up the risks to the pregnancy of allowing tests to go ahead when the chances are high that the pregnancy is perfectly healthy given Daniella's age.

Screening tests aren't mandatory—they're optional. I suggested to Will and Daniella that they ask to see the obstetrician in charge of the clinic to talk about their position, before they make a decision to forego all tests.

Checklist of specialist tests

Screening tests

• Nuchal scan: a special ultrasound scan carried out at 11–13 weeks that screens for high risks of chromosomal defects (see p.184)

• Triple test: A sample of the mother's blood at 15–18 weeks screens for hormone levels indicating a higher risk of Down syndrome (see p.184)

• AFP Test: A blood test at 15–18 weeks screens alphafetoprotein levels, which may show a risk of Down syndrome. This test is being used less often

Diagnostic tests

• Chorionic villus sampling: cells from the developing placenta are examined at 11–13 weeks to check the baby for chromosomal abnormalities (see p.186)

• Amniocentesis: fetal cells from the amniotic fluid are removed at about 18 weeks and checked for chromosomal abnormalities such as Down syndrome (see p.185)

• Cordocentesis: in this test, fetal blood from the umbilical cord is tested for abnormal chromosomes or infection (see p.187)

CHAPTER 8

Caring for your unborn baby

If you're observant and aware, you and your partner can be in touch with your unborn baby throughout pregnancy. Your baby can hear you talk and sing, and can feel you touch him through your abdominal wall. And while not all babies have a trouble-free development, modern medical techniques mean that even these babies have the best possible chance.

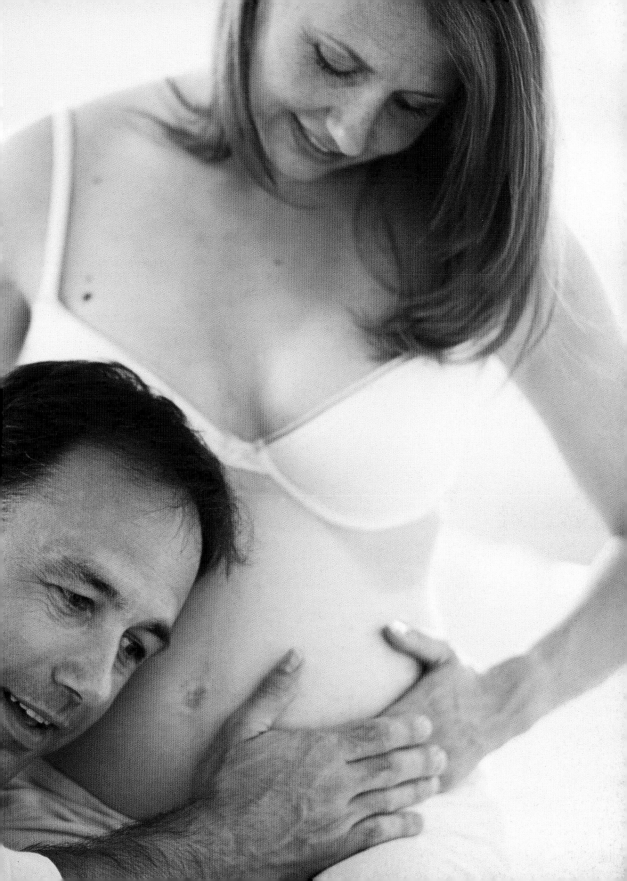

In touch with your baby

It's never too early to start getting in touch with your baby. What you say, do, think, or feel, even the way you move, may be carried through to your baby in your womb.

Talk and sing Get in the habit of talking out loud to your baby and singing to her. Some children have recognized lullabies played to them when they were in the womb.

Touching Stroking your baby through your tummy is another way of keeping in touch. It will usually soothe her and may continue to do so after she is born. In the final months, you may be able to feel her foot or hand through your skin.

Thinking Be aware of your baby. Think positive, happy thoughts about her. If you're upset about something, don't shut her out.

Moving Keep your movements as relaxed as you can. The gentle movement of your womb as you walk soothes her. Rocking and swinging will remain a favorite relaxing activity after she's born.

Feeling When you feel happy and excited, so does your baby. When you feel depressed, so does she—so reassure her that you still love her. Share feelings with her consciously.

Being aware of your unborn baby at all times is the first stage in bonding with her and making sure you have a good relationship in the future. Keeping in touch means you'll be aware of what's best for your baby's physical and emotional health.

WHAT YOUR BABY EXPERIENCES

Even while she's in your womb, your baby feels, hears, sees, tastes, responds, and even learns and remembers. She's not, despite what doctors used to think, an unformed, blank personality. She has firm likes and dislikes. She enjoys soothing voices, simple music with a single melody line (lullabies, flute music), rhythmic movements, and the feeling of your stroking her through your skin. Her dislikes include loud voices; music with an insistent beat (hard rock); strong, flashing lights; rapid, jerky movements; and being cramped when you sit or lie in an awkward position.

Sight Although your baby is protected by the walls of your womb and abdomen, very strong light can get through to her; she can detect sunlight if you're sunbathing, for instance. What she sees is probably just a reddish glow, but from about the fourth month, she'll respond to it, usually by turning away if it's too bright. The limits of her sight at birth (she'll be able to see faces within 12 in/30 cm of her own) may be a result of the limits of her "home" before she was born.

Sound Your baby's sense of hearing develops at about the third month, and by midterm she's able to respond to sounds coming from the outside world (see above). She's suspended in *amniotic fluid*, which carries sounds well, although what she hears will be muffled just like sounds are when you're under water. She's also able to make out the emotional tone of voices and moves her body in rhythm to your speech. She'll be soothed if you use a soft, reassuring tone.

The sound of your heartbeat is a constant presence in her world, and this seems to have a lasting influence on her. In one study, newborn babies who were played a tape of mothers' heart sounds gained more weight and slept better than a control group of babies who did not hear the tape.

A MOTHER'S INFLUENCE

Your unborn baby first experiences the world through you, her mother. Your baby senses not only things happening outside the womb (see above), but also your feelings. She can do this because our various emotions trigger the release of different chemicals into our bloodstream—anger releases adrenalin, fear releases *cholamines*, elation releases *endorphins*. These chemicals pass across the placenta to your baby within seconds of your feeling that particular emotion.

Babies don't like their mothers to feel negative emotions, such as anger, anxiety, or fear, for long periods. But short bursts of intense anxiety or anger (caused by a moment of panic or an argument with your partner) don't appear to have any long-term effect on your unborn child. They may even be good for her, as they may help her start to learn how to cope with stressful situations in the future. On the other hand, research suggests that long-term festering anger or anxiety, such as you might feel if you have relationship problems or an unsupportive partner, or you're living in poor conditions, can be harmful for your baby. These effects may include a problematic birth, a low birthweight, being a colicky baby, and future learning problems. Fortunately, studies also show that if a mother is generally happy and positive about being pregnant and doesn't shut out her unborn baby, any periods of negative emotions seem to have far less effect.

A FATHER'S INFLUENCE

As the expectant father, you are the second most important influence in your unborn baby's life. Your attitude toward your partner, the pregnancy, and your child is crucial. If you're happy and looking forward to your baby's birth, your partner is much more likely to be content and to enjoy her pregnancy. Your baby, in turn, is much more likely to be a happy, healthy child. Try to talk to your unborn baby as often as you can—research has shown that newborn babies can recognize the voices of their fathers as well as their mothers.

WHAT YOUR BABY DOES

Even while still in the womb, your baby is a little personality, with many ways of interacting with her world.

Movement She moves constantly while she's awake. She'll kick and wriggle her body in response to what's happening outside—for instance, if you sit in a position she finds uncomfortable.

Hearing From the sixth month your baby responds to sounds. She moves in rhythm to your voice, and she may jump and kick when you raise your voice.

Seeing She doesn't like bright light, especially if it flashes. She'll move away, put her hands up to her face, or become agitated.

Feelings She'll have changes in mood to match yours when the chemicals your emotions release into your bloodstream cross the placenta into her body.

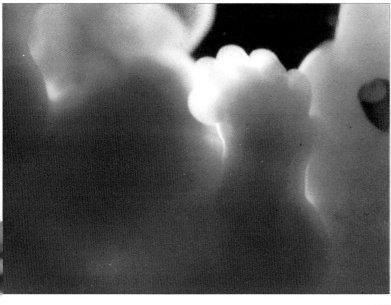

Her secure world
If she finds the world she experiences through you a reassuring place, she's likely to develop a generally trusting, positive personality. If she finds the uterus stressful, she may develop a generally anxious approach to life.

Your baby's movements

You can feel your baby's movements because they're transmitted through the wall of your womb to the sensitive nerve endings in your abdomen.

The reason you don't feel any of your baby's movements until several weeks after they actually begin is partly because they're very weak at first, and partly because your womb doesn't transmit them. Only when your womb has grown enough to touch the wall of your abdomen are you able to feel any movements inside it.

If your baby is kicking or squirming more than usual, sit down in a comfortable, quiet place and calm her down. Playing her gentle, relaxing music, singing her a lullaby, or humming to her will often help. The sound will be pleasant to her, and you'll become more relaxed yourself, so she'll tend to do the same. Reading to her, or just talking, is also soothing, as is gently stroking your stomach.

The moment you feel your baby move inside you for the first time is a huge thrill—proof that she actually exists. Even though you may have had an ultrasound scan, which showed your baby moving around in the womb, she'll seem much more real when you feel her for yourself. If she's your first baby, you'll probably first notice her movements inside your womb at about 18–20 weeks. If you've already had a child, you may feel movements at 16–18 weeks or even before. The earliest noticeable movements of the baby—known as "quickening"—make a delicate sensation that's been likened to the fluttering of wings. First-time mothers often mistake this feeling for indigestion, gas, or hunger pangs, but the experienced mother knows what to expect, so is quicker to identify these feelings as movements of her baby.

WHY YOUR BABY MOVES

Your baby stretches and flexes her growing limbs as they develop. This activity is vital to help her muscles grow properly and starts around the eighth week, when she begins making tiny movements of her spine. In those early weeks you might not notice her movements, but by about the end of the sixteenth week, you may feel the vigorous kicking of the now fully formed limbs, although you might not recognize them.

Your baby will kick, push, punch, squirm, and do somersaults, and you'll often see as well as feel her movements. She'll move more and more as she grows, and is at her most active between weeks 30 and 32. The typical baby averages 200 movements a day at week 20, rising to 375 a day at week 32, but the number of movements a day can range from 100 to about 700 over a period of several days.

After week 32, it will become harder for your baby to move as she grows to fill the uterus. Although restricted, she'll still be able to give plenty of sharp kicks. When her engaged head bounces on your pelvic floor muscles, you'll feel a jolt.

Changing position and emotional reactions Your baby needs to exercise and coordinate her growing muscles, but she also moves around for other reasons.

She may, for instance, shift her position because she feels like a change, or because you're sitting or lying in a position that's uncomfortable for her. Or she may be trying to find the thumb that she'd been happily sucking before she moved.

She may also be moving around in response to your emotions. Hormones, such as adrenalin, are released into your bloodstream when you're physically or emotionally stimulated. Pleasure, excitement, anger, stress, anxiety, or fear also stimulate the production of chemicals that will pass across the placenta and into your baby's bloodstream. These hormones affect your baby, so if you get angry or very anxious, she may become agitated and start kicking and squirming. If you can, sit down in a quiet place and practice your relaxation techniques (see p.258). This will help to calm both you and your baby.

COUNTING THE KICKS

Just like the rest of us, your baby will feel and be more active on some days than on others, but her daily pattern of movements will become more consistent after about week 28. From then on you can keep tabs on your baby's movements. On average, most women can feel around nine out of every 10 of their baby's movements, although for some women the proportion is only six out of every 10.

Whether you feel a movement or not depends on its direction and strength, and the position your baby is in when she makes it. For instance, if she is facing and kicking in toward your spine, you won't feel the sort of short, sharp jab that you get if she kicks out toward your belly or up toward your ribs.

FETAL MOVEMENT RECORDING

There are several ways of counting your baby's movements, and your prenatal clinic may give you their own "kick chart" to fill in, or you can make your own "count-to-ten" kick chart like the one shown (right), which you can draw up on a piece of graph paper. You don't have to keep a kick chart, but it can be a useful way of checking your baby's well-being.

Making a kick chart Down the left of the chart, mark out a 12-hour period, from 9 a.m. to 9 p.m., during which you're going to count the number of movements your baby makes. Mark in the days and weeks across the top, with a column of squares for each day of the week.

Each day, choose a two-hour period during which you'll count the number of movements your baby makes until you reach 10. Mark the time of the tenth movement on your chart. For instance, if you start on the Monday of the 29th week of pregnancy, and you count 10 movements by quarter to three in the afternoon, fill in the 2:30 square. You don't have to count any more that day. If on any day you count fewer than 10 movements in two hours, fill in the actual number in the space at the bottom on the chart. Go to the hospital or call your doctor or midwife if there's any change in your baby's usual movements.

If you notice any significant change in the pattern of your baby's movements as your due date approaches, tell your doctor. If you feel fewer than 10 movements for two days in a row, call your doctor or the hospital. If you don't feel any movements at all in one day, get in touch with your doctor or the hospital immediately. It's especially important to monitor movements after 40 weeks to ensure that your baby is doing well. Even if the kicks seem to have stopped, don't panic. Your doctor or midwife can quickly assess your baby with ultrasound and electronic fetal monitoring and decide whether anything needs to be done.

KICK CHART

Time	39th week							40th week						
	M	T	W	T	F	S	S	M	T	W	T	F	S	S
9 am														
9:30														
10 am														
10:30														
11 am														
11:30														
12 pm														
12:30														
1 pm														
1:30		▓												
2 pm														
2:30	▓													
3 pm										▓				
3:30			▓											
4 pm											▓			
4:30														
5 pm									▓					
5:30														
6 pm														
6:30														
7 pm														
7:30														
8 pm														
8:30														
9 pm														

If fewer than 10 movements in two hours, record total here.

9														
8				▓										
7														
6														
5														
4														
3														
2														
1														

Monitoring your baby's movements

This is a useful way of checking your baby's well-being, especially if you're overdue. Only you can tell if your baby is moving in a way that's normal for her. If there's a significant drop in the number of her movements, contact your doctor, midwife, or the hospital.

Fetal problems

I know this is something that every mother worries about, but I can't stress strongly enough that such problems are very, very rare, so please try not to be too anxious. The cause of many fetal defects is still unknown. Some may be caused by a defective gene (see p.24) while others could be due to the harmful effects of drugs, radiation, infections of a baby in the womb, or metabolic disturbances.

There are a number of different kinds of defects, but most are very rare. The parts of a baby's body that are most actively growing at the time when the damaging factor happens are the most likely to show the defect. Some malformations are incompatible with life, and no treatment is possible. The defects that are especially important to recognize just after birth are those that endanger life but, with prompt intervention, can be treated successfully. The good news is that an increasing number of problems are now picked up by ultrasound scans before birth (see p.180), and many can be treated just after birth or later in infancy.

Imperforate anus This means that the anus is sealed, either because there's a thin membrane of skin over the anal opening, or the anal canal that links the rectum with the anus has not developed. The rectal pouch may be connected to the vagina, urethra, or bladder, and a baby with this problem will need immediate surgery. This condition is rare, but every baby is carefully checked at birth, so treatment can be given if necessary.

Umbilical hernia In most babies, the gap in the muscle sheath in the abdominal cavity, where the umbilical cord entered his abdomen, normally closes up in time. Sometimes, though, a soft swelling called an umbilical hernia forms when the abdominal contents bulge through this weak spot in the abdomen. The hernia usually disappears eventually, although a few babies may need surgery later in childhood.

Congenital heart disease Hole in the heart (ventricular septal defect) is the most common form of congenital heart disease. In this condition there's a hole in the baby's *septum*, the thin dividing wall between the right and left ventricles (pumping chambers) of the heart, so the ventricles are connected instead of being divided. A newborn baby doesn't usually show any signs of the problem. It may take as long as four weeks for the blood vessels in the lungs to relax sufficiently to allow pressure differences to develop between the ventricles ,and this means that there may be much left-to-right shunt of blood through the hole for a month or so. Until then, there probably won't be any symptoms. Signs to look out for are a bluish tinge to the skin, especially

NEONATAL HEART SCANS

A *congenital* condition is one that's present from birth. Congenital heart disease can be diagnosed by a form of ultrasound scan called *echocardiography*.

A congenital heart condition, such as hole in the heart (*ventricular septal defect*—see main text), sometimes isn't detected until a baby is about four weeks old. Echocardiograms are used to confirm the diagnosis and how serious the problem is so the right treatment can be given.

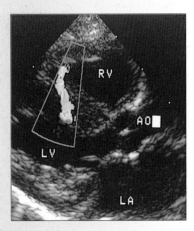

Echocardiography
The scan above shows a baby's heart with a ventricular septal defect. Echocardiograms are taken by an ultrasound scan and displayed as a series of lines on the screen. By using color enhancement, the flow through the defect is shown as red. The abbreviations used are: Ao = aorta (main artery); RV = right ventricle (pumping chamber that pumps blood into the lungs to be oxygenated); LA = left atrium (collecting chamber that collects reoxygenated blood from the lungs); LV = left ventricle (pumps reoxygenated blood back to the body).

around the mouth, floppiness, and breathlessness. One of the first signs may be breathlessness while feeding. Not all babies need surgery; in some, the hole closes by itself.

Some types of congenital heart disease can be picked up by an ultrasound scan before birth. If your baby is found to have a serious heart problem, your doctors may advise you to give birth in a hospital that's equipped with special facilities for dealing with such conditions.

Congenital dislocation of the hip The hip can dislocate when the ball at the head of the thighbone doesn't fit snugly into the socket of the hip joint. In the newborn infant this is a potential, rather than an actual, problem. It's much more common in girls and in breech babies.

When your midwives do their routine check of your newborn baby (see p.293), they'll check his hips for excessive mobility, or for a characteristic "clunk" felt when his legs are spread apart and his thighs are flexed. If there's any doubt, they'll get specialist advice. Early followup and treatment such as manipulation and splinting may prevent trouble later, but some babies with severe dislocation may need surgery.

Spina bifida In this condition the vertebral bones of the spine do not fuse and the *meninges* (the coverings of the brain and spinal cord) bulge through at some level in the spinal column. The area may be covered with skin, or only by a bluish membrane. It may contain nerve roots, or the spinal cord itself may be exposed. In many cases, the place where the bones of the vertebrae are not fused is covered with skin and is only marked by a small, dark, hairy mole. Happily, spina bifida is becoming less common. There's careful monitoring of those more at risk, and we know much more about the importance of taking folic acid before conception and during the early weeks of pregnancy (see p.20).

Because the various coverings that normally protect the cord aren't there, meningeal infection can happen very easily. This can be prevented by immediate surgery to cover the defect. Spina bifida can be picked up by ultrasound, and babies with a good prognosis can be sent to a special clinic where the necessary surgery can be performed without delay. But for babies with severe defects, the outlook is not encouraging. Problems may include paralysis, incontinence, mental retardation, and the appearance of *hydrocephalus* (see below).

Hydrocephalus (water on the brain) Hydrocephalus means there's too much *cerebrospinal fluid* inside the baby's skull. It often accompanies other neurological defects, such as spina bifida, and it's caused by restricted circulation of cerebrospinal fluid in the brain. Hydrocephalus is most common following brain hemorrhage in an unborn baby. The baby's head swells, and soft tissues between the skull bones and the fontanelles become wide and bulging. If this happens before birth, due to congenital

CLEFT LIP AND CLEFT PALATE

These conditions happen when the upper lip or the palate, sometimes both, don't develop completely.

In a cleft lip, sometimes known as a harelip, the halves of the upper lip fail to join properly as the baby is developing. Similarly, in a cleft palate the halves of the baby's palate fail to join.

Babies with these problems can usually breastfeed, but bottlefeeding may be more difficult. and you will need a special nipple. You also have to be careful when feeding a baby who has a cleft palate, because the cleft may permit milk to enter his nose and cause him to gag.

It's important to see a plastic surgeon as soon as possible to plan treatment, although some hospitals are now performing immediate closure of the cleft lip at birth. If a cleft palate is closed too early, though, it may mean a major operation during early adulthood, as the palate might not be able to develop fully. Most recently surgeons are using devices to stretch the tissues first, and then perform the surgery at a later date.

TRISOMIES

Trisomy is a chromosomal disorder. There are three chromosomes where normally there would only be a pair, and this defect exists in all the cells of the affected person.

The most common trisomy is Down syndrome (see p.24), also known as trisomy 21, in which there are three number 21 chromosomes.

The baby is born with small features, a tongue that tends to stick out, and slanting eyes with folds of skin at their inner corners. The head is flat at the back, and the ears are unusual. The baby may be rather floppy, with hands and feet that are usually short and wide and have a single transverse crease across the palms and soles. He may also have congenital heart disease.

Down syndrome sufferers are usually mentally handicapped, although the degree of handicap varies, and many Down syndrome children are near normal.

Children with Down syndrome are very rewarding. They're affectionate, outgoing, and have a great sense of humor. With careful attention and early education, many do well and some manage to live independently.

Other trisomies include trisomy 13 (Patau syndrome) and trisomy 18 (Edwards syndrome), both of which produce a number of severe physical and mental abnormalities. Both these conditions are much rarer than Down syndrome.

malformations, it will obstruct labor, or cause a baby's head to get very large after birth. If doctors suspect hydrocephalus before birth, they will make frequent ultrasound checks and measure the circumference of the baby's head.

Neural tube defects such as spina bifida and hydrocephalus may be diagnosed by ultrasound (see p.180) or amniocentesis (see p.185) well before a baby is born.

Cerebral palsy This is caused by damage to the brain before, during, or after birth—for instance, because of a poor supply of oxygen to the brain in late pregnancy or a difficult labor. Other causes include infection of a mother's uterus, or meningitis or a severe injury to the baby's head after birth. Premature babies are particularly vulnerable.

Cerebral palsy causes muscular paralysis, stiffness, and coordination problems. It cannot be detected before birth, and the symptoms aren't usually obvious until a baby is several months old and his development appears to be delayed. He may not be walking, sitting, or making normal progress as expected; he may have stiffness in his arms or legs, or a persistent abnormal posture. The degree of disability varies widely. If the limbs tend to be stiff and fixed in certain postures, a child is termed "spastic." If he is prone to frequent, purposeless writing movements, he is said to be "*athetoid.*"

Cerebral palsy is an incurable condition, but it is not progressive—it doesn't get worse as the child grows older. And it's quite common for a child with cerebral palsy to have normal intelligence and social capabilities. Physiotherapy will help to prevent the deformities caused by stiffness and spasms, and develop muscular balance and control; speech therapy will help to ease any communication problems. As with all disabled children, the emphasis should always be on what the child can do, not on what he cannot.

Respiratory distress syndrome (RDS) In this condition, a baby's lungs are lacking in *surfactant*, a substance that keeps open the minute air sacs in the lungs through which oxygen is absorbed into the blood. It happens because the baby's lungs are immature, or because crucial lung cells are temporarily not working properly because of a lack of oxygen. Respiratory distress syndrome is most common in small premature babies and in babies of diabetic mothers whose condition is not sufficiently well controlled. It's very rare in full-term babies.

Now that doctors are better able to detect immaturity of a baby's lungs before birth and the management of early deliveries and resuscitation has improved, RDS happens more rarely. It can also sometimes be prevented or made less severe by treating the mother with steroids before delivery. Infants born with RDS need to be cared for in an intensive care unit and are given surfactant to mature their lungs.

Pyloric stenosis In this condition the ring of muscle (the *pylorus*) linking the stomach to the small intestine thickens and narrows. It's much more common in boys, but the cause is unknown.

Symptoms begin when the baby is two to four weeks old. Food builds up in the stomach, which contracts powerfully in an attempt to force the food through the narrow pylorus. Because this is impossible, milk is vomited up violently after a feeding. This is known as projectile vomiting because the vomit may be thrown for up to a couple of yards. The baby may suffer constipation and dehydration. A simple operation widens the pylorus, giving a complete cure.

Epispadias and hypospadias About one in 1000 male babies has an abnormality of the penile opening of the urethra. In *epispadias*, the opening is on the upper surface of the penis; the penis may curve upward. In *hypospadias*, the opening is on the underside of the glans (head) and the penis may curve down. In extreme, but rare forms of hypospadias, the urethral opening lies between the genitals and anus, and the genitals may appear female. Surgery is straightforward and usually successful. Neither epispadias nor hypospadias causes infertility.

CLUB FOOT (TALIPES)

This means that a baby is born with the sole of one foot, or both feet, facing down and inwards or up and outward.

The exact causes of the many kinds of club foot are not fully understood, but the condition can run in families. On rare occasions sufferers spontaneously recover.

Most babies, though, need treatment to correct the defect. The usual remedy is for the child's foot to be manipulated regularly over a period of many months. Between manipulations, the foot is held in place by some form of bracing such as a splint or a plaster cast. Some babies may need surgery, and this is usually successful.

FETAL DEFECTS PER 10,000 BIRTHS

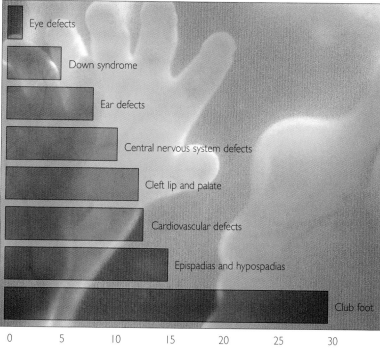

- Eye defects
- Down syndrome
- Ear defects
- Central nervous system defects
- Cleft lip and palate
- Cardiovascular defects
- Epispadias and hypospadias
- Club foot

0   5   10   15   20   25   30

Incidence of fetal defects
This chart summarizes typical occurrences of birth defects. It may be worrisome to think about, but the chart shows just how rare most of these are. The most common is club foot, which affects both boys and girls. Epispadias and hypospadias, the second most common, are defects of the urethra and affect only boys. Cardiovascular defects affect the heart and circulatory system, including congenital heart disease, and the defects of the central nervous system include spina bifida and hydrocephalus.

Fetal surgery

EFFECTS ON PARENTS

If your unborn baby has to have surgery, it's going to be a very stressful time. But most parents cope extremely well.

When an unborn baby is diagnosed as having a serious illness or defect, doctors may suggest fetal surgery. This is a hard decision for parents, and they'll be given expert counseling to help them decide whether or not to go ahead. Fetal surgery is advancing rapidly but is still very much at the experimental stage. In some experienced clinics, simple procedures like exchange transfusions are performed routinely. The most complicated techniques, though, are only attempted if there's nothing to lose.

If the surgery is successful, the rewards are immense, and the mother's fertility doesn't seem to be affected much. Many women conceive again and have normal pregnancies. With less successful surgery, a woman could suffer miscarriage or premature birth, or have to have a cesarean section. She may also have complications after the operation, which can be extremely stressful for all concerned.

Thanks to the development of specialized surgical techniques, it's now possible to correct some defects when a baby is still in the womb. Some procedures are still experimental, but they may be the baby's only chance, and many parents see this as a risk worth taking.

There is only a small number of pioneering surgeons involved in the highly specialized field of fetal surgery, and the number of defects they can help is limited, but research is continuing. New methods are constantly being tried and evaluated, and as the diagnosis of fetal defects improves, it's getting easier for doctors to decide if surgery is appropriate.

ULTRASOUND-GUIDED SURGERY

In the more straightforward types of fetal surgery, thin needles are inserted through a mother's abdomen and womb and into the amniotic sac. Ultrasound allows the surgeon to see the baby and manipulate the needles (only one at a time is used) to take blood or tissue samples or give the baby any drugs or blood transfusions that are necessary.

Using ultrasound-guided techniques, surgeons are able to treat a growing number of life-threatening conditions. Rhesus and other incompatibilities between the immune systems of mother and baby may be corrected through intrauterine blood transfusions. Drugs to correct fetal heartbeat irregularities and destroy tumors may be injected into the baby; minute drainage tubes (shunts) that prevent further buildup of fluids may be inserted to drain excess fluids from the baby—for instance, from the brain in cases of hydrocephalus—and to clear urinary tract blockages. Ultrasound is also used to guide the tiny forceps and scalpels with which surgery can be carried out.

Intrauterine blood transfusions In some cases of Rhesus incompatibility (see p.202), in which a mother's blood is Rhesus- (Rh-) negative and her baby's Rh-positive, the baby may become dangerously anemic. If this happens, he'll be given one or more blood transfusions into one of the blood vessels in the umbilical cord to keep him going until he can be delivered safely. Fresh Rhesus-negative blood will be injected slowly, in amounts related to the baby's estimated weight and the seriousness of the anemia.

Blood transfusions made to a baby in the womb have a good success rate, but in some severe cases, Rh incompatibility causes miscarriage or stillbirth, despite numerous transfusions. Until recently, if transfusions were unsuccessful, there was nothing more that could be done. Research is underway, though, to find out whether injecting the baby with donated Rh-negative bone marrow will stimulate him to become Rh-negative and so remove the incompatibility.

A more uncommon type of incompatibility between a mother and her baby results in the mother's producing antibodies that destroy the baby's blood platelets. These platelets help blood to clot, and without them the baby could be in danger of suffering a hemorrhage and dying. This situation can now be prevented by giving the baby transfusions of platelets and, in severe cases, donor antibodies that counteract those of his mother.

Shunts for urinary tract problems Some unborn babies suffer a condition called *hydronephrosis*. In this, one of the baby's kidneys becomes swollen with urine because the ureter that drains it is narrow or blocked. If left untreated, this can lead to severe kidney damage; if it affects both kidneys, it can cause kidney failure. Hydronephrosis can sometimes be corrected by the insertion of shunts by means of fetal surgery.

OPEN FETAL SURGERY

This is an even more extraordinary technique, used to correct some fetal defects that cannot be treated by ultrasound-guided surgery. It involves opening up a woman's womb and partially removing her baby so he can be operated on. Open fetal surgery has been used to repair *diaphragmatic hernias*—when a baby has a hole in his diaphragm that allows his intestines to protrude into his chest cavity and damage his lungs—and to remove certain types of tumors.

The operation Ultrasound-guided techniques are always carried out under local anesthetic, but for open fetal surgery, both mother and baby need a general anesthetic. When the anesthetic has taken effect, the surgeon makes an incision in the mother's abdomen to expose her womb, and uses an ultrasound scan to find the exact position of the placenta. The amniotic fluid is then drawn off and kept warm. Next, an incision about five inches (12 cm) long is made in the womb and amniotic membranes, taking care to keep well away from the placenta to avoid damaging it. The baby is eased gently out through this opening, just far enough for the surgeon to be able to repair the defect.

After the operation Once the surgeon is finished, the baby is carefully replaced in his mother's womb, along with the amniotic fluid. A small amount of antibiotic is added to the fluid to prevent infection. The incisions in the amniotic membranes and the womb are closed with absorbable stitches and surgical glue, and the incision in the abdomen is stitched together.

The mother rests in bed after the operation, and she and her baby are intensively monitored. Although generally healthy, most babies who undergo open fetal surgery are born before term, usually by cesarean section.

PROSPECTS FOR A BABY

Fetal surgery is used to help babies who have defects that are easier to correct before they are born than afterward, or who will die without it.

In general, the earlier in pregnancy fetal surgery is carried out, the better a baby's chances of survival. There are two main reasons for this. First, wounds heal relatively quickly in a developing baby. Second, organs that cannot grow until the defect is repaired have time to complete their normal development. For instance, if a baby's lungs cannot grow properly because of a diaphragmatic hernia, they'll need time to mature so that he'll be able to use them when he's born.

The exact time when a baby canbe operated on depends on a number of factors—most importantly, when the defect can be diagnosed. Blood and antibody problems can usually be detected in the earliest weeks of pregnancy, and often, as in many cases of Rh incompatibility, they may be predicted. Most physical malformations cannot be diagnosed until the organ or organs they affect have grown enough for the defect to be apparent. As a result, surgery to correct defects of this type isn't usually carried out until after about week 18.

The Rh-Negative mother

Case study

Name   Elizabeth Duncan
Age   27 years
Past medical history   Nothing abnormal
Obstetric history   One daughter age
two years; normal birth, no postnatal
complications; child's blood group
Rhesus- positive

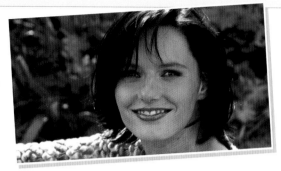

Elizabeth's blood group is Rhesus-negative and her partners, Chris, is Rhesus-positive. This means that their second baby has a 50:50 chance of being born Rhesus-negative if Chris passes on a recessive Rhesus-negative gene. Their first baby was Rhesus-positive so Elizabeth may have developed anti-Rhesus-positive antibodies. If this second baby is Rhesus-positive, the baby's red blood cells may be damaged by the antibodies. To prevent any damage, Elizabeth will need to have special care throughout her pregnancy.

About 85 per cent of people have the Rhesus factor in their red blood cells and they are Rhesus positive. The other 15 per cent who lack the factor are Rhesus negative. A Rhesus-negative mother who's carrying a Rhesus-positive baby may develop antibodies to her Rhesus baby's Rhesus-positive blood cells and injure them.

AN INCOMPATIBLE MOTHER AND BABY

Elizabeth's first pregnancy went without a hitch. This is usual with first pregnancies where the mother has Rhesus-negative blood and the baby is Rhesus-positive (an incompatible pregnancy).

However, when cells from the baby's blood mix with blood cells from the mother—for example, during delivery—the mother's blood becomes sensitized. When the Rh factor from the baby's blood enters the mother's bloodstream, it acts as an *antigen* and stimulates the production of anti-Rhesus-positive antibodies. These will attack and destroy the blood cells of her next Rhesus-positive (incompatible) baby. This causes *hemolytic* disease of the newborn (see p.342) and infants affected with blood conditions ranging from mild jaundice to serious, possibly fatal, anemia. Fetuses that develop the disease can often be saved by intrauterine blood transfusion (see p.200).

DO ALL WOMEN BECOME SENSITIZED?

Not all Rh-negative women with Rh-positive babies become sensitized, but there's no way of predicting which women will. All women who are Rhesus-negative should be offered an Anti-D injection at 28 weeks of pregnancy and after delivery of a Rh-positive baby. Women who are Rhesus negative are also given an Anti-D injection after the following:

• an abortion
• chorionic villus sampling
• an amniocentesis or cordocentesis, especially if there's blood on the needle after it is withdrawn from the uterus
• heavy vaginal bleeding after miscarriage

DESENSITIZING ELIZABETH

Within 48 hours of delivering her first baby, Elizabeth was injected with Anti-D (Rh immune-globulin) to help prevent the destructive antibodies from forming. If she'd miscarried, she would have also needed the injection, because her blood and her baby's would have mixed.

CAREFUL MONITORING

It's likely that Elizabeth won't have developed antibodies because she was given Anti-D after the birth of her first baby. In this case she won't need any further tests. However, if antibodies have already formed, the Anti-D injection will be ineffective. Therefore, Elizabeth's blood

Elizabeth's baby

Elizabeth's baby is likely to be fit and healthy, thanks to the Anti-D injections and the special care she'll have during her pregnancy.

• Immediately after the birth, Elizabeth's baby will have a Coombs test to check for the presence of maternal anti-Rhesus-positive antibodies.

• If the baby is affected by Rh incompatibility, his bilirubin levels will rise quickly after birth because his liver can't get rid of it.

• He may need an exchange transfusion—blood can be withdrawn from the baby via the umbilical vein and replaced with donor blood that's compatible with his mother's blood. If severe hemolytic disease had been predicted before he was born, he may have been successfully treated by a transfusion while in the womb.

• A high level of bilirubin will make him look yellow. This can be treated by placing him under ultraviolet "bili" light, which converts bilirubin into a harmless substance.

will need to be monitored throughout her pregnancy. At each visit, Elizabeth will have a specimen of blood taken to examine for increasing levels of antibodies. Only if they increase beyond a certain point is her developing baby in any danger. If this happens, she'll have a Doppler scan (see p.187). This will show whether her baby has a healthy blood flow and indicate when a blood transfusion through the umbilical cord may be needed.

In the second or third trimester, a test for the presence of *bilirubin* (a byproduct of red blood cell destruction) can be done by cordocentesis (see p.187). This lets doctors check how severe the condition is and decide if blood transfusions are needed.

BIRTH EXPECTATIONS

If her antibody count remains low, Elizabeth won't need further special care during her pregnancy. If the count rises moderately, her baby may be induced early to prevent serious consequences. Elizabeth will need to deliver in a hospital with an experienced obstetric department and NICU (Neonatal Intensive Care Unit). In a very few cases, the baby has to have a blood transfusion to replace its own blood cells that have become damaged during pregnancy.

RHESUS DISEASE IN PREGNANCY

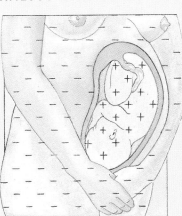

Rhesus disease only happens when a woman who has Rhesus-negative blood (symbolized by red minus signs in the picture) is pregnant with a Rhesus-positive (symbolized by blue plus signs in the picture) baby. Most Rhesus-negative mothers carry their first babies without any problems—just as Elizabeth did. If they then develop antibodies to Rhesus-positive blood (symbolized by green triangles in the pictures below), any babies that they have later could be at risk.

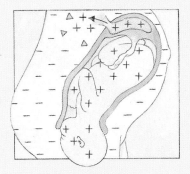

Mother is sensitized
If the mother is not given an Anti-D injection within 48 hours of delivery, she may develop antibodies to Rhesus-positive blood.

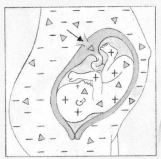

A future pregnancy
If she becomes pregnant with another Rhesus-positive baby, her antibodies may attack this baby's red blood cells.

CHAPTER 9

Common complaints

Very few women go through pregnancy without suffering a few ailments, but most are uncomfortable rather than serious. Knowing what might happen is half the battle and also allows you to tell the difference between those that are just a nuisance and those that could be serious.

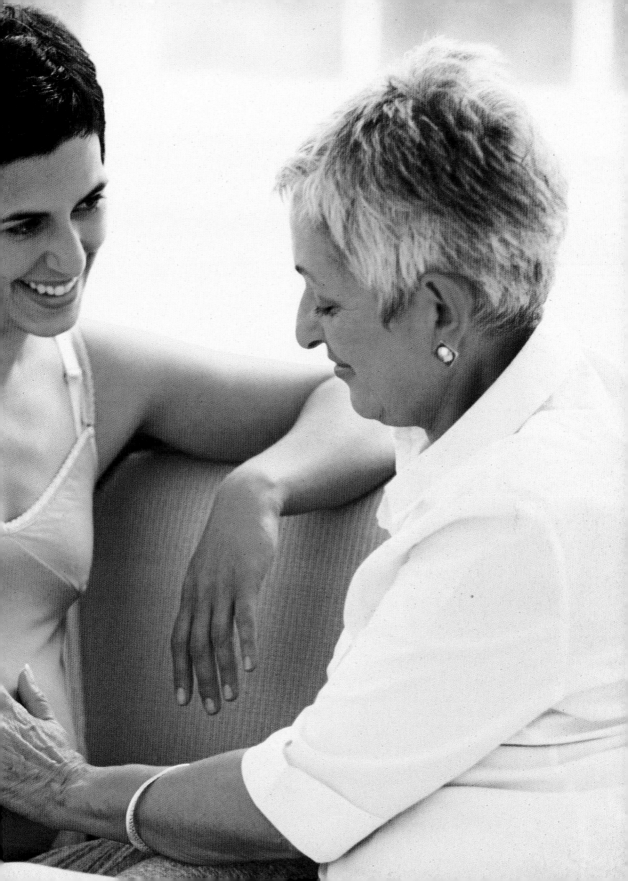

Common Complaints

Complaint	Why it happens
Backaches are usually felt as general discomfort across the lower back, often with pain across the buttocks and down the legs. You can get it when you've been standing for too long with bad posture, or after lifting something heavy, especially during the third trimester.	High progesterone levels soften the ligaments of the pelvic bones so they stretch to allow your baby to be born. But the ligaments of the spine also relax, putting extra strain on the joints of the back and hips.
You might also get an intensely painful low backache when you rotate your spine and pelvis in opposite directions, such as when you turn over sideways in bed.	The baby is resting against your sacroiliac joint, which is located some 3 in (7½ cm) in from the top of your buttocks. Rotary movements of the spine and pelvis open and close the sacroiliac joint, causing pain.
Carpal tunnel syndrome feels like pins and needles, mainly in your thumb and index finger, with numbness and sometimes weakness. Occasionally your whole hand and forearm can be affected, and this can happen from conception onward.	Pressure on the nerve that passes from the arm to the hand along the front of the wrist. The pressure is caused by swelling of the carpal tunnel (a ring of fibers around the wrist under which the nerve passes) because of water retention.
Constipation is when you have dry, hard stools that are difficult to pass. This may happen from conception onward.	Progesterone relaxes the muscles in the intestinal walls, so there are fewer contractions to push the food along. This means that much more water than usual is absorbed from the stool in the colon, making it hard and dry. Stools may be less frequent, too.
Cramps are a sudden pain in your thigh, calf, and/or foot, followed by a general ache that lasts for some time. They tend to be more common in the third trimester, and usually wake you from sleep.	Cramps may be caused by low calcium levels in the blood, or they can be due to salt deficiency. Check with your doctor.

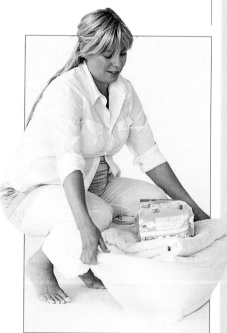

Protecting your back

When lifting anything heavy, whether a pile of laundry or a toddler, always use your thighs to do the work. Don't treat your back as a crane.

When you're pregnant, you may have a number of minor complaints that are irritating but not serious. Most are caused by a combination of hormonal changes and the extra strain that your body is experiencing. They can be treated very simply, and are nothing to worry about. A few, though, can be serious, so it's important to be aware of the symptoms and be prepared to do something right away if you're worried.

What can be done

Risk to baby

Massage may help (see p.152). Do exercises to strengthen your spine. Make sure your mattress is firm. Lift heavy weights correctly (see bottom left, opposite). Try to improve your posture (see p.160), and don't wear high-heeled shoes. If the pain runs down your leg toward your foot, check with your doctor in case it's a slipped disk.
Osteopathy can be helpful, in even the most severe cases. Backaches usually ease off in the fifth month when your baby tips forward—although you may not be able to wait that long!

None.

You will be given physiotherapy treatment. A splint on the wrist at night may help, as may holding your hand above your head and wiggling your fingers. Acupuncture may help too. Sleep with your arm on a pillow. Symptoms usually disappear soon after delivery.

None.

Drink lots of water. Eat as much roughage in the form of fruit, vegetables, and fiber as you can. Walk briskly for 20 minutes once a day or more. Don't take a laxative without consulting your doctor. Natural fiber laxatives are best because they simply increase the amount of water in the stool, making it soft. Figs and prunes will also do the job.

None.

Massage the area very firmly. Flex your foot up and push into the heel.

None.

Relieving foot cramps
Keeping your foot flexed up, carefully make circling movements with your lower leg.

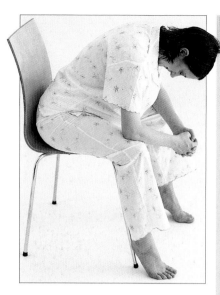

What to do if you feel faint
If you feel faint, sit down and bend your head toward your knees. When you feel better, get up slowly.

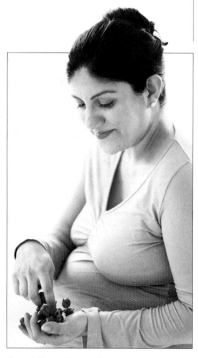

Avoiding heartburn
Eat smaller meals so your stomach doesn't get too full. Try snacking on nutritious foods such as fruit and nuts and eating little but often.

Complaint

Diarrhea can happen at any time during your pregnancy. You'll have soft, watery stools and need to go to the bathroom frequently.

Faintness is a feeling of dizziness or vertigo that comes on suddenly, making you unsteady on your feet. You may feel faint if you stand up too quickly, or you've been on your feet for too long, especially in hot weather.

Heartburn is a burning sensation just behind your breastbone, and you may also bring up some stomach acid into your mouth. It can happen when you lie down, cough, strain when passing a stool, or lift something heavy.

High blood pressure (hypertension) is an increase in blood pressure. It can be mild or severe, and there may be no, few, or many symptoms, including headaches, visual disturbances, and vomiting. You may also have water retention (see p.212) with swelling of your feet, hands, and ankles. High blood pressure can happen at any time, but it's more likely near your due date. It's more common in women having their first baby, especially if they're over 35, and also in women having more than one baby. Your midwife will keep a close watch on your blood pressure because a rise may be a warning of preeclamptic toxemia (PET or preeclampsia, see p.226).

Why it happens

Usually because you have an infection from bacteria or a virus.

A combination of a lack of blood supply to the brain, often caused by pooling of the blood in the legs and feet when standing, and the demands of the uterus for an increased blood supply.

Early in pregnancy, the muscular valve at the entrance to your stomach relaxes under the influence of progesterone. This allows stomach acid to flow up into your esophagus, causing a burning feeling. Later in pregnancy, your baby can press up on your stomach, forcing the contents back into the esophagus.

It's not clear why some women get high blood pressure in pregnancy. In some mothers, cells from the placenta produce chemicals called *vasoconstrictors* that may cause the blood vessels to constrict. This may raise the blood pressure and cause the kidneys to hold on to sodium, leading to water retention.

What can be done

Drink plenty of water—about 12–14 glasses a day—to replace the fluid you lose and make sure that your blood pressure remains normal. Check with your doctor, who will test your stools for infection and give you treatment if necessary.

Try not to stand for long periods. Always sit or lie down when you feel dizzy. Don't get up suddenly from sitting or get out of a hot bath too quickly. Keep cool in hot weather. If you feel dizzy, bend your head down toward your knees or lie down with your feet higher than your head.

Eat small meals so that your stomach is never too full. Sleep propped up with several pillows. Drink a glass of milk at bedtime to help to neutralize stomach acid. Your doctor may prescribe antacids, and these are safe to take throughout your pregnancy. Chewable antacid tablets are a great source of calcium and help heartburn.

If you suffered from high blood pressure before you were pregnant, tell your doctor. Keep an eye on your weight. Tell your doctor if you often have headaches and nausea.

Your doctor will test your blood pressure and urine, and look for any swelling (edema—see Water retention, p.212) of your hands, face, and ankles at each prenatal visit.

If your blood pressure goes up at any stage of your pregnancy, you'll almost certainly have to see your doctor more often and you may be watched in the hospital for 24–48 hours.

If the rise is severe, you'll need to go into the hospital, where you can be monitored continuously. If your baby appears to be suffering, your labor may be induced or you may have a cesarean section. Your blood pressure will return to normal once your baby has been born.

Risk to baby

If diarrhea goes untreated for a long time, the dehydration and loss of calories it causes can put your baby at risk. If diarrhea is profuse and protracted, you may need to go into the hospital for intravenous feeding.

None, unless you fall very heavily on to your stomach.

Pregnancy-induced hypertension (see Preeclampsia, p.224) can slow your baby's growth rate because blood flow to the uterus is reduced. Your baby may also be short of oxygen. Both these factors may lead to low birthweight. There is a severe form called eclampsia (see p.224), which can be life-threatening, but thanks to good prenatal care this is now very rare in the West.

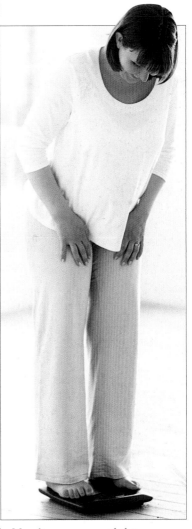

Monitor your weight
A sudden weight gain can be a symptom of preeclampsia, so tell your doctor if you notice any change.

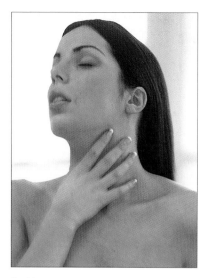

Self-massage
If you feel tense, massaging your face, especially your temples and neck, is a wonderful way to relax and can also help you get to sleep at night.

Complaint	Why it happens
Insomnia is the inability to sleep at night, making you tired and irritable during the day. It can happen at any time from conception onward.	Your baby lives on a 24-hour clock, and his metabolism keeps going even when you want to sleep. This can affect your body's responses. Other causes of insomnia include night sweats and a desire to empty your bladder more often than usual, particularly during the third trimester.
Mood swings are rapid, uncharacteristic changes in mood, often with unexplained crying and anxiety attacks. They are common from conception onward, but are especially likely to happen in the third trimester.	Changes in your hormone balance during pregnancy have a depressant effect on the nervous system, causing symptoms similar to those you may have before a period. Identity crises and the way you feel about the changes in your body may have a profound effect on you when you're pregnant, and mixed feelings about pregnancy and parenthood can cause sudden shifts in your moods.
Morning sickness is a feeling of sickness and nausea, sometimes with vomiting. Contrary to its name, it can happen at any time of the day, but generally when you haven't eaten for a long period, or after a night's sleep. Feelings of nausea are most common in the first trimester and then usually lessen.	The main cause is low blood sugar, but pregnancy hormones may irritate the stomach directly.
Hemorrhoids are dilated rectal veins (see Varicose veins, p.212) that may protrude through the anus. They don't usually develop until the second trimester.	Your growing baby presses down on your rectum and can prevent the blood from flowing back to the heart. The blood therefore pools, causing the veins to dilate to accommodate the dammed-up blood.

What can be done	Risk to baby
A warm bath and a hot milky drink at bedtime may help, as may a relaxing massage (see p.152). Watch TV or read until you feel sleepy. Find a comfortable position, and try to stay cool. Instead of sleeping pills, your doctor may prescribe an antihistamine-type medication (e.g., Benadryl) to help you sleep and be safe during your pregnancy.	None.
These are natural feelings and moments of depression, anxiety, and confusion are common even in the easiest of pregnancies. Trying to analyze such feelings may only serve to prolong them. (See also Emotional Changes, p.154.)	None.
Food will help you avoid feeling nauseous, so eat little and often. Eat high-carbohydrate foods such as whole-wheat bread, potatoes, rice, and cereals, and avoid fried food and coffee, which trigger nausea. Keep glucose candy in your car, desk, or handbag. To prevent sickness in the morning, put a glass of water and a plain cookie by your bed at night, and have them as a snack 15 minutes before you get up. Cigarette smoke and other strong smells may also trigger nausea. Drink extra fluids such as fruit juice or skim milk—if you can keep them down. Eat small, frequent meals (one plate of food over four hours).	In its severe form (called *hyperemesis gravidarum*), vomiting can deplete you of fluid and minerals, leading to low blood pressure. Tell your doctor if you vomit more than three times a day or if you lose weight for three days. In very severe cases, you may need to go to the hospital for treatment to replace the fluids that you have lost.
Eat plenty of fiber to keep your bowels regular and your stools soft—this will help you avoid straining. Don't lift weights, since this increases pressure in the abdominal area and in the rectal veins. Have coughs treated promptly for the same reasons. Aromatherapy may relieve cough symptoms.	None.

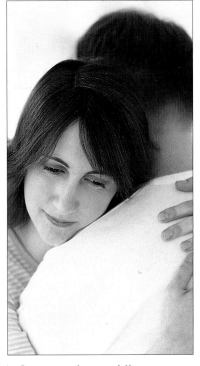

A reassuring cuddle
A comforting hug from your partner can be just what you need when you're feeling anxious and upset.

Complaint	Why it happens
Rib pain can be felt as extreme soreness and tenderness of the ribs, usually on the right side, just below the breasts. The pain may be worse when you sit down, and it tends to happen mainly during the third trimester.	It's caused by compression of the ribs as your womb rises in your abdomen. Also, your baby can bruise your lower ribs with his head, or by excessive punching and kicking.
Tender, painful breasts that feel heavy and uncomfortable, with a tingling sensation in the nipples, is often one of the first signs of pregnancy. Your breasts may feel tender throughout, but become more so toward term.	Hormones are getting your breasts ready for lactation. The milk ducts are growing and being stretched as they fill with milk.
Thrush is a yeast infection. Typically you'll have a thick, white, curdy discharge from your vagina, with dryness and intense itching around your vagina, vulva, perineum, and, sometimes, your anus. You may also have pain when passing urine. Thrush can happen at any time.	It's caused by an infection with the yeast *Candida albicans*, which is always in your bowel. Infection happens when the yeast grows uncontrolled by other bacteria, perhaps after a course of antibiotics. Thrush is more common in pregnancy probably because increased vaginal blood flow can cause a leakage of sugar into body fluids. Excess sugar intake often aggravates the condition.
Varicose veins are swollen veins just below the skin. Although most common in the legs or anus, they can also develop in the vulva.	See Piles p.210.
Water retention happens when there's more fluid than usual in your body tissues. This causes swelling (edema), especially of the feet, face, and hands. Your rings may become tight.	Standing all day, especially in hot weather, can cause fluid to pool in the ankles. High blood pressure (see p.208), which often happens in pregnancy, can force fluid from the bloodstream into the tissues, causing edema. Pregnancy hormones can cause retention of sodium by the kidneys, which in turn causes the body to retain fluid.

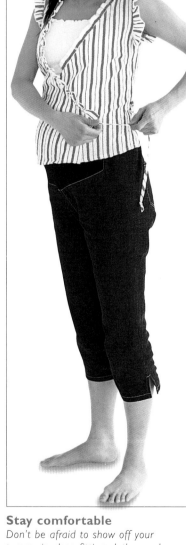

Stay comfortable
Don't be afraid to show off your tummy in close-fitting clothes as long as they're stretchy and comfortable.

What can be done	Risk to baby
Wear clothes that don't compress your ribs. Improve your posture. Prop yourself up on cushions when you lie down. The pain stops when the baby's head drops into the pelvic cavity before birth.	None.
Wear a good supportive bra from early in pregnancy. If your breasts are large, wear a bra at night, too (see p.163). Wash your breasts gently once a day with a mild soap and pat dry. Put baby lotion or oil on your nipples if they're sore.	None.
Tight underpants and pants can encourage infection. Choose cotton instead of synthetic fibers. Your doctor will prescribe cream or suppositories that you should place in your vagina at night, as directed. You'll also be prescribed a cream that you gently rub into the skin around your vaginal opening and anus, and on the thighs. This will stop the itching.	None.
Don't stand for too long. Put your feet up. Wear pregnancy support hose. Gentle massage may help to prevent varicose veins, but do not massage the area if you develop them.	None.
Don't stand for long periods. Put your feet up when you can. Avoid salty foods. Your doctor will check your hands, face, and ankles for any swelling at each prenatal visit. Diuretics are not recommended during pregnancy.	Potentially dangerous (see Preeclampsia, page 224).

Take time to relax
Remember to make time to put your feet up—this will help prevent water retention and varicose veins—but don't lie on your back for too long.

The mother who has MS

Case study

Name Kathy Dixon
Age 29 years
Past medical history Developed multiple sclerosis at the age of 23 years
Obstetric history 14 weeks pregnant

When Kathy developed multiple sclerosis a year after her marriage to Tom, both were devastated. Each had dreamed of having children. Kathy and Tom came to believe that Kathy's MS made it harder for her to conceive, possibly even infertile. They also worried that it wasn't good for women suffering from MS to become pregnant because it could make the condition worse, with serious relapses and increased disability.

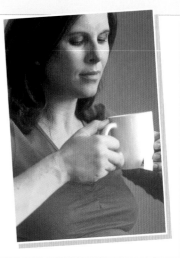

Kathy has always longed to have children, but because of her multiple sclerosis, she and Tom believed that they had no chance of having a family. They talked matters over with their elderly family doctor, who continued to advise them against getting pregnant. Recently, however, they heard about a new obstetrician who had different views.

A NEW PICTURE

Since Kathy's walking was still steady, her eyesight was hardly affected, and she had no troublesome urinary symptoms or vertigo, she and Tom decided to go for a second opinion. They went to see a modern obstetrician who'd seen several MS patients through successful pregnancies. He enlisted the help of a neurologist throughout prenatal care, and this way, both mother and baby received the best care.

To their delight, Kathy and Tom were given an entirely new and encouraging picture by the obstetrician, who told them that their general practitioner's advice was out of date. He explained to them that MS does not affect a woman's fertility in any way and has no effect on pregnancy, labor, or delivery. In a study of 36 pregnant women with MS, the only problems noted were two cases of mild vomiting. There's no increase in spontaneous abortions, complications in pregnancy or delivery, malformations, or stillbirths.

A GOOD PROGNOSIS

Kathy did wonder whether pregnancy would make her MS worse. I reassured her that many research studies suggest that pregnancy is a protection for women with MS. This is probably because the natural state of immunosuppression that happens in pregnancy to prevent a woman from rejecting her baby also suppresses the inflammation that causes nerve and brain damage in MS. On the other hand, there's a slightly increased risk of a flareup for three to six months after the birth. Between 40 and 60 percent of women have a relapse during this time—20 percent of these suffer from permanent side effects while 80 percent go back to their pre-pregnancy state of MS. Pregnancy does not appear to affect the long-term course of MS.

I told Kathy that the management of her labor and delivery would follow normal medical routine. She could be given pain relief—gas, injection, or epidural anesthetic—and this would have no effect on her MS. A cesarean would not affect her MS, nor would forceps if they proved necessary.

MS AND THE BABY

Tom was concerned that Kathy's MS might be passed on to their child. I explained that in an area with a high prevalence of MS, one person in 1000 out of the normal population would be likely to develop the disease. One study has shown that among children of people with MS, the figure could rise to one in 100. Dietary and genetic factors may be involved, although nothing has as yet been proved. Most people feel that the risk of their child's having MS is not great enough to stop them from choosing to conceive.

MS MEDICATION AND THE DEVELOPING BABY

Kathy was worried that the drugs she's given for MS might harm her developing baby. I told her that in the first 12 weeks of pregnancy, drugs are avoided, even if she does have MS, unless her life or the life of her baby is in danger. Drugs to stop painful muscle spasms would be discontinued before she conceives, as would long-term anti-inflammatory therapies. Drugs that help to control urinary frequency or incontinence would also be stopped. Very powerful drugs like steroids, which are only given if either the mother or the baby's life is in danger, are hardly ever needed during pregnancy.

AFTER THE BIRTH

Kathy wanted to know whether MS would affect her ability to feed and care for her baby. There are no medical reasons for her not to breastfeed, and she should insist on doing so. It's extremely important for her to rest, though, so she'll need to have help with her baby and express milk so someone else can give night feedings. She was also worried that having a baby to care for might increase the sense of insecurity she already has because of her MS. I told Tom that he would be the best person to calm Kathy's fears on that score.

HAPPILY PREGNANT

Kathy and Tom thought about what they'd been told, and read as much as they could find about Multiple Sclerosis and pregnancy in pamphlets and on the Internet. They were stunned that after all the years they'd spent hoping for a miracle, there didn't appear to be much of a risk for Kathy after all. They decided to try for a baby.

Kathy is now 14 weeks pregnant. She's going to routine prenatal clinics and seeing her neurologist once a month. Kathy's doctors have told her that there's no need for special testing or monitoring of her pregnancy. She's being given iron to prevent anemia, and her doctors are on the lookout for warning signs of a urinary tract infection, which needs to be treated promptly if it happens. So far, her pregnancy is going normally and her MS remains unchanged.

PREGNANCY ADVICE

One of the chief symptoms of MS is fatigue. Tiredness is also a feature of pregnancy so an MS mother can easily become profoundly fatigued. An MS mother must accept that she'll have to rest at times during the day. People around her, especially her partner, will need to support her in this and make sure she gets enough rest. Here are the guidelines I gave Kathy:
- stop doing things if you get breathless
- put your feet up when you can
- learn to catnap in your spare time
- take two naps a day of at least 30 minutes each
- go to bed early—say, not later than 9:30 p.m.

Kathy's baby

There's every expectation that Kathy's baby will develop normally and be born in a straightforward way without the need for any special medical intervention.

- She cannot inherit MS from her mother by transmission across the placenta, and the risk of transmission through genes appears to be very small.

- Kathy should be able to breastfeed her baby and express milk for bottlefeeding.

- If Kathy checks with her doctor before starting drug treatment again, her baby won't be at risk from drugs in the breast milk.

- Kathy should rest while feeding to save her energy. I suggested she practice breastfeeding with a doll before the birth while lying on her bed or sofa with the doll resting on a pillow under each arm.

CHAPTER 10

Medical emergencies

Medical emergencies in pregnancy tend to happen in the first and third trimesters. In the first trimester, there may be a miscarriage. In the third trimester, there may be complications such as preeclampsia, or problems with the placenta. Be reassured that most babies are delivered safely.

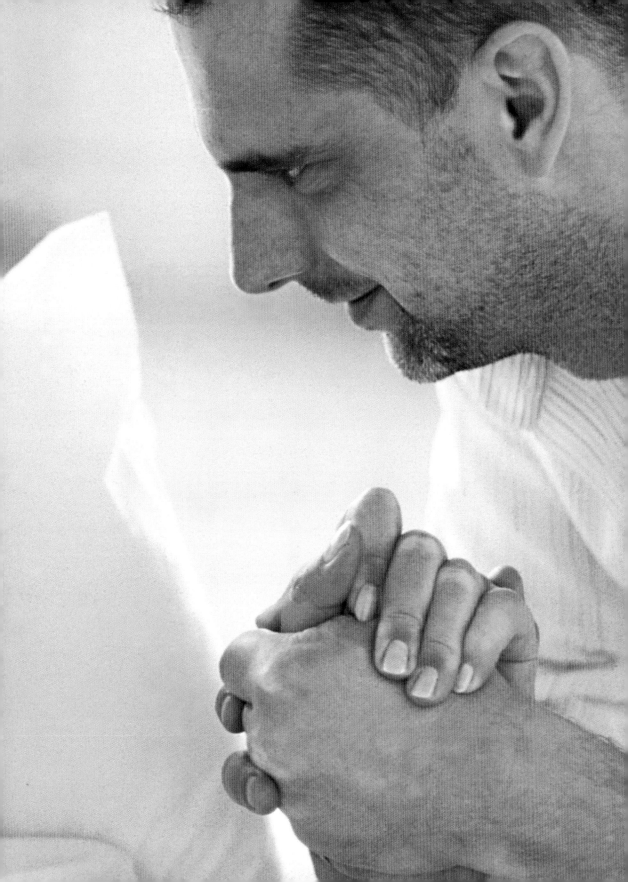

VAGINAL BLEEDING

Don't disregard vaginal bleeding at any stage of pregnancy – it should always be taken seriously. Bleeding may be a sign of an abnormally placed placenta, placenta praevia (see p.222), or warn that a miscarriage is imminent. Both of these conditions need prompt medical treatment.

- About one-quarter of all pregnant woman suffer some vaginal bleeding in the first trimester. More than half of them go on to give birth to a healthy baby at term. If you have any bleeding, call your doctor or midwife, who will probably refer you to the Early Pregnancy Unit at your local hospital. These are walk-in clinics, where you can be scanned quickly to check for your baby's heartbeat. If it's confirmed, there's a very good chance (more than 80 percent) that all will be well. Women with a history of repeated miscarriage may go to these units regularly to boost their confidence. Studies show that reassurance alone has a positive effect.

- If you start to bleed at any time during the second or third trimester, call your maternity unit and go there as soon as you can. There may be serious problems with your placenta, or you could be going into premature labour (see pp.298 & 299), but there are other less serious causes. It's important to be seen right away just in case.

Medical emergencies

Most women carry their babies to term without any problems or emergencies. It's a good idea, though, to be aware of the danger signs just in case, so you know when to call for medical help.

MISCARRIAGE

Spontaneous miscarriage is when a baby dies or is expelled from the womb before the twenty-fourth week. After the twenty-fourth week, this is called a stillbirth. About one-third of all pregnancies end in miscarriage in the first few weeks, but one quarter of these happen before a woman even knows or suspects she is pregnant, so she is unaware anything has happened.

Miscarriages are more likely the older you are and the more pregnancies you've had. They are most common in the first trimester and the usual symptom is bleeding, which happens in 95 percent of cases. If you notice bleeding at any time in your pregnancy, call your doctor.

Many early miscarriages are due to a seriously abnormal fetus failing to implant in the wall of the uterus, while 70 percent are due to chromosomal abnormalities. Causes linked to the mother include abnormalities in her uterus, such as large fibroids, and hormonal imbalances. Some miscarriages are also caused by bacterial and viral infections. Cervical incompetence (see p.223) accounts for only one percent of spontaneous miscarriages. Causes linked to the father include abnormal sperm, or incompatible blood type, which causes a mother to produce antibodies to her partner's blood. These antibodies then attack and kill her fetus. Doctors divide spontaneous miscarriages into several categories:

Threatened miscarriage Miscarriage is possible but not inevitable. A mother suffers vaginal bleeding and sometimes pain. This happens in about 10 percent of all pregnancies and may be confused with the slight bleeding that can come at the time of the first missed period.

Inevitable miscarriage A woman has vaginal bleeding and pain because her uterus is contracting. Unfortunately, if her cervix also dilates, she will lose her baby.

Complete miscarriage The fetus and placenta are expelled from the uterus, sometimes without any symptoms. Ultrasound examination can confirm this.

Missed miscarriage The fetus and placenta die, but remain in the mother's womb for some time, even months, before being expelled. The symptoms of pregnancy disappear, but there's no other indication of fetal death until much later.

Incomplete miscarriage There's a miscarriage, but some of the products of conception, such as the amniotic sac or the placenta, remain in place.

Recurrent miscarriage A woman suffers a miscarriage on three or more occasions. This may happen at the same stage of pregnancy or at different stages, and the reasons may be the same or differ each time.

Treatment If you're bleeding in the second or third trimester, call the hospital and go there as soon as you can (see box on p.218). If you bleed in the first trimester, call your doctor and stop any physical activities, such as strenuous exercise and sexual intercourse. If the bleeding and pain stop, you're quite likely to go on to deliver a healthy baby.

If a miscarriage seems inevitable, there's little that doctors can do to prevent it. Complete and incomplete miscarriages are very often treated in the hospital. After an incomplete miscarriage, the uterus will be cleaned out by a procedure called *dilatation and curettage* (D and C) under anesthetic. Painkillers are given, along with drugs to stop the bleeding. If a lot of blood is lost (at least a pint/500 ml), a transfusion may be needed.

There's no urgency in treating a missed miscarriage, but if, after a time, a spontaneous miscarriage hasn't taken place, a D and C procedure will be carried out. If a baby dies later in pregnancy, prostaglandin pessaries or an oxytocin injection are given to stimulate delivery (see also p.312).

After suffering a miscarriage because of cervical incompetence (see p.223), some women can be treated by stitching the cervix shut at the beginning of the next pregnancy, though this is not always successful.

Other possible reasons for recurrent miscarriage are genetic or hormonal disorders, which often can be pinpointed (see pp.42–47). Long-term infections, such as listeria, may sometimes cause repeated miscarriages, but these can be difficult to diagnose and treat. Other contributing factors can be poor nutrition; chronic disease, such as renal disease; tumors in the uterus (particularly fibroids) or abnormalities such as partial or complete *septums* (see column, right) that can usually be corrected by surgery; and immune disorders.

This last happens when a mother's immune system identifies the fetus as foreign and attacks it—Rhesus blood incompatibility (see p.202) is one example of such a situation. Other immune problems can sometimes be treated by using medication, which acts to suppress the mother's immune reaction. Alternatively, the fetus can sometimes be injected with antibodies, either via the umbilical cord or directly into the fetus itself if the cord is underdeveloped.

UTERINE SEPTUMS

In all mammals, the uterus (womb) develops from two separate tubes in the embryo.

In some, such as monkeys, horses, and human beings, the tubes join to make a single uterus. In others, such as cats and dogs, the tubes develop into two separate uteri.

If the tubes don't join completely, this can leave a partition, or septum, in the uterus. A uterine septum doesn't always mean having a cesarean section—only if the baby is lying in an awkward position.

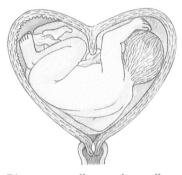

Bicornuate (horn-shaped) uterus
The baby is forced to lie across the uterus from the second trimester onward.

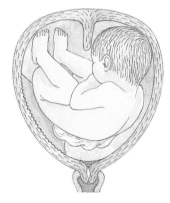

Subseptate uterus
The septum restricts the baby's movements, which can hinder birth.

219

The mother who has miscarried

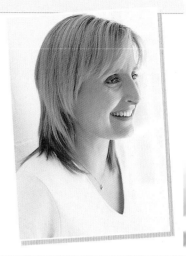

Liz was deeply distressed by her miscarriage. What made the situation even harder to bear was that there didn't seem to be a cause, and nobody seemed to understand her intense feelings of grief, despair, and anger. Liz is now pregnant again and is naturally worried about what might happen this time.

FIRST REACTIONS

When she miscarried nine months ago, Liz felt very alone as she battled with her feelings of guilt, despair, and anger. Her doctor couldn't look her in the eye or talk openly about her lost baby. Her family and friends were sympathetic, but their attempts to comfort her were a little clumsy. Some people said it was all for the best, because there must have been something wrong with the baby. Others reassured her that she could soon have another one. Her unborn baby was not as real to them as it had been to Liz, and they did not understand her intense sense of loss.

She began to wonder if her reactions were normal—perhaps she wasn't justified in grieving for a baby who'd never really existed? I reassured Liz that it is natural for a mother to mourn the loss of her child, even if the child has not been born. Her emotions as well as her body needed time to readjust. I also encouraged her to share her feelings with her partner, so that they could grieve together.

ACCEPTING THEIR LOSS

At first Alan was reluctant to share his feelings with Liz, and she felt she had to force him to talk to her. She knew that it would be impossible to care for another baby until she had given up this one, and this was something that they had to do together. I encouraged them to share their anxieties and frustration, talk through their feelings, and cry together. It was important that they didn't deny their grief. I also suggested that it might help if they had a private memorial ceremony—perhaps something as simple as planting a tree in memory of their miscarried baby.

WAS SOMETHING WRONG WITH THE BABY?

After her miscarriage, Liz was taken to the hospital and examined to make sure there were no fragments of the placenta left in her uterus, where they could cause infection. Following her doctor's advice, she gathered up everything her body had expelled and took it with her so that the fetus could be tested for chromosomal abnormalities. None were found.

Liz was reassured by this at first, but then began to blame herself —perhaps the miscarriage was her fault. I explained that one in three first pregnancies ends in miscarriage. There are thought to be two reasons for this. First, an immature uterus might need to mature by having a trial run before it's ready to carry a pregnancy to term. Second, defects in the sperm or egg can produce an abnormal fetus.

ARE THERE CHANCES OF ANOTHER MISCARRIAGE?

Research on miscarriage in early pregnancy shows that a woman who's had one miscarriage is more likely to miscarry again. The risk seems to increase if a woman conceives too soon after the miscarriage. Fortunately, I'd warned Liz and Alan about this, so they waited for four months before trying to conceive again.

PREDICTIVE TESTING

A simple predictive test, carried out before pregnancy, can help to identify women who are more likely to miscarry again. During the menstrual cycle, if there's too high a level of LH (luteinizing hormone) before ovulation, the risk of miscarriage is increased. LH controls other hormones involved in pregnancy, including estrogen. When Liz's LH levels were tested, they were normal.

REPEATED MISCARRIAGE

Some women do miscarry repeatedly, but even for them, the chance of a successful pregnancy after three previous miscarriages is about 60 percent. Women who've had several miscarriages are tested for uterine abnormalities, hormone imbalances, and disorders of the immunological system. Recent research has focused on a woman's immunological system and on hormone imbalances as causes of repeated miscarriage.

IMMUNOLOGICALLY INDUCED MISCARRIAGES

The immune system is designed to repel foreign bodies because they can be harmful. Pregnancy normally overrides this, so that the woman's body protects the baby rather than rejecting it. But for unknown reasons, the override fails in some mothers—the immune system reasserts itself and the baby is aborted. One still-experimental treatment is to immunize women so that they don't produce antibodies hostile to their babies.

HORMONALLY INDUCED MISCARRIAGES

Women suffering from polycystic ovary syndrome—a condition usually characterized by multiple ovarian cysts—seem to have more miscarriages. This syndrome is caused by a hormone imbalance that causes the body to make too much testosterone and overstimulate the ovaries so that immature eggs are produced. Women with PCOS who are thinking of getting pregnant will be tested for hormone imbalances and abnormal ovulation. They may be given fertility drugs such as clomiphene (see p.46), although this will not protect them against miscarriage.

PREGNANT AGAIN

Now that Liz is pregnant again, she's being extremely careful in every aspect of her life. Most importantly, she's given up blaming herself for the miscarriage and is taking a positive attitude toward her new pregnancy. I told Liz that although she can't be sure what the outcome will be, she knows her body is better prepared for pregnancy than it was last time. Alan is "sure it's going to be all right this time," but he doesn't want to make plans for the future as he did before.

Liz's baby

Liz is fit and healthy and doesn't appear to have any condition that makes her likely to miscarry again. Liz's baby has every chance of developing perfectly normally.

In several ways, Liz's baby will actually benefit both before and after birth—because of her mother's history of miscarriage.

• Liz's baby will be well nourished because her mother is paying such careful attention to what she eats and to relaxation and exercise routines.

• The baby should be comforted by the positive feelings that Liz is directing toward her.

• When she's born, Liz's baby will be greeted with relief and delight because she's making up for a previous disappointment. She represents success.

• Because of her previous history, Liz will be given extra care during her pregnancy. The health of her baby will be closely watched for any signs of distress so that any problems can be averted.

ABNORMAL POSITION OF THE PLACENTA

If the placenta has implanted in the wrong position, it can obstruct a baby's birth.

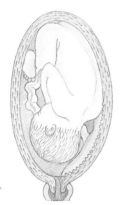

Side position
In partial placenta previa, the placenta implants on the side and extends to the cervix, but doesn't cover it. A cesarian section will be required.

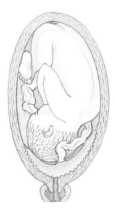

Blocking the cervix
In complete placenta previa, the placenta implants centrally, completely covering the cervix and making it impossible to open. Delivery by cesarian section is necessary.

PLACENTAL SEPARATION

The partial or complete separation of the placenta from the uterus can cause bleeding from the placental bed. Blood builds up and eventually escapes around the membranes and through the cervix into the vagina. This is known as placental abruption (*abruptio placentae*) and happens in about one in 200 pregnancies. Causes of placental abruption include smoking (risk rises with the number of cigarettes smoked per day); uncontrolled high blood pressure; trauma; and illicit drug use. Obstetricians divide placental separation into three types according to the severity. If severe placental abruption happens before the third trimester, a baby may die, but it can survive less severe separations.

In mild separation, your blood loss may be slight. You'll need bed rest, with ultrasound examination to monitor the situation. If it happens late in pregnancy, your labor may have to be induced.

In moderate separation, one-quarter of the placenta separates and between one and two pints (500 ml to one liter) of blood is lost. A blood transfusion is needed and, if your pregnancy is at or nearing term, you'll usually need a cesarean section.

Severe separation is an acute emergency, when at least two-thirds of the placenta shears off the uterine wall, and up to four pints (two liters) of blood are lost. This causes severe shock, disturbance of blood coagulation, and full kidney shutdown. A rapid blood transfusion will be given, and if the pregnancy is near term, a cesarean may be carried out to try to save the baby.

PLACENTA PREVIA

This happens when the placenta is implanted in the lower segment of the uterus instead of the upper part (see column, left). It lies in front of the baby as she comes to descend the birth canal at the start of labor. The baby cannot pass down the canal without dislodging the placenta and interrupting her own blood supply. Placenta previa is a major cause of bleeding after the twentieth week and of hemorrhage in the final two months of pregnancy. It's more common in women who've had several children, but the cause is unknown.

The greater the proportion of the placenta lying in the lower uterine segment, the greater the likelihood of complications during delivery. Even though the growth of the placenta in both size and weight slows down after the thirtieth week of pregnancy, the lower segment of the uterus is increasing in length quite rapidly. There may be shearing stresses between the placenta and the uterine wall, leading to episodes of bleeding.

This extremely dangerous condition can be diagnosed well ahead of delivery by ultrasound (see p.180). Early symptoms include bleeding, with bright red blood, which may happen after sex. The doctor will advise a mother with these symptoms to go into the hospital for ultrasound examination and bed rest, with blood transfusions if necessary. She should continue to rest in bed, if possible, until the thirty-seventh week, when the baby will be delivered by cesarean section (see p.308).

There may be a postpartum hemorrhage after the birth, but this is usually anticipated, and drugs to prevent it will be given as soon as the baby is born. In a very few cases, hemorrhage will continue despite treatment, and then a hysterectomy may be a possibility. For these reasons, placenta previa should only be treated by obstetricians qualified to cope with these complications. The mother deliver in a well-equipped hospital, with a blood transfusion service on hand.

PLACENTAL INSUFFICIENCY

During pregnancy the baby receives oxygen and nourishment, and gets rid of carbon dioxide and waste products, via the placenta and the umbilical blood vessels. A healthy placenta that can perform all these functions effectively is crucial for the baby's continuing health and well-being.

Assessment and treatment There's no reliable way of checking whether your placenta is functioning properly. But doctors may suspect insufficiency if your uterus is growing too slowly, or if your baby's development is less than normal.

Ultrasound is the most reliable way to measure your baby's growth. If it shows that your baby is not growing as expected, your doctor may need to do more scans and make a biophysical profile that takes account of your baby's breathing and body movements, the tone and quantity of amniotic fluid, and a non-stress test. You may also choose to keep a kick chart to check the baby's activity levels (see p.195)—by 28 weeks there should be 10 kicks per hour—but this is less useful than scans or fetal heart recordings. Placental insufficiency may mean that labor needs to be induced or even that you have to have a cesarean section.

INCOMPETENT CERVIX

Fortunately, this condition is rare, unless the cervix has been damaged during a previous pregnancy or surgery. When you're pregnant, the cervix normally remains tightly shut and is sealed with a plug of mucus. This means that your baby is safely held in the womb until labor begins, when the cervix begins to dilate.

Occasionally, though, the cervix begins to open before it should, usually in the third or fourth month—a condition termed cervical incompetence. This allows the amniotic sac containing the baby to sag through into the vagina and rupture, with a sudden loss of amniotic fluid followed by miscarriage. Unfortunately, an incompetent cervix is usually diagnosed only after a woman has suffered a first miscarriage.

If cervical incompetence is thought to be the cause of previous miscarriage, a soft, nonabsorbable thread will be inserted around your cervix to tighten it (see column, right). After bed rest in the hospital, you'll be able to go home, but you'll need to get plenty of rest during the remainder of your pregnancy. The thread will be cut about seven days before term, and your baby will be delivered vaginally in the normal way.

REASONS FOR PLACENTAL INSUFFICIENCY

The placenta may be unable to support a baby sufficiently for a number of reasons:

- the placenta may have developed abnormally

- blood flow through the placenta may be restricted, or placental tissue may be lost because of a blood clot

- the placenta may separate, or partly separate, from the uterine wall

- the placenta may be too small

- the placenta may be poorly developed

- the pregnancy may go beyond the due date, so that the placenta becomes relatively inadequate for the baby (see p.260)

- if a mother has diabetes (see also p.140), this can adversely affect the placenta.

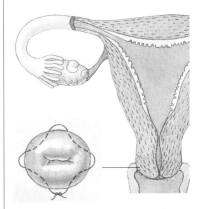

Securing the cervix
The cervix is kept closed by passing a thread all the way around it—like the strings of a purse. The thread is normally cut about seven days before the expected delivery date.

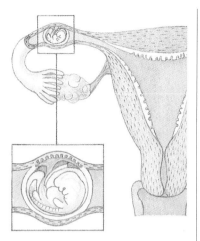

Tubal implantation
About one in every 300 pregnancies is ectopic. In 99 percent of ectopic pregnancies, the blastocyst (see p.32) implants in the fallopian tube. Very rarely, the blastocyst may implant in the abdominal cavity, the cervix, or on one of a woman's ovaries.

PREECLAMPSIA

Preeclampsia is a potentially serious condition. It can affect as many as one in 10 women, especially first-time mothers and women carrying more than one baby. It's unique to pregnancy and starts in the placenta, so the baby may grow more slowly than normal. We don't know quite why it happens, but it does tend to run in families.

Symptoms Preeclampsia itself doesn't really have any symptoms, but your midwife or doctor may suspect its presence if you have significantly raised blood pressure and protein in your urine. Both of these symptoms should be picked up at a prenatal check, which is why it's very important to have your blood pressure taken at each visit. You may also have *edema*—swelling of the ankles and wrists—although you can have edema without preeclampsia. The pregnancy can't be restored to normal, but delivery of the baby and placenta ends the problem.

Treatment You'll be admitted to the hospital, or asked to go to a special outpatient clinic, so that arrangements for the birth of your baby can be made before you suffer any serious complications. Your blood pressure, kidney and liver function, and blood clotting will all be monitored closely, as they may be affected by the condition. Very rarely, preeclampsia can develop into eclampsia. This is one of the most dangerous complications of pregnancy, causing coma and convulsions. It's nearly always preceded by preeclampsia, which acts as an early warning signal, and can be prevented by delivery of your baby.

ECLAMPSIA

The word eclampsia derives from the Greek words meaning "like a flash of lightning"—the condition seems to strike from out of the blue, with seizures and, eventually, coma. Eclampsia is a potentially life-threatening condition for both mother and baby and used to be quite common. Fortunately, it's now extremely rare in the Western world because doctors can diagnose the condition in its earliest phase (preeclampsia, see above) and they are constantly alert for the warning signs.

Symptoms Eclampsia is a medical emergency because the blood vessels in the uterus go into spasm, cutting down the blood flow to the baby so that the level of oxygen in her blood becomes dangerously low.

Your own life is threatened because the spasms lead to kidney failure. Brain oxygen levels are also lowered, causing heightened brain sensitivity, which shows as seizures. Tissues become waterlogged because of fluid retention, and hemorrhages can happen in tissues such as the liver. The earliest signs are drowsiness, headache, dimness of vision, as well as rising blood pressure and protein in the urine (see p.177), edema (see p.212), and right upper abdominal pain. Urgent delivery of the baby is usually required to enable proper treatment of the mother.

Treatment If eclampsia does develop, doctors try to increase the blood flow to the mother's brain, sedating the brain and reducing high blood pressure. They deliver her baby, usually by cesarean section. As soon as the baby is born, the condition begins to subside, although the mother will continue to have close monitoring after the birth.

ECTOPIC PREGNANCY

In an ectopic pregnancy, the fertilized egg implants somewhere other than in the cavity of the womb, usually in a fallopian tube. The rapidly growing embryo causes the tube to distend, and the invading placenta weakens its walls, causing bleeding. Eventually the tube bursts under the strain.

Before a fallopian tube bursts, there are usually certain symptoms around the sixth week of pregnancy that signal all is not well. If you should notice any of these, it's important to report them to your doctor immediately. Doctors define two forms of ectopic pregnancy:

Unruptured After a positive pregnancy test, warning signs of an ectopic pregnancy may be pain in the abdomen, usually only on one side, sometimes accompanied by vaginal bleeding, fainting, and pain in the shoulder (on the same side as any pain in the abdomen). Sometimes an ectopic pregnancy is detected by an ultrasound scan after a small amount of bleeding from the vagina early in the pregnancy. Although there's some leakage, there is no rupture as yet, and it may not be detected until eight to 10 weeks' gestation. This kind of ectopic pregnancy can sometimes be treated by injecting a drug into the embryo, causing it to die and then be reabsorbed, which can save the fallopian tube. Otherwise the pregnancy can be removed by *laparoscopy* (see p.45).

Ruptured This happens when the tube bursts, leading to severe pain and shock, with extreme paleness, weak but rapid pulse, and falling blood pressure. A woman suffering this acute form of ectopic pregnancy will be admitted to the hospital immediately for emergency surgery. The pregnancy will be removed from the fallopian tube and the tube itself may also have to be removed.

Ectopic pregnancy is becoming more common in developed countries. We don't know why, although some doctors think there could be a link with increases in pelvic inflammatory disease, which causes scarring and blockage of the fallopian tubes. On the other hand, there may just appear to be more ectopic pregnancies because doctors are better able to diagnose them, thanks to ultrasound.

Outlook Almost 60 percent of women who've had an ectopic pregnancy become pregnant again, 30 percent avoid further pregnancy voluntarily; the rest are infertile. If you have had a previous ectopic pregnancy, tell your doctor because you will need special care during your current pregnancy.

POSTNATAL INFECTION

Postnatal infection, which used to be known as childbed fever, is now very rare. Before antibiotics were available, it was one of the main causes of death in mothers.

Postnatal infection is an infection at the site of the placenta, sometimes caused by remnants of the placenta remaining in the womb. The first symptoms are a high temperature, acute stomach pains, and bad-smelling lochia (see p.354).

If you should develop any of these symptoms, tell your doctor at once. Any remaining placenta will be removed and you'll be given antibiotics to treat the infection.

A mother with preeclampsia

This condition, which is unique to pregnant women, has the following symptoms: a rise in blood pressure, swollen ankles, feet, and hands, and protein in the urine. Although nothing can be done to prevent the onset of preeclampsia, good prenatal care can make sure that the condition does not get worse.

AMIE'S HISTORY OF PREECLAMPSIA

There are quite a few statistics I can draw on to reassure Amie. First, preeclamptic toxemia (PET) is most common in first pregnancies, so in a way she's been exposed to the highest risk already. Second, her PET was very mild. Her symptoms were slight edema—swelling of the hands, fingers, feet, and face—and a marginally raised blood pressure that needed no treatment. She didn't have the other important sign of PET, the appearance of protein in the urine. Best of all, the PET came on only four weeks before the birth. In the end, Amie had a perfectly normal vaginal delivery and her baby was completely healthy.

Statistics show that the later PET starts in pregnancy, the lower the risk of its happening in a second pregnancy, but it's impossible to predict for certain.

SOME FACTS ABOUT DIET AND PET

Amie's very eager to know if she can do anything to make it less likely that she'd have PET again, but there are no self-help measures that are guaranteed to work. What we do know is that PET isn't caused or prevented by what you eat; by how you feel about your pregnancy; by whether or not you exercise; by how hard you work; or by how much rest you take.

Amie eats healthily and has heard that a high-protein diet might protect her against PET. I had to tell her that there's nothing to support this theory. Some people say that calcium and fish oil supplements may help, but the evidence isn't strong enough for me to recommend that she add any supplements to her diet.

WHAT IS PET?

Preeclampsia is an illness that happens only in pregnancy, possibly affecting mother and baby, and is most common toward the end of pregnancy. We don't really know what causes PET, though it seems to run in families—the daughters of women who have had preeclampsia are slightly more likely to get it themselves.

PET AND THE PLACENTA

What's known for certain is that preeclampsia starts in the placenta. Toward the end of pregnancy, the placenta gets as large as a dinner plate, about two inches (5 cm) thick, and needs a large and efficient blood supply from the mother to keep her baby growing healthily. In preeclampsia, the placenta seems to run short of an adequate blood supply, and this has potentially serious consequences for mother and baby.

WARNING SIGNS ON THE MOTHER'S SIDE ARE:

• her blood pressure starts to rise
• valuable protein leaks out into the urine as her kidneys can't function as efficiently as before
• fluid starts to collect in her hands, feet, and face
• her blood-clotting mechanism may be affected.

It's likely that if PET did come back in her second pregnancy, it would be milder than before. Nonetheless, I advised Amie to take a close interest in everything that goes on at her prenatal clinic and in the results of her prenatal tests. I also suggested that she get her partner, Ed, involved because there might be moments when she's confused or alarmed and she'll need to talk to him. She'll also need him for moral support at her prenatal visits.

GOOD PRENATAL CARE

I told Amie that by far the most important preventative measure is for her to make sure she has excellent prenatal care throughout her pregnancy. Because she's had the condition before, she may need more frequent prenatal visits than usual, and she'll need regular checks if any signs of PET are detected. I reassured her that because of her past history, she'll be given very careful attention by her doctors.

BASELINE TESTS

While there are no screening tests that can predict Amie's risk of developing preeclampsia during her pregnancy, there are some baseline tests that she could have done in the first half of her pregnancy. These can be repeated at regular intervals to give early warning of the onset of PET. So, apart from the normal checks on blood pressure, urine, and weight, she needs to make sure she has tests for:

• kidney and blood-clotting function
• ultrasound scans to track the baby's growth
• Doppler scans to measure the efficiency of blood flow to the placenta.

HOSPITAL ADMISSION

I reassured Amie that at the first sign of PET, in even its mildest form, she would be admitted into the hospital for 24-48 hous so that her doctors and midwives could assess the severity of PET, as well as her progress and that of her baby. If necessary, her baby could be delivered before complications set in. Preeclampsia is progressive. It doesn't get better, so once admitted Amie shouldn't expect to be allowed to go home until after her baby's been born. If PET is mild, however, it is possible to have frequent out-patient follow-up.

DRUGS

Doctors may prescribe drugs to bring down a mother's blood pressure if it's found to be too high. Though these drugs don't affect the underlying disease, they can reduce the risk of some of the complications that are linked with it.

It's also possible that Amie may be given small daily doses of aspirin during her pregnancy, which could prevent or delay the onset of PET. Aspirin works directly on the clotting blood cells, known as platelets, which are involved in PET.

WHAT CAN HAPPEN WITH PET

If PET is getting worse, if the baby shows signs of distress, or if the mother's condition is deteriorating, there's only one treatment: urgent termination of the pregnancy—sometimes by cesarean if the situation demands. However, last time Amie had a perfectly normal delivery, and chances are she'll have the same this time.

Also, I reassured Amie that even if she did have a cesarean, it doesn't mean subsequent deliveries will be in the same way. Women who've had one cesarean section can attempt a normal delivery next time. I suggested to Amie that if she did need a cesarean, she could have an epidural, rather than general anesthesia, in order to be awake for the delivery and to include Ed in theprocess. This wouldn't be possible if Annie were asleep under a general anesthetic.

INVOLVEMENT OF EXPERTS

It was important for Amie and Ed to talk to their doctor about their worries at the first prenatal visit. Maternal-fetal medicine specialists are trained to care for women at risk of or with preeclampsia. Research shows that the most important factor in a happy outcome to a PET birth is the involvement of doctors are familiar with the condition and can take action at once if there are any warning signs.

CHAPTER 11

A sensual pregnancy

The very high levels of female hormones in your body when you're pregnant mean that you may find you enjoy all aspects of sex, from massage to lovemaking, far more than ever before. You may also experience some sexual problems, but most can be resolved easily as long as you and your partner are open with one another.

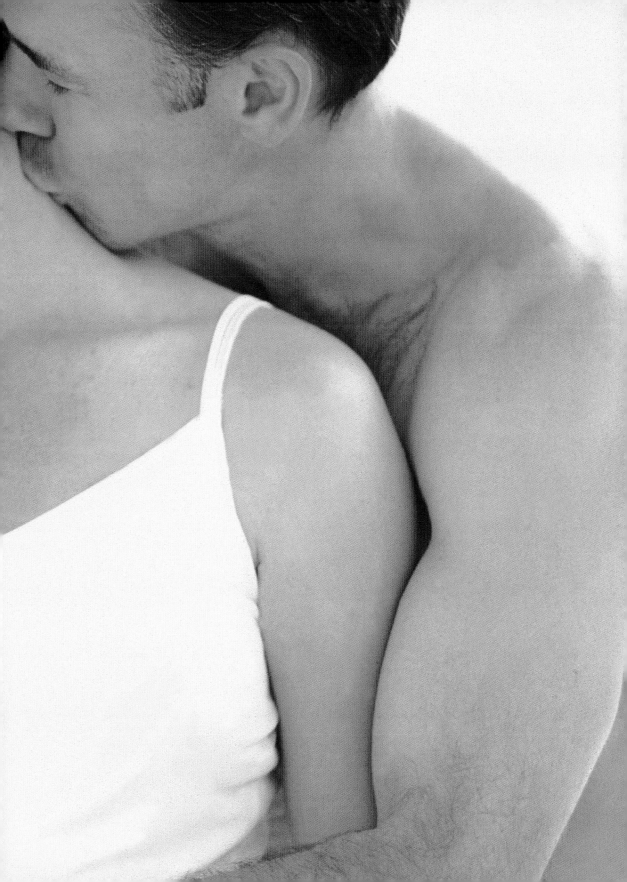

YOUR HORMONES

You may go through all kinds of physical, emotional, and psychological changes during your pregnancy, which can affect how you feel about sex. These changes are mostly due to the vastly increased levels of hormones circulating in your body.

The most important hormones involved in maintaining your pregnancy are progesterone and estrogen. In the early days of a pregnancy these are produced by the *corpus luteum* in the ovary. Once the embryo has implanted in the uterine lining it, and the developing placenta, take over as the primary sources of progesterone and estrogen.

The increase in the amounts of progesterone and estrogen circulating in the body is swift and dramatic. The level of progesterone rises to 10 times the amount before conception, and you produce as much estrogen in one day as a nonpregnant woman does in three years. In fact, during the course of a single pregnancy, a woman produces as much estrogen as a nonpregnant woman could over 150 years.

Progesterone and estrogen bring a sense of well-being, giving you shining hair, supple and glowing skin, and an aura of tranquility and contentment.

A sensual pregnancy

It's perfectly safe to enjoy lovemaking during your pregnancy, unless there are medical reasons why you should abstain. Every pregnant woman has the potential to enjoy sex—and some enjoy it even more than they did before conception.

How much you want and enjoy sex can vary during pregnancy, not only from one woman to another, but also in the same woman at different times throughout the 40 weeks. Most women feel less interested in lovemaking during the first trimester (especially if suffering from tiredness and nausea). Desire generally increases in the second trimester and declines again in the third.

When you do have sex, you may find it far more exciting and satisfying than it was before you conceived. In fact, some women have their first orgasm or multiple orgasms while pregnant.

This enhanced sexuality is mainly due to the very high levels of female hormones and pregnancy hormones circulating throughout the body during pregnancy (see column, left). These cause changes to your breasts and sexual organs, making them more sensitive and responsive than usual. Also, being pregnant is such an affirmation of being female that you may find yourself feeling much more feminine and sensual.

SEXUAL EXCITEMENT DURING PREGNANCY

One effect of the high estrogen levels during pregnancy is an increase in blood flow, especially in the pelvic area. Because of this, the vagina and its folds, the labia, become slightly stretched and swollen. This stretching and swelling, which normally happens only when you're sexually excited, makes the sensory nerve endings hypersensitive, and you become aroused much more rapidly than usual.

One of the first things that happens when you get pregnant is that your breasts start to get bigger—one of the classic signs of pregnancy is sensitive, enlarged breasts and tingling, even painful, nipples. The increased sensitivity of the breasts makes them a focus of sensory arousal, and you may feel the most exquisite pleasure when your partner kisses and caresses your nipples and breasts. This sexual foreplay can also arouse the clitoris and the vagina, which will swell very readily.

The increased blood flow makes your vaginal secretions quite profuse, so you'll find you're ready for penetration much earlier than usual. Penetration is particularly easy because of the plentiful vaginal fluid, and you may climax quite quickly if your clitoris is stimulated at the same time. You may find the intensity of your orgasms reaches new heights and the time taken to "come down" from an orgasm is much longer. The labia minora and the lower end of the vagina can remain swollen for anything up to two hours after orgasm, particularly in the last trimester.

As well as stimulating the whole genital tract, the pregnancy hormones stimulate the production of a hormone within the brain called *melanocyte-stimulating* hormone (or MSH). This causes areas where the skin pigmentation is deeper anyway to get darker—as in the darkening of the nipple area. Darkening of the nipples can act as a sexual signal to a man, making his partner's breasts very attractive to him.

WHEN TO MAKE LOVE

You can make love whenever you want to, provided you don't try to get too athletic and there are no medical reasons for you to avoid sex (see p.236). Good sex in pregnancy is not only very enjoyable, but also helps to prepare you for childbirth by keeping your pelvic muscles strong and supple. It helps strengthen your bonds with your partner, too, which will help you cope much better with the stresses of parenthood.

There's no physical reason why a woman having a normal pregnancy shouldn't continue enjoying making love with her partner. If both partners are happy, sex can continue right up to when you begin labor. In a low-risk pregnancy, the uterine spasms that you have with orgasms are perfectly safe, and in late pregnancy they help prepare the uterus for the rigors of labor.

It's not true that sex can cause an infection during pregnancy and harm the baby. Infection is virtually impossible because the cervix is plugged with a tough mucus that prevents bacteria from getting into the uterus. Also, the baby is completely enclosed inside the amniotic sac, which resists rupture even when under great pressure and cushions him against all external forces (including the weight of a partner during intercourse). That said, extremely athletic sex is not a good idea, because it may cause soreness and abrasions, and a pregnant woman should be free of these unnecessary discomforts.

Lovemaking positions You'll find that the missionary position becomes awkward and uncomfortable as your pregnancy goes on, but there are other sexual positions you can use to enhance your enjoyment—without in any way diminishing that of your partner. Side-by-side positions are often pleasurable; so are rear-entry positions, because in these positions your abdomen is not under any pressure from the weight of your partner. Sitting positions can be very enjoyable in the later months of pregnancy, allowing you to adjust your position but still see your partner's face and feel close to him.

If you are feeling sexy, but you don't really want intercourse, you and your partner could explore other forms of sensual and sexual pleasuring, such as erotically stroking and kissing each other, massage (see p.232), mutual masturbation, and oral sex.

BUILDING YOUR RELATIONSHIP

The physical and emotional changes that happen when you're pregnant can't help but have an impact on your sexual relationship with your partner. Love and understanding will help you to overcome any problems that may arise.

As pregnancy advances, you may find that you have to change your sexual habits. It's best to be open to these changes and see them as a chance to build on and enhance the physical side of your relationship. For instance, you might be prompted to explore (perhaps for the first time) the pleasures of new lovemaking positions and of other forms of sexual activity such as mutual masturbation and oral sex.

Try to understand any changes in your own and your partner's sexual desires. Be ready to talk to each about your needs, but don't let your sex life become the dominant feature of your overall relationship. Concentrate on loving rather than lovemaking, and if at any time you or your partner don't feel like sex, rediscover the intimacy and joy of simply being with the one you love.

GOOD FOR YOU

Use sensual massage as a source of pleasure in itself, or as part of your foreplay.

Sensual massage is a nice way of keeping up a close physical relationship with your partner during your pregnancy, especially if intercourse isn't possible for medical reasons, or if you find it uncomfortable or undesirable. If you make the massage as sexy as you can, and masturbate each other while you do it, both of you will probably be able to reach orgasm without penetration. If you're still having intercourse, use sensual massage as a loving, prolonged, and highly effective method of foreplay.

Sensual massage

A loving, sensual massage can be relaxing and highly erotic for you and your partner, and reinforces the feelings of love and tenderness you have for each other, particularly if making love is difficult for some reason. Begin with loving hugs, cuddles, and stroking, then take turns massaging each other all over, from head to toe. Use slow, sensuous hand movements and plenty of massage oil.

A SHARED PLEASURE

Massage is a way of discovering what gives you sensual pleasure, so let yourself be open to the experience and see what happens. You may both be pleasantly surprised at how sexy it feels to have certain parts of your bodies, ones you'd never thought of as erotic, caressed by your partner.

Preparing for massage   Choose a time when you're not likely to be disturbed (switch on the answering machine and turn off your cell phone). Spend a little time getting your bedroom ready, making sure it's warm and comfortable. If your bed is too soft for giving a massage, put a mattress, a comforter, or a pile

SENSUAL MASSAGE

Back massage
Working slowly and sensuously, gently knead the back of her neck and then her shoulders between your palms, thumbs, and fingers. Massage her lower back with the heels of your hands.

Leg strokes
Put both hands on her ankles, fingers pointing in opposite directions. Slide your hands up to her thighs and back down again, going gently over the backs of her knees.

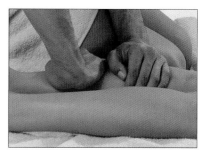

Make sure you are well supported, then lie back and enjoy being massaged

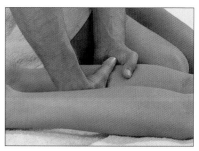

Leg massage
Hold her leg with both hands, thumbs uppermost. Pressing firmly, slide your hands up to the back of the knee. Work down again without pressure.

of folded blankets on the floor and cover them with a large, clean towel or sheet. Dim the lighting, light some scented candles if you like them, and play some gentle music to create a soothing, relaxing atmosphere.

Lubricating the skin It's best to use specially made massage oil or lotion—you'll find that hand cream or ordinary body lotion is absorbed into the skin too quickly, and baby oil leaves an oily film on the skin. Warm the oil before you use it (the simplest way is to put the bottle in a bowl of warm water) and make sure your hands are warm and your fingernails are short and smooth. When you're giving the massage, pour some oil into your hands and smooth it onto your partner's skin. Never just pour the massage oil directly on to your partner; it doesn't feel good, and it's wasteful and messy.

Touching intimately Lightly coat your fingertips with massage oil and delicately trace the outlines of each other's lips, cheeks, jaws, ears, and neck. Then, using plenty of oil, work your fingers and the palm of your hands sensuously over breasts, chest, sides, and abdomen, and across the shoulders and down the arms. Stroke firmly up the inside of each thigh in turn, using the lightest of finger pressure on the return stroke. Always handle her breasts carefully since they will be tender.

GOOD FOR YOUR BABY

Your baby may also respond with pleasure as your body is stroked and caressed, and she'll share some of the benefits you gain from massage.

- From about the fifth month onward, your baby may feel stroking movements through your abdomen, which she'll find very comforting and soothing.

- Learning to massage your own and your partner's body during pregnancy will help you to soothe your baby through touch after her birth.

- Continue to massage your baby after she's born: babies find massage soothing, too.

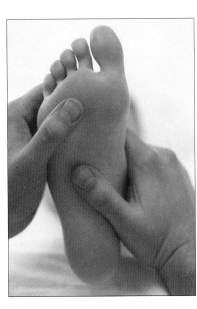

Foot massage 1
Using both your thumbs, gently circle over the whole area of the sole. Apply as much pressure as feels comfortable.

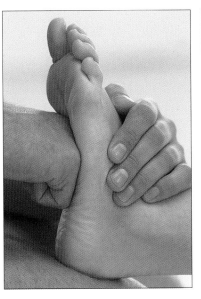

Foot massage 2
Holding the foot with your left hand, press your right fist into the sole of the foot. Using small movements, circle over the whole area.

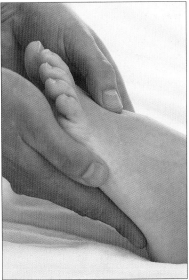

Foot massage 3
Support the foot with one hand. Using the thumb of your other hand, press down the grooves between the tendons at the top of the foot. Work from the ankle to the toes.

Making love

Keep on making love as late into pregnancy as you wish, as long as there are no medical reasons for abstaining (see p.236). Your baby is safe in your uterus. He's not harmed by normal sexual activity (see column, left), and probably enjoys sex as much as you do as your hormones reach him via the placenta (see p.192).

In the early months, use any lovemaking position you like, but as your abdomen gets bigger, you may find some positions uncomfortable. After about 24 weeks, it's best to avoid lying on your back for any length of time, so don't use the missionary position, with your partner on top—there are lots of other exciting options. These may also be the best choices when you first start making love again after the birth (see p.364).

WOMAN-ON-TOP POSITIONS

You may find these the most comfortable from the second trimester onward. As your abdomen grows, you can lift yourself farther off his stomach by supporting yourself on your bent legs. This also prevents too much pressure on your abdomen and breasts. In these positions, too, it's easier for you to control the depth of penetration and the speed and rhythm of lovemaking.

These positions allow a great deal of intimacy. You and your partner have your hands free to caress and stroke each other and he can easily reach your breasts with his mouth. Alternatively, you can brush his chest with your breasts to stimulate him further.

KNEELING AND SIDE-BY-SIDE POSITIONS

Many of these involve entering from behind, and are useful in pregnancy, particularly if you don't feel comfortable on your back, or you don't want to take too active a part in lovemaking.

Kneeling positions allow your partner freedom of movement and let him vary the amount of penetration. Side-by-side positions are comfortable and permit plenty of kissing and caressing. The "spoons" position, so called because the partners nestle together like a pair of spoons, is also good to try if you feel any soreness or discomfort when you start making love again after you've given birth, especially if you've had an episiotomy.

SITTING POSITIONS

These are good in the middle and late months. They don't allow a lot of movement but are comfortable for both partners and ease pressure on the abdomen. Also, the depth of penetration can be controlled. Your partner sits on a sturdy, comfortable chair or the edge of the bed and you sit on his lap, either facing him (if your abdomen is not too big), facing to one side, or facing away.

Your partner can use his hands to caress your body and breasts and to stimulate your clitoris. His range of movement is limited, so you control the sexual tempo.

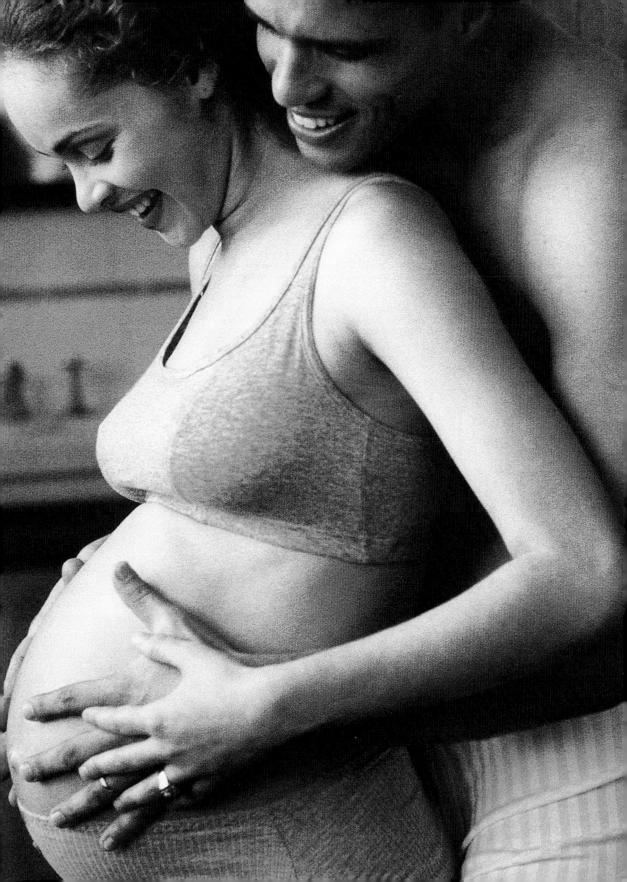

Sexual problems

If yours is a high-risk pregnancy, you may need to avoid sex at certain times or even completely.

Your doctor will warn you if there's any risk that sexual activity will be a danger to your pregnancy, and advise you on what (and when) is safe. Make sure that your doctor explains the problem fully so you're completely clear about what you can and cannot safely do.

The most common reasons and times for restricting intercourse during pregnancy are:

- whenever there's any sign of bleeding. The bleeding may be harmless, but you should check with your doctor immediately

- if placenta previa is suspected or confirmed (see p.222)

- in the last trimester if you have a multiple pregnancy

- in the last 12 weeks if you have a history of premature labor or if you're showing signs that you might go into premature labor

- if your water has broken.

When you're pregnant, there are many physical and emotional factors that can lessen your enjoyment of lovemaking. Fortunately, there are very few that actually prevent you from having sex, and these are relatively rare.

For many women, the most common reason for taking less pleasure in sex is the feeling that your body is becoming less and less attractive to your partner as your pregnancy goes on. Your abdomen swells as your baby grows, and you may view your disappearing waistline, spreading hips, swelling breasts, and widening thighs and upper arms with alarm. Some women become shy and defensive about their appearance, believing that their femininity is gone, and start to feel embarrassed about being seen naked.

In fact, the opposite is probably true, and most men find their pregnant wives very attractive. Talk to your partner about your fears—he'll probably be astonished that you feel unsure about your appearance.

LOSS OF LIBIDO

While you may find your sex drive increases during pregnancy, it must be said that some women don't feel like making love very often during the first trimester. Morning sickness, which can make you feel thoroughly wretched and unattractive in every way, is one reason for this. Tiredness is another enemy of the libido, and because pregnancy can be exhausting, you may sometimes feel you just don't have enough energy to enjoy sex with your partner. Both morning sickness and tiredness are common problems in the first trimester, but usually lessen, or disappear, in the second.

Once free of the discomforts of morning sickness and exhaustion, most women find that their interest and pleasure in sex increase in the second trimester. Toward the last weeks of pregnancy, though, libido may wane again as tiredness increases. Sadly, many women feel like beached whales at this time and don't enjoy their rounded beauty. Some may feel shy about stripping bare and making love.

Hormone levels can swing quite violently during pregnancy, and you'll probably find yourself emotionally volatile, switching from feeling very contented to sadness and tearfulness, and then to great elation. This is perfectly normal, but of course it can be difficult for your partner to understand and can disrupt your sexual relationship.

If you do have problems, try to be open with your partner and be honest about your feelings. If you don't want to make love because you feel physically ill or excessively tired, tell him the truth, so that he doesn't feel rejected.

DISCOMFORT

The hormone-controlled changes in your breasts and genitals make them more sensitive and responsive to touch. This increased sensitivity can heighten your sexuality, but can also sometimes cause discomfort. This is especially true of the breasts in early pregnancy, and you may find that they're very tender for the first couple of months. Explain this to your partner and ask him to avoid touching them during love play.

The engorgement of your genitals may also cause some slight discomfort, particularly later in pregnancy, as they remain swollen and aching after orgasm. This can create a feeling of unrelieved fullness, which may make sex less satisfying. Some women find they can overcome this lack of satisfaction by masturbation, especially if they tend to have better orgasms through masturbation (by themselves or by their partners) than via intercourse.

A common source of discomfort comes when the baby enlarges. Eventually, your abdomen is so swollen that it's increasingly difficult for you to make love in the missionary position. Instead, try other lovemaking positions (see page 234).

WHEN TO STOP

Stop having sex if you're bleeding at any time, and check with your doctor as soon as possible to find out why this might be happening. The bleeding is probably not serious, and may simply be because of changes in the cervix that make it soft and easily damaged by deep penetration, but you'll need medical advice. If the bleeding is caused by the sensitivity of the cervix, it's best to avoid deep penetration when you next make love.

It's not a good idea to have sex if the mucus plug that seals the cervix has become dislodged (a show, see p.271). And you should also abstain after your water has broken. Both of these are signs that labor is about to begin, although you can have a show seven to 10 days before contractions start. Both usually happen near term, although they can be earlier and could be a sign that you're going into premature labor (see p.298).

ANXIETIES

In any relationship, it's difficult to enjoy relaxed, happy lovemaking if either or both of you are feeling anxious, tense, or nervous. During pregnancy, there are lots of things to feel anxious about, including fears about the safety of having sex, and the difficulty some couples or individuals have in adjusting to the idea of imminent parenthood.

Worries about the safety of sex during pregnancy are usually unfounded. As for anxieties about your relationship, the best thing to do is talk frankly and fully with your partner about how you feel about moving from partnership to parenthood. As long as you keep talking most problems can be solved.

If your sex life is causing you concern, and you and your partner cannot resolve it between you, don't hesitate to seek professional advice and counseling.

SEX WITHOUT INTERCOURSE

When you don't want, or can't, have intercourse, there are other ways of enjoying sexual pleasure.

Extended foreplay Sensual massage and passionate kissing and caressing can stop short of or lead to orgasm, as you want.

Mutual masturbation You and your partner can give each other sexual pleasure, and bring each other to orgasm, without having intercourse. To make the experience more sensual and also to avoid harming the delicate skin of your genitals, have your partner smear his hands and fingers with a suitable lubricant such as saliva.

Oral sex Fellatio and cunnilingus, as well as or instead of mutual masturbation, are perfectly safe when you're pregnant. The vaginal secretions generally have a much stronger odor during pregnancy than at other times, though, and some men find this distasteful.

CHAPTER 12

Getting ready for your baby

From the thirty-sixth week, nesting begins in earnest. You'll find there's plenty to do—getting your baby's room ready, choosing equipment and baby clothes, and finalizing your choice of names. You'll also want to make preparations for the birth and to decide what kind of childcare you'll need if you're going back to work.

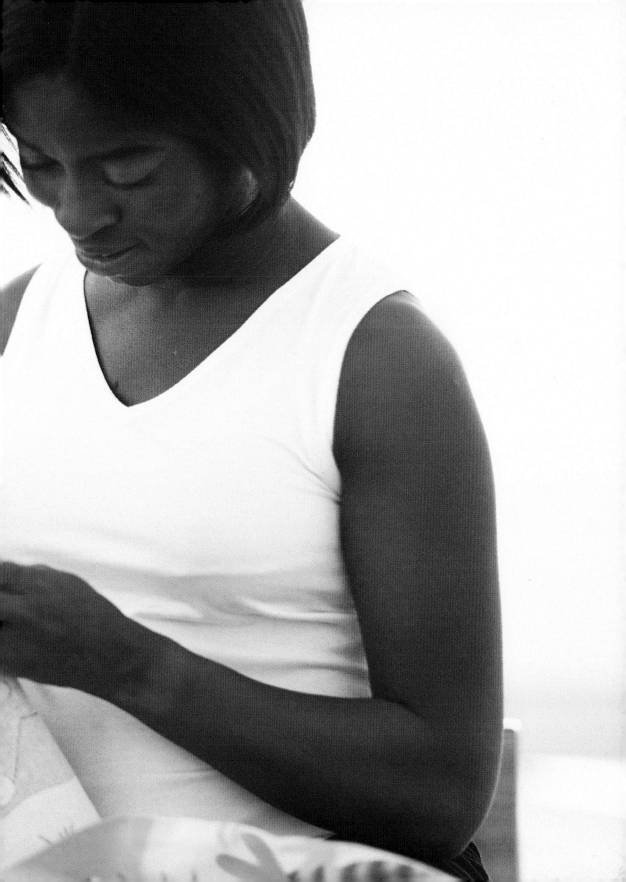

Preparing for your baby

Getting everything ready for your new baby can be great fun, and you'll feel very excited once her room is prepared and you have a stock of tiny baby clothes. So you don't get overtired, start doing things a little at a time, rather than rushing to do it all at once. Get your partner involved, too—the preparations will help you both to bond with your unborn child.

YOUR BABY'S ROOM

Since you first became pregnant, you may have had lots of ideas about how to arrange your baby's room. It's a good idea to prepare the room before the birth—once you have your baby, most of your time and energy will be taken up by her care. Make safety and comfort for both of you your main priorities.

SLEEPING

You'll probably want your baby to sleep close to you in your room for the first few weeks of her life. But it's a good idea also to have somewhere that's a special space for your baby—this may be either a whole room, or an area in another child's room. Make sure you have enough space for sleeping, feeding, bathing, diaper-changing, and dressing. A baby's room doesn't have to be expensively decorated, and if you keep it simple there'll be fewer changes needed as she grows up. You can usually find most of the things you'll need secondhand, or you can sometimes adapt existing furniture to your needs (see below). Whether your baby has her own room or shares yours at first, she needs to be kept warm. Try to keep a constant temperature of around 60–70°F (16–20°C); if necessary, install a thermostatically controlled heater.

FURNITURE AND STORAGE

A chest of drawers with a sturdy frame and legs is ideal both for storing your baby's clothes and as a changing table. Attach the dresser to a wall, if possible, so that if a child climbs on it or opens too many drawers, it will not tip over. It should be high enough (about hip-height) to allow you or your partner to use without bending too much. Make sure the surface can be cleaned easily, and, if it's wooden, check that there are no cracks or splinters. Choose a chest with at least three spacious drawers. Keep diaper-changing equipment in the top drawer or on wall shelf units nearby—these can be used later for books and toys. Put a plastic-covered changing mat with raised sides on top of the chest and have a small pedal bin, lined with a plastic bag, nearby for dirty diapers. Keep a straight-backed chair in the room so that you or your partner can feed your baby in comfort. If possible, place a small, sturdy table nearby so you have somewhere to put drinks, bottles, and so on.

LIGHTING

You're bound to want to check your baby while she's sleeping at night, so it helps to have lighting that you can put on without disturbing her sleep. Install a dimmer switch for the ceiling fixture and adjust it so you can put on the light without waking your baby. You could also use a night-light or shaded lamp, but be very careful not to leave any electrical cords trailing over the floor.

FLOORS AND WALLS

The floor in your baby's room needs to be nonslip, warm, and easy to clean. Don't use small rugs or mats— you may trip or slip on them. Vinyl floor coverings are hard-wearing and easily washed, and cork tiles are warm and practical. Paint the walls with a nontoxic, washable emulsion paint, or if you prefer wallpaper, make sure it can be wiped clean.

WINDOWS AND CURTAINS

Keep your baby's room well aired, but make sure the windows are draftproof and above your baby's reach. Put up lined curtains or room-darkening shades or blinds to block out light during daytime naps. Always choose fire-resistant materials. Blinds should have a safety mechanism so your baby can't be strangled by the cords.

WHAT'S GOOD FOR BABY

A brightly colored environment with lots of sounds is very stimulating for a young baby.

A bright musical mobile placed low over her crib will give your baby lots of pleasure. Hang another mobile above her changing table. Hang plastic-coated photographs or a small mirror in the crib—she loves to look at faces close up. Give her rattles, and toys that make a noise when thrown, batted, or shaken. Molded soft toys are good for sucking.

Toys for the newborn
Choose brightly colored, lightweight toys that can't be swallowed or pinch your baby's fingers.

SAFETY PRECAUTIONS

- Put a safety lock on each window in your baby's room, and install bars if the window is close to the floor.

- Use fire-resistant fabric for bedding, upholstery, and curtains.

- Place childproof covers over all electrical outlets.

- Screen fireplaces or space heaters with a fire guard.

- Coat walls and furniture in nontoxic, lead-free paint or varnish.

- Put childproof safety catches on all cupboards and drawers, especially in the kitchen. You can also get locks for the refrigerator, freezer, and oven.

- Install smoke detectors.

- Make sure all electrical cords are well out of your baby's reach.

- Use nonslip mats in the bathtub and on the bathroom floor.

MEETING YOUR NEEDS

Choosing equipment

You don't need much equipment at first—just something in which to transport your baby, somewhere for him to sleep, and something to bathe him in.

Babies grow quickly and some items of equipment may be more expensive than they're worth for the short time they're in use. Try to choose equipment that has a long life—a crib that becomes a child's bed, for example. Baby equipment is rarely worn out, simply outgrown, and there's no need to buy everything new— check for secondhand items in your local paper or on your baby clinic notice board. Ask friends and family, too; most people are only too happy to lend or pass on baby items.

TRAVEL

You'll need something to carry your baby around in as soon as he arrives. Before you buy anything, think very carefully about how much space you have for storage, and the kind of lifestyle you lead. A simple baby carrier is perfect for the first few months.

Strollers The newest models can be used from birth until your child is about three. Most have a seat that reclines in several different positions so a young baby can lie flat or an older baby or toddler can sit up and watch the world go by. Some also include a car seat, shopping basket, canopy and so on. Some parents like to use a baby carriage for a young baby, but although a carriage is comfortable and sturdy, you do need to have plenty of space to store it when it's not in use.

Adaptable transportation
The latest models can be used from birth to around three years and combine a stroller with a removable car seat.

Make sure that your stroller or carriage has handles at a comfortable height so you don't strain your back. Good brakes are essential: you must be able to apply them without letting go of the handle.

Your baby will quickly outgrow a cradle, so it is better to choose a crib that later converts into a bed. Make sure the height can be adjusted so you don't have to bend low to lift your baby.

Car seats The law demands that your child be safely restrained in a car, so make sure you have an appropriate safety seat before taking your baby home from the hospital, and check that it's securely anchored.

The seat must meet current safety regulations, and it's never a good idea to buy car seats secondhand in case they've been damaged.

Baby carrier
Your baby will enjoy the warmth of your body and the sound of your heartbeat when carried next to your chest.

242

Portable baby chair Your baby will enjoy sitting in one of these so he can see what's happening around him, and a bouncing chair will be fun when he kicks his feet. These are easy to carry around, but always make sure the base is wide and sturdy so that he can't tip himself over, and always strap him in securely.

SLEEPING AND BATHING

At first your baby will fit snugly into a bassinet, cradle, or even a drawer! The important thing is that his bed is the right size and is comfortable. Choose a thin, close-fitting, waterproof mattress and cotton sheets. He must not have a pillow. Crib bumpers aren't a good idea, either, since they keep air from circulating and may make your baby too hot. It's much more important to keep your baby's room draft-free and at an even temperature. Warm, light cotton cellular blankets are probably best for bedding. Remember that if your sleeping baby seems to be chilly, don't just add an extra covering—this will trap cold air inside, making him colder. Pick him up and cuddle him until he's warm, then dress him in warmer pajamas.

His crib Once your baby is too big for his first bed, choose a new or secondhand crib. Make sure it's sturdy and has nontoxic paint or varnish. The space between the bars should be no wider than 2½ inches (6 cm) so your baby's head can't get trapped. The sides of the crib should be high enough to keep him from climbing over, and have safety catches on the drop side to keep it from being released by accident. Choose a close-fitting, waterproof mattress, with no gaps between the edges of the mattress and the frame. Don't tie any toys to the crib that the baby could get its head stuck in, and keep ties short. Don't use crib bumpers at this stage, either, since an adventurous baby may try to use one as a step to help him climb over the bars of his crib.

Changing You won't need a changing table if you have a sturdy tabletop or chest of drawers and a plastic changing mat in your baby's room. As for washing your baby, you can always use the sink, but if you want a special bath with a stand, make sure it's stable and at the right height for you to use comfortably.

MEETING YOUR BABY'S NEEDS

Safety is the most important thing when choosing equipment for your baby, as any number of items can take care of his basic needs.

- Choose blankets and quilts without any fringes or loose ends that your baby could choke on.

- Use closely woven blankets that don't trap fingers and toes..

- If you use a baby carrier, choose one with a neck support and wide straps that will support your baby's weight.

His first bed
A bassinet will make a snug first bed for your newborn baby.

- Make sure cribs, strollers, and baby carriages don't have any sharp edges or sharp screws.

- When choosing a stroller, make sure there's adequate protection for your baby's head.

- Make sure there's nothing on the stroller that will pinch his fingers or toes.

- Wherever you put your baby down to sleep, make sure he is lying on his back.

Bathtime
Choose sturdy, practical equipment for bathtime. Yellow ducks are visually stimulating for your baby and lots of fun!

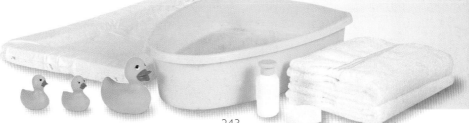

Baby clothes

SHOPPING TIPS

Don't wait until the last minute to buy your baby's clothes; shop while you still feel comfortable enough to enjoy it.

- Don't try to get everything all at once, and ask your partner or a friend to help you carry any heavy bags.

- Your baby doesn't care what color and style her clothes are, so choose machine-washable garments in colors that won't run.

- Don't buy too many clothes for the first months in advance, since you don't know how fast your baby's going to grow or what the weather will be like. But don't skimp on the number of essential items. You always need more than you think.

- Choose medium-priced items from reliable stores. Cheap baby clothes fall apart at the seams, fabrics become rough and irritating, and they may have to be thrown out after only a few washes.

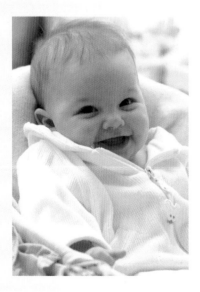

Most of us overprepare for a new baby, especially if it's our first. Don't forget that babies grow fast, and very small garments will soon be outgrown. On the whole, it's better to buy larger sizes (except for pajamas, which should fit snugly), since clothes that are too close-fitting may make your baby hot and rub his skin. Babies have no idea what they are wearing, so keep all clothing simple and comfortable.

Choosing clothes and accessories Baby clothes are getting better all the time in terms of fabric, design, and washability, so shop around to get a feel for what's available before making a final choice. You'll see lots of things you don't need and would never use, so don't waste your money on unnecessary items. Ask a friend or relative with a baby what she found useful, and you may find she can pass you on things her baby has grown out of. Don't be embarrassed about accepting such gifts.

You'll need several changes of sheets, stretch suits, T-shirts, and shawls so that you can have a few in the wash without running out. Choose patterned fabrics or sheets and clothing, rather than solid pastels, so that every little stain doesn't show. Natural fibers are best, as they allow sweat to evaporate, but remember that bedding and clothes with a high percentage of cotton may shrink once they're washed, so buy at least a size bigger than you think you'll need. Choose T-shirts with wide necks, as babies hate having tight things pulled over their heads. Don't buy any clothing with buttons or zippers that are close to the neck. Also, think about what's convenient for you. Even if you prefer cloth diapers, keep a supply of disposable diapers on hand for times when you need to make a quick change with as little fuss as possible.

Essential baby items

1 bonnet—the type will depend on the season	diapers or 2 dozen cloth diapers and 1 packet of diaper liners
6 cotton T-shirts with wide or envelope neck	2 diaper pails
	2 soft new towels
2 plain cardigan sweaters, jackets, or loose sweatshirts	8 muslin squares
	1 packet cotton balls
2 pairs cotton socks or slip-on bootees	baby lotion
2 shawls	1 packet safe diaper pins or plastic fasteners
6 stretch suits	
gloves or scratch mittens	blunt-edged scissors
6 pairs of plastic pants	diaper rash cream
1 box smallest-size disposable	

CHOOSING CLOTHES FOR YOUR BABY

Choosing clothes for your baby can seem like a daunting task at first because there are so many different items now to choose from. The most important thing is to be practical in your choice, bearing in mind some of the points below.

Cotton fleece jackets are warm and more practical than lacy sweaters

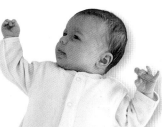

YOUR BABY'S NEEDS

Comfort and safety, rather than style, are the main priorities when choosing your baby's clothing.

- Look for soft, machine-washable fabrics. Cotton is ideal. Synthetic fabrics don't always absorb sweat, and wool can irritate the skin of some newborn babies.

- In warm weather, two layers are usually ample. In winter, add more layers but do not wrap her up too much with tight clothes.

- A baby's gestures are jerky and expansive, so make sure garments are loose and easily stretched.

Outdoor wear

When choosing clothing for outdoors, warmth is the most important thing. Don't be distracted by color or fashion. Your baby's head, feet, and hands are vulnerable to the cold, so make sure they're covered.

Stretch suits are ideal for keeping baby warm all over; fastenings in the crotch and inside leg will make diaper-changing easy

A baby's nightie should be long enough for warmth, with a wide neck opening

Envelope-neck shirts should be made of soft cotton or thermal material

Going to bed

Babies move in their sleep—not as much as adults, but it's something to consider. Choose clothing that allows your baby to move freely and does not entangle her limbs

Breast or bottle?

**Unless there are good reasons
not to, it's always better to
breastfeed your baby if you
possibly can.**

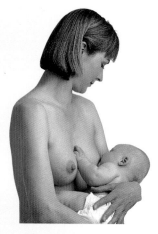

Breastfeeding means that your
baby gets the ideal food; breast milk
is always available and doesn't require
special equipment or preparation.
Many women enjoy breastfeeding,
and it's better for your body: for
instance, it helps your uterus return
quickly to its normal size.

Breastfeeding has drawbacks, but
these can be easily overcome. The
quantity and quality of your milk
depend on your health, so eat well
and take care of yourself. Feeding
can lead to sore nipples or breast
infections (see p.356), which need
prompt treatment. It can be tiring, so
make sure you get lots of rest.

Bottlefeeding Infant formulas are
very nourishing, but they are still
only second-best to breast milk.
Bottlefeeding costs more and, if you
take your baby out for any length of
time, you have to carry equipment
and a supply of formula with you.
Bottlefeeding may be necessary if
you need to take certain
medications after delivery.

Breastfeeding is better for your baby than bottlefeeding. But if
for some reason you can't breastfeed your baby, don't
worry—modern milk formulas are good, and she will be
adequately nourished.

The best possible preparation for breastfeeding your baby is to
make sure you and your partner are aware of all the benefits it has
(see below). Make sure you know what's involved, and that you're
physically and mentally ready for it. Physical preparations are
simple and straightforward—all you need to do is keep yourself
well nourished, avoid hazards that could affect your milk supply,
and make sure you care for your breasts properly. Your healthcare
provider or childbirth instructor should be able to answer any
questions you have.

If you decide on bottlefeeding (see pp.332 & 334), you'll need
to buy supplies of formula, bottles, and nipples, as well as
sterilizing equipment, before your baby is born.

BREASTFEEDING

Breast milk is the perfect food for a baby. It contains all the
essential nutrients (fat, protein, carbohydrate, vitamins, and iron)
that a baby needs; it's never too rich or too watery; it's clean,
readily available, and always at just the right temperature. And
like the colostrum that's produced by your breasts before your
milk comes in (see Producing milk, p.326), it contains antibodies
that help protect your baby from common infections such as
gastroenteritis.

Breastfeeding is a fulfilling and enjoyable experience that will
enhance the loving relationship between you and your baby.
What's more, despite occasional snags such as sore nipples or
engorged breasts, it's good for you, too. The extra calories you
use in producing breast milk help to use up the fat reserves you
gained during pregnancy, so you get back to your prepregnancy
weight more easily. When you breastfeed, the hormone oxytocin,
which makes your milk glands contract when your baby suckles
(see p.326), also causes contractions in your uterus, helping it to
return to its normal size more quickly.

There's also some evidence that women who have breastfed are
less prone to breast cancer and to osteoporosis (brittle bones).
From a purely practical point of view, breastfeeding is quick, easy,
and convenient. It's virtually free, and you don't need to carry
around any special equipment.

Breastfeeding does have some drawbacks, though. Until your
milk supply is sufficiently well established for you to collect and
store it for later feeding by bottle (see p.327), you're the only
person who can feed your baby. If you prefer privacy when
breastfeeding, you may find it difficult when away from home.

Breastfeeding can lead to sore or cracked nipples and other breast problems (see p.356); illness, tiredness, stress, and menstruation can reduce your milk supply; if you're taking any medication or drugs while breastfeeding, these can pass into your milk and possibly cause harm to your baby; and some foods that you eat, such as oranges, may upset your baby's stomach.

Most problems and difficulties you may have in getting your baby to breastfeed tend to lessen after the first couple of weeks. So if you find breastfeeding your baby frustrating at first, stick with it for a while. Once the initial difficulties have passed and you've both settled down, you'll probably find it easy, immensely rewarding, and enjoyable.

BOTTLEFEEDING

Although modern infant formula milk provides adequate nourishment for your baby (as you can see from the chart below), it doesn't contain the protective antibodies found in colostrum and breast milk. Other disadvantages are that it's harder to digest than breast milk (but because of this, your baby will need feeding less frequently); it gives more formed bowel movements with a stronger smell than those of a breastfed baby; formula may lay the foundation for a milk allergy later on; preparing it is time-consuming; and you may find it harder to lose weight because you're not using up calories in producing milk. Also, you have to buy the equipment and the formula, and if you go out, you need to take a supply of bottles with you.

BABY'S EXPERIENCE

Your baby will greatly enjoy being breastfed, and breast milk is specifically designed to give her the best start in life.

Breast milk is nutritionally superior to formula, easy to digest, and, like colostrum, protects against many common infections, particularly those of the gastro-intestinal and respiratory tracts. Even if you only breastfeed your baby for the first few weeks, the antibodies in your colostrum and milk will do her a great deal of good, and the close contact between you will strengthen your relationship.

Formula If you're unable to breastfeed, your baby will, of course, thrive and grow on formula milk. Whenever you bottlefeed, give your baby lots of skin and eye contact, and talk or sing to her to help to intensify the bonding between you.

Comparison of milks and formulas			
NUTRIENT (PER 100 MILLILITERS)	HUMAN MILK	COW'S MILK FORMULA	SOY-BASED FORMULA
Energy (Cal)	68	66	65
Fat (g)	3.8	3.7	3.6
Protein (g)	1.25	1.45	1.8
Carbohydrate (g)	7.2	7.22	6.9
Vitamin A (mg)	60	80	60
Vitamin D (mg)	0.025	1.0	1.0
Vitamin C (mg)	3.7	6.8	5.5
Iron (mg)	0.07	0.58	0.67

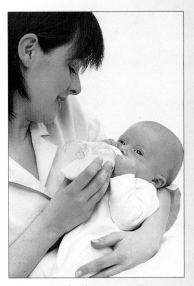

Creating intimacy
As you bottlefeed your baby, keep your attention focused on her. Maintain eye contact, and smile and talk to her.

Choosing a name

POINTS TO THINK ABOUT

Here are a few things to bear in mind when you're choosing a first name for your newborn baby.

- Will the name be suitable for your child at all stages of life?

- Is it obvious how the name is spelled and pronounced?

- Does the name sound right when put together with the middle name(s) you like and your last name?

- Do the initials of the full name make a word when they're put together?

- Are you happy with any associations with the name—famous people or people you know, for example?

- Is there any reason why your child might be teased because of the name you've chosen?

Naming your baby can be surprisingly difficult. There are so many things to think about—will the name you've chosen go with the family name? Is it likely to go out of style? You may be influenced by many different associations and considerations, but the main thing to remember is that the name you choose is for your baby, and hopefully it will please him throughout the whole of his life.

FASHION

This does influence lots of parents, either consciously or unconsciously. A name can suddenly become very popular—often because of a particular celebrity—and then fall out of fashion equally suddenly, so dating the children bearing it.

It's very difficult to predict which will be the "in" names in any given year, although some are always popular and many parents define what is fashionable or unfashionable by their own social set. The annual publication *The Top Ten of Everything* lists the most popular names for boys and girls in any given year. And the Social Security Administration (www.ssa.gov) has lists of the most popular names for both sexes, stretching back over a century.

You may be influenced by whether a name is traditional or modern. Some people prefer old, familiar names and shrink from new, invented, or imported names; others see no reason to use names from the past, and choose something that is meaningful to them and part of the age in which they live.

ASSOCIATIONS

Parents often choose names because of their association, rather than their particular meaning. Meaning tends to play a much smaller role in the Western world than it does in some other parts of the world.

Personal associations can have a positive or negative influence. Some people like to name a child after a friend or a family member—a much-loved grandparent, for example. You won't want to use names you associate with someone you don't like. Godparents are sometimes honored, and public associations might include royalty, pop singers, and movie and television stars. Place-names, too, have begun to be used if they have particular meaning for parents (Brooklyn, Phoenix), but take care when combining these with surnames (e.g., "Brooklyn Bridge") to avoid your child being teased.

Characters in books and films can also inspire parents. The 1956 movie *High Society* starred Grace Kelly as Tracy Samantha Lord, which led to a surge of popularity for Grace, and the use of Tracy, Samantha, and Kelly as first names for girls. Today some parents like to name their children after characters in popular television series such as soap operas.

For many people, a name can conjure up a particular image or character, and they may expect children to fit or suit a name. As this can influence the way a child is treated, and consequently how the child responds, children may well grow into the names they're given.

Other names, such as Patience or Faith, can reflect the parent's desire for the child (usually female in the Western world) to possess particular virtues, and were first introduced by the Puritans (see column, right).

Some first names are inspired by where a baby is conceived or something that happens during pregnancy, or around the time of the birth. These can include time of birth—Noël or Natalie for a Christmas baby; month names such as May, June, or occasionally Octavia for an October birth; a favorite record that was played during pregnancy, at or after birth; Dawn or Eve for the actual time of birth.

FAMILY TRADITIONS

Names that have been passed down through a family from generation to generation were at one time the automatic choice for many parents, especially for a first-born. If the traditional name was masculine, it was sometimes feminized for a girl (Thomas, Thomasina), especially if there was no male heir. These customs have lapsed in recent times, leading to many traditional family names being dropped, although they are sometimes used as a child's middle name.

Some families, particularly among the aristocracy in Scotland, and in the American South, used the mother's maiden name as the first-born son's given name. This appears to be dying out, although the maiden name is still given as a middle name. Because of this custom, surnames such as Russell, Howard, and Cameron have become normal as first names, particularly for boys. Couples who are not married or in which the woman prefers to keep her maiden name sometimes like to give the mother's surname as the child's middle name.

Many parents choose names for their children that work together, although few go as far as the Victorians (see column, right). Some parents like all their children's names to start with the same initial, although this can cause confusion with letters and official documents.

NATIONALITY

Many parents choose names that reflect where they come from, even though they no longer live there. This can lead to problems of spelling and pronunciation, so the spelling may be simplified—from Gaelic to English, for example (Síle—Sheila; Aodán—Aidan). In other cases, first names that are perceived as being "national" may not be used in their country of origin. Colleen, for example, comes from the Celtic *caitlín*, meaning "girl" or "wench," and is popular for girls of Irish origin in North America and Australia, even though it's not used as a given name in Ireland.

NAMING FASHIONS

There are trends in name-giving just as there are in other things. Many of today's first names have been used for centuries.

Norman After they conquered Britain in 1066, the Normans introduced a fixed name system. Norman names included Alan, Henry, Hugh, Ralph, Richard, Oliver, William, Alice, Emma, Rosamund, and Yvonne. These were names given to the aristocracy and later copied by those lower on the social scale, so Norman names rapidly replaced most Old English names. Of these, some such as Edward and Edith survived.

Biblical In the sixteenth century there were many names used primarily by Catholics. These included Mary, and saints' names such as Sebastian, Benedict, and Agnes. The Protestants turned to the Bible for inspiration, and Adam, Benjamin, David, Joshua, Michael, Samuel, Abigail, Dinah, Hannah, Rachel, Ruth, and Sarah became popular. The Puritans in the seventeenth century used "virtue" names—Faith, Charity, Grace, Hope, Patience, and Prudence.

Victorian At the end of the nineteenth century, there was a vogue for using gemstones or flowers as first names for girls. Thus Amber, Pearl, Ruby, Lily, Ivy, and Rose became popular. Sometimes, all the girls in a family would bear the name of different flowers or gems.

Contemporary The twentieth century saw the rise of exotic spellings, such as Jayne, Nikki, and Debra, and of combinations, such as Raelene and Charlene. Since the 1960s, many descriptive words, such as Sky, Free, Rainbow, and River, have been given as first names.

NAMING TWINS

There's a tradition of giving twins names that are related. The names may reflect an association; begin with the same initial (Paul, Patricia); sound alike (Suzanna, Hannah); or have a similar rhythm (Benjamin, Jonathan).

But there are lots of reasons why your twins won't thank you if their names are too closely associated for comfort.

First, and most important, people will be much more likely to get them confused if there's a strong link between their names. Names are used as labels and twins, perhaps more than other children, need individual labels that belong solely to them.

Second, official forms, examination papers, and letters can easily become confused, especially if initials are shared.

Third, if the names are closely linked by association, twins are likely to be in for a lot of name teasing or punning.

MEANINGS

The meaning or origin of a name tends to be less important than its associations for most modern Western parents. Many Western first names have had a more convoluted history than those of other cultures. This is because these names, along with other traditions and customs, have been transferred from one society to another, often by invasion followed by integration, migration, or contact between different cultures. For this reason, many names have become divorced from their original meanings, but some Western parents do still choose names primarily because of what they mean.

FORM OF A NAME

The way our names are pronounced and spelled, and the shortened forms we prefer, are very important to most of us. It's irritating if your name is constantly misspelled or mispronounced, and it can be annoying if someone uses a short version you don't like, or the formal version that wasn't actually bestowed.

Diminutives The pet forms of names (Megan, Kate, Jamie) are often used, and sometimes given, in preference to the full versions (Margaret, Katherine, James). Even if you intend to always use the diminutive, it's worth considering giving your child the full formal name, since there may be times when it's more appropriate. On the other hand, if you intend always to use the full version of a name (Patricia, Edward) it's good to consider how your feel about any pet forms (Pat, Patty, Patsy, Trish, Tricia; Ed, Eddie, Ted, Ned) since your child's name will almost certainly be shortened by friends.

Sound You may like a name because of its sound—it could be that the name is naturally harmonious, or perhaps it sounds good alongside your last name. Most parents take particular care to select a happy partnership, with surnames balanced by given names. Indeed, some parents bestow names in the order they feel sounds best (Elizabeth Anne, Arthur James), but call their child by the middle name (Anne, James).

Spelling and pronunciation It's worth giving your child a name that everyone can spell and pronounce easily to avoid confusion and irritation for your child in later life. In the last 50 years or so, there has been an increasing tendency for exotic spellings of ordinary first names (Jayne, Kathryn, Jonothon). Some names have more than one pronunciation (Helena), while others are confusing (Phoebe), and still others have more than one spelling (Clare, Clair, Claire).

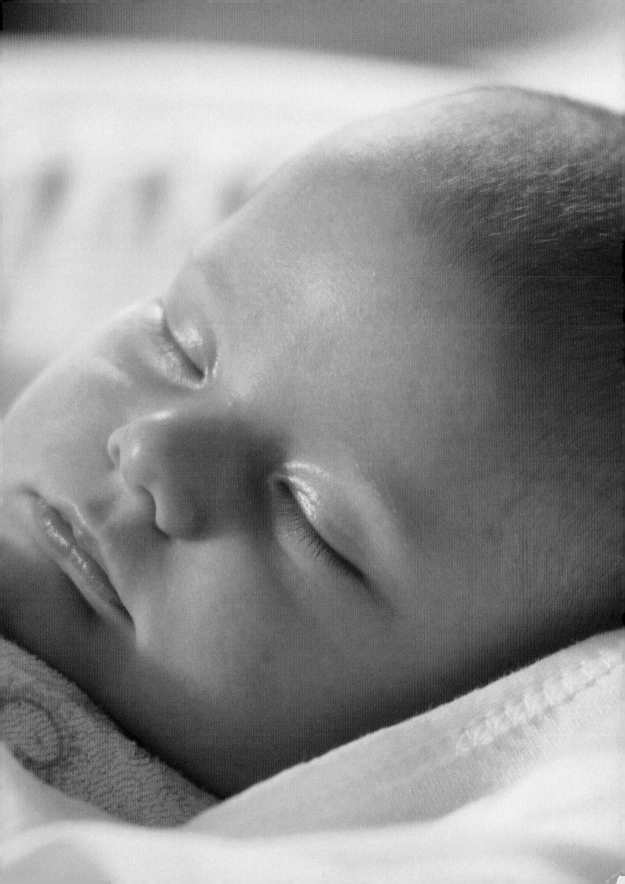

Preparing siblings for a new baby

Involving your older child
Talking to your older child about the arrival of your new baby, and encouraging her to take an interest in her new brother or sister's development, will help her feel involved and avoid feelings of neglect.

Any child who's enjoyed the undivided attention of both parents for any length of time—say, a year or longer—will suffer what child psychologists call dethronement when a new baby arrives. This is not simply about having to take second place with Mom and Dad for a while, nor putting up with less attention than before. It's about feeling displaced and rejected. Nearly all toddlers suffer a deep sense of loss of parental love when a new sibling arrives. It's not surprising that their psychological disturbance shows in changes in their behavior after the new arrival.

To a small child, the arrival of a new baby topples him from the top of the heap, from being first in his mother's considerations, the apple of her eye and the focus of her love, nurture, and attention. A child feels this displacement very dramatically and, of course, responds as only a small child knows how: by using all the tactics at his disposal to regain his parents' love and attention.

The result can be "regression," which means the toddler goes back to earlier, happier times, when he couldn't feed himself, perhaps, or when he wet and soiled his diapers, or before he'd learned to talk. This may look to adults like some sort of rebellion, but a toddler can't help this behavior. So the worst thing you can do is punish him for it. In fact, the opposite is essential— he needs some extra-special time alone with Mom and Dad, extra-special loving care, plenty of rewards, praise and physical affection with games, kisses, cuddles, and lots of jokes and laughter.

Armed with this knowledge of how your toddler is likely to react to the arrival of a brother or sister, you can ease him through this painful time with some careful preparation and planning.

Involving your older child in the pregnancy Be honest with your child from the start. Tell him that a new baby is on the way and he's going to have a new brother or sister. You might even ask him what his favorite names are. Make a list, put them up in the kitchen, and talk about them from time to time.

Encourage your child to put his hand on your tummy as it gets bigger to feel the baby kicking. You could also tell him that your baby loves the sound of his voice and that he should talk to her through your tummy. Ask him to sing her songs and nursery rhymes through your tummy.

Incidentally, this isn't all hot air. Your developing baby does remember the voices of those around her and will bond with them after birth. So she'll respond instantly on hearing her brother's or sister's voice once she's born, if she's heard it constantly during your pregnancy.

Helping your older child to understand what's happening Show him what's happening in your tummy month by month using the pictures in this book (see pp.72–89). Copy them on large sheets of paper so that it's all very clear. Point out how the baby is developing and put up the drawings around the wall at a height where your toddler can see them easily. Perhaps you could then make up stories about each stage of the new baby's development saying things like, "Now your new baby's heart is beating." "Now your new baby can move his hands and legs and we can feel him kicking." "Now your new baby can suck her thumb." "Now your new baby is getting ready to be born," and so on.

Try to encourage your toddler to take ownership of his new sister by using the word "your," as in "your baby," "your new sister." If you do, very soon he'll develop a sense of ownership and of a desire to take care of his new brother or sister. If you and your partner always talk about "our new baby," he may feel excluded and frozen out.

It'll help your toddler to feel included if you involve him in the preparations for the new baby—helping to make up the crib and setting out equipment, for example. You might even suggest that he could try out the baby bath first, saying something like, "Wouldn't you like to see what the baby bath feels like before your sister uses it?"

All toddlers like to help and love to imitate your actions. So give your toddler small jobs to do and be very appreciative of all his efforts. You can show him all the new baby's tiny clothes and encourage him to feel special by saying how much bigger he is and how much he's grown since he needed them.

AFTER THE BIRTH

If you're going to be in the hospital for several days, try to arrange for your child to visit you and the baby as soon as possible after the delivery.

When your toddler visits, have eyes only for him. Ideally, your new baby should be asleep in the bedside crib. Make a fuss of your toddler until he asks about the new baby. Only then show him his sister, but not for long, not with any fuss, and not paying too much attention to her. Make his visit short so that you can attend to your baby once he's gone.

Bringing the baby home Try to help your toddler to feel secure and bond with the new baby.

- When you greet him, make sure someone else holds the baby so that you are free to cuddle him.

- For the first few minutes, give him all your attention.

- Give your child a present from the new baby, something he's really been looking forward to.

- In the first weeks, set aside some time when the two of you can be together without any interruptions.

- Involve your child in the new baby's bathtimes, changing, and feeding times. Get him to fetch and carry and imitate your loving sounds with lots of ahhs and ooohs and words like "softly" and "gently." Describe everything that your new baby is doing so that he can get to know her and relate to her.

- A newborn baby has a well-developed grasp reflex. Put one of your child's fingers into her hand—she'll grasp it very tightly, and he'll interpret this as love from his newborn sister.

FATHER CARE

In many households, the father is the main helper when his partner arrives home with their new baby. Some men immediately involve themselves in caring for their partner and child, but others need to be encouraged.

What you need from your partner more than anything else at this time is understanding, sympathy, and a readiness to let his routine relax and go along with you and the baby. It's best to have a serious discussion about this before your baby is born. Otherwise, your partner may find it hard to adapt and feel neglected, inadequate, and bereft of your affection and attention.

You may find it best to divide the work between you. For instance, your partner could take over the cleaning, shopping, and laundry, leaving you free to concentrate on taking care of yourself and the baby. Or you might prefer to share all the household and childcare work.

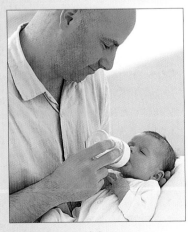

Help at mealtimes
If you're breastfeeding, express milk into a bottle (see p.327) so that your partner can also have the pleasure of feeding the baby.

Arranging childcare

In the last weeks of pregnancy, it's a good idea for you and your partner to talk about how you are going to organize things at home once your baby is born. If your partner is able to take time off work and able to play a full part, you'll be able to cope without too much difficulty; if not, you'll need someone else to give you some help and support, especially in the first few weeks.

The first few days of motherhood will be harder than you think. Labor and birth are physically and emotionally draining; you'll feel you have very few reserves left, and you'll be very tired. You'll realize, once at home with your baby, that one job or activity succeeds another almost without a moment's pause, and in the middle of all this, you're still learning about being a mother. Even if you've read every baby book in print, you'll find that your baby conforms to no typical schedule or plan, and that you have to work out your life around your baby's routine. Trying to impose a routine on your baby only causes you more work; it's best to take your lead from him. As far as sleep is concerned, you need to get it when you can—new babies don't know night from day and need the same attention during the night as they do in the day.

During the first few weeks at home with your baby, try to get someone else to do the household chores, or simply cut back the amount you do to the bare minimum, until you get used to the schedule your baby follows naturally.

SOURCES OF HELP

So that you don't become overtired, and even depressed and weepy, you'll need some help to tide you over at least the first few days, and preferably the first week or two. Don't be too proud to ask for or accept help—if you don't say what you need, you may come to regret it. Having help does not make you an inadequate mother. The best possible solution is to have someone living in your house, so that your day can be split into shifts. That way, you can at least make sure that you get enough rest and time to pay attention to what you're eating.

Family and friends Your mother and your mother-in-law are probably the people you trust most in the world when it comes to childcare. They've had children and are experienced at caring for babies, and they'll give you lots of helpful support and advice. If possible, ask one of them, or another close relative who has the flexibility and time, to come and live in your house around the time you go into labor. That way, your helper can establish herself in your home with your partner and other children if you have them, and be ready to help you settle in when you come home with the baby.

Such a helper is invaluable. You'll feel confident that the household is ticking along normally. She can take over all the organizational tasks, do the cooking, laundry, and shopping, and so on. This also takes some of the responsibility from your partner so you can both devote more time to your baby. And if your helper has had children of her own, she'll probably have lots of valuable information and advice for you.

Nannies   Nannies can either live with you or come on a daily basis. If you decide that you'd like a nanny, it's best to arrange for her to be settled in with your family before your baby is born so you can get to know each other. Having a newborn baby in the house is quite a traumatic event, and it's important to have a helper who'll fit in with your routines and lifestyle. It's also vital for you to feel confident about her abilities and happy with her relationship with your baby.

You can find a nanny through personal recommendations, advertising, or through a reliable nanny agency. In-home care of this kind can be expensive, but if you have more than one child it becomes economical.

However you recruit your nanny, you'll need to see her at least twice before you hire her. Make sure you get two good references, and follow up these references with a telephone call to tease out any "between the lines" information. The first time you meet, suggest you relax over coffee or lunch together, or maybe go shopping. Follow this up with a formal interview. Both you and your partner should be involved in the process, because you'll probably see different aspects of her character.

Draw up a contract of employment with a formal job description in which you cover all the tasks you expect her to undertake, and include the approaches and attitudes you expect. Your nanny should be prepared to alter her usual practices in order to fit in with yours. Remember that you are her employer and as such you are responsible for her welfare. She has the same employment rights as an employee in any other line of work.

Au pairs   These are young women (or occasionally young men) from other countries who help you with your baby in exchange for room, board, a small wage, and an opportunity for academic study. They are expected to be proficient in English, but you are required to provide them with training in child safety and development. You may not ask an au pair to work more than 45 hours per week. Remember that an au pair is an employee, and federal law requires you to pay him or her a certain minimum wage. You will also have to follow other rules laid out by the Department of State. It's probably easiest to hire an au pair through a reputable agency that can help you understand all the legal requirements.

MATERNITY NURSES

If you want short-term, live-in help, you could hire a maternity nurse. She'll join your household just before or after your baby is born and will help with all the babycare.

As well as providing welcome help with your baby, maternity nurses are invaluable teachers. They'll show you how to see to your baby's daily care: how to change diapers; how to breast- or bottlefeed him, how to know when he's had enough, and how to take the baby carefully off your breast to avoid soreness and cracked nipples, for example.

But it's up to you and your maternity nurse to work out what kind of regimen you would like. You may decide, for instance, that you'd like to have a night's sleep without interruption so the nurse will be on duty all the way through the night. You'd then take over at, say, 7 a.m. so that she can get some rest. Later in the day, she could do the baby's laundry, make up bottles if necessary, keep the baby's room clean, and tend to all the baby's needs and some of yours, too.

As a rule, a maternity nurse does not stay with you for more than four weeks, but you can arrange for her to stay for longer if your finances can accommodate it. Maternity nurses are expensive, but will get you off to a good start if there's no one else to help.

The working mother

Case study

Name Vicky Dyson
Age 29 years
Past medical history Nothing abnormal
Obstetric history One son age six; normal
birth

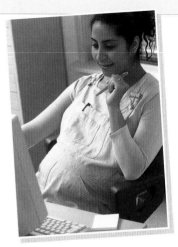

Vicky, a junior partner in a firm of accountants, is very eager to keep working
while pregnant. She passed her accountancy exams while she was expecting
her first child, so she knows she can cope. She also knows that she can
combine work and mothering, having worked since shortly after the birth of
her son. Her challenge now is to combine pregnancy with work, be a mother
to a schoolboy, and keep up a good relationship with her partner. The keys are
managing her time well and being sensitive to her own needs.

*Vicky has decided to continue with a very
demanding job while she has her second child.
To do this, she has to fit the pieces of her life
together like a jigsaw puzzle—when to leave
work, when to return, childcare arrangements,
her family, and her health. She needs to make
her own well-being and her baby's top priority
in all her plans.*

VICKY'S WORK SITUATION

Vicky's colleagues and senior partners are all men, and
she fears they might resent her taking a lot of time off
either before or after the birth. I suggested that she tell
her senior partners that she's pregnant right away and
arrange to talk to them, sometime within the next three
months, about when she might leave work and when she
might return (see p.64). I also advised her to make sure
she eats well so she has all the energy and nutrition she
needs to keep working while her baby develops. She'll
need some extra rest so, if she can, she should take a
nap in the afternoon—or at least rest with her feet up.

WHEN TO LEAVE

No two pregnancies are alike, so Vicky can't know how
she'll feel this time around. I advised her not to commit
herself to staying at work beyond the thirty-second week,
but perhaps she could make an informal arrangement to
do so if she feels well enough.

WHEN TO RETURN

This is a more complicated decision, since there are so
many things to take into account. Vicky's menstrual cycle
may take only three months to get back to normal, but
her muscles and various organs will need more time.
The process takes a year altogether. Vicky has to make
special feeding plans if she wants to go back to work
before her baby is four months old. She doesn't want to
give her baby milk substitute, so she'll have to express
her breast milk and freeze it (see At the office, opposite,
and p.327). Vicky will need to allow time to build up a
stock of milk initially, then a further six weeks for her
baby to get used to the new arrangement.

I suggested that Vicky could arrange a provisional date
for her return to work, but bear in mind that she may
feel quite different after the birth. She'll need to check
with her doctor as she nears her return date.

CHOOSING A CAREGIVER

When choosing a caregiver, she'll need to investigate all
the available options well in advance—daycare centers,
nannies, au pairs, and so on—until she finds a caregiver
who's just right for her family.

MAKING TIME

Once she's back at work, running her home, caring for
her family, and mothering her new baby, Vicky will
probably feel that time is very precious—and that she
doesn't have enough of it.

She must have some time alone with her new baby every day, and her son, Jack, will also need lots of attention and reassurance at this stage. The best way to give him this is to make sure he has his own special time with her, so that he doesn't feel shut out. Vicky will also want to have time alone with her partner, Peter, so that their relationship doesn't suffer. She and Peter, with or without the children, will also want to see their friends. Above all, Vicky will need some time to herself—even if it's only one free hour a week when nobody is making any demands on her. Many mothers feel guilty about taking time to be alone or doing something for themselves, but it's really important if you're going to be relaxed and happy.

FINDING A ROUTINE

I suggested that Vicky would be likely to feel less overwhelmed if she has a routine to work to, and that the rest of her family would also feel happier if their days were structured. For example, Vicky's time with her baby could be when she gets back from work. She could encourage Peter and Jack to bring her a cup of herbal tea, make sure she's comfortable, then leave her with her baby while they play together. Her special time with her son could be his bedtime, when she reads him a story and listens to him talk about his day. She and Peter could then have an evening meal together and chat, before their baby needs her late-evening feeding.

EXPRESSING HER MILK

I explained to Vicky that she'll need to keep up a good supply of breast milk by feeding her baby or by expressing it regularly. Leaving milk in the breast discourages further milk production, and supplies soon dwindle. Vicky feels sure that she'll have enough milk for her to be able to express some just after feedings so that she can gradually stockpile milk for future use.

AT THE OFFICE

I told Vicky she will probably find that her breasts will become full twice a day, so she will have to make time to express it at work.

Vicky told me that she intended to use a breast pump. Although most of the people at work are men, there's a comfortable, clean ladies' room where she can express her milk in private, and a refrigerator in her office where she can store her milk until she goes home in the evening, so she doesn't think she'll have too many problems. She knows that all containers must be sterilized and that breast milk can only be kept for up to 48 hours in the refrigerator—it can be stored for up to six months in the freezer.

Since Vicky will be at work all day, her caregiver will be responsible for defrosting each day's supply of breast milk. This should usually be done in the refrigerator, although if you do need to defrost breast milk quickly, you can place the container under running lukewarm tap water. Leftover milk must be thrown away and never kept or refrozen for later use.

Vicky's baby

Since her mother is working, Vicky's baby will also have to adjust to a routine.

• She'll have to accept bottles of expressed milk, something she'll find easier if she's introduced to it before she's five weeks old.

• If she refuses to accept milk from a bottle, it's worth trying bottles with a different type of nipples.

• Six weeks before Vicky returns to work, she'll have to start weaning her baby off the breast for her daytime feedings. She can start by replacing one daytime feeding with a bottle until she's used to it.

• She'll have to accept the person who cares for her all day while Vicky is at work. Vicky's baby will develop close bonds with her caregiver, who'll be an important person in her life. But this won't affect her relationship with her parents.

• When Vicky gets home from work, her breasts will be full of milk and her baby will be ready for a feeding; this is a good time for them to spend together.

• She'll be quick to figure out that Mommy is there all night and may become a wakeful baby, as two of my own sons did.

GETTING ENOUGH SLEEP

A good night's sleep is one of your top priorities in the late stages of pregnancy.

If you can, get eight hours of sleep a night, but you may find you suffer from irritating insomnia. Although your metabolism slows down at night, your baby's doesn't, and he may be active and kicking through the night hours. If you can't sleep, there are a number of things you can try:

- take a warm (not hot) bath before going to bed to relax you and make you sleepy and calm

- a hot milky bedtime drink helps you drop off; also, read a calming book, listen to music or the radio, or watch television

- deep breathing and relaxation exercises are excellent treatments for insomnia, so find a bedtime routine that suits you

- instead of worrying about your lack of sleep, get up in the middle of the night and do something—perhaps a job that you've been putting off for some time—or go into your baby's room, look at things, touch them, rearrange them, and feel happy at the thought of your baby

- if you have worries that keep you from sleeping, visualize each one as being written on a piece of paper. Then mentally crumple it up and throw it away.

The late stages of pregnancy

Very little goes wrong in the last few weeks of pregnancy. From week 32 onward, your doctor and midwife will be mainly keeping an eye on the continued growth of your baby and your own health. For example, if you stop putting on weight, it could be a sign that your baby isn't growing, or an increase in blood pressure could warn of preeclampsia (see p.224). You'll need to have checkups more often than before, probably every three weeks from week 32 to week 36, and then every two weeks up to week 40.

One of the problems of later pregnancy is that it's harder and harder to get comfortable. As your abdomen grows larger, sitting or lying in your usual positions can become difficult. If you lie flat on your back, the weight of your growing baby will press down on your major blood vessels and nerves that lie against the spine and cause numbness and tingling pain, even dizziness and shortness of breath. Experiment with your sleeping position in bed and make sure that you can make yourself as comfortable as possible. You may find that it helps to use some cushions or soft pillows to support your body (see below).

TENSE AND RELAX TECHNIQUE

Good relaxation techniques combine the release of tension in the mind and body with deep, regular breathing. You'll find it helpful to practice these techniques so that toward the end of pregnancy, they've become second nature. A good way to relax your whole body completely is to use the tense-and-relax technique. This is a

Resting on your side
In late pregnancy, it's often most comfortable to lie on your side, propped up with lots of cushions or pillows.

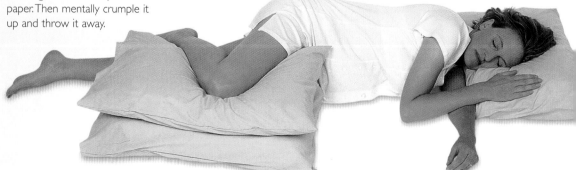

pleasant way to relax during pregnancy, and will also serve as a good preparation for labor, when it's a great help to be able to relax most of the muscles in your body, so that your uterus contracts without the rest of your body tensing.

What you do is tense and relax different parts of your body one after the other. Your partner can help by touching you where he can see you are tensing up: you respond to his touch by relaxing. Practice this technique twice a day for 15–20 minutes if you can, before meals or an hour or more after eating. You'll find it really helps you feel better.

Find a comfortable position, either lying on your back or propped up with pillows. Close your eyes and then try to clear your mind of any stressful thoughts, anxieties, or worries by breathing in and out slowly and regularly and concentrating all your attention on your breathing actions. Let pleasant, relaxing thoughts flow through your head, and if anything worrying or nagging tries to surface, prevent it from doing so by saying "no" under your breath, then go back to concentrating completely on your deep breathing.

When your mind is totally relaxed and your breathing deep and regular, begin the tense-and-relax routine. Think about your right hand: tense it for a moment, palm facing upward, then relax it and tell it to feel heavy and warm. Work up through the right side of your body, tensing and relax-ing your forearm, upper arm, and your shoulder. Then repeat the process on the upper left side of your body. Next, roll your knees outward, and then in turn tense and relax your buttocks, thighs, calves, and feet. Press your lower back gently into the floor or cushions, then release and relax.

Finish off by relaxing your head and neck. Relax the muscles of your face, particularly your forehead, and smooth away any frowns.

Sitting in a chair
When you sit in a chair, sitting up straight will help strengthen your back muscles. If you need extra support, put a cushion at the small of your back.

YOUR BABY'S POSITION

As a baby reaches full maturity at about 37 weeks, he usually becomes heavier and tips head-down. But some babies remain breech (see p.307) until term.

If a baby is in the breech position at term, he may be delivered by cesarean section (see p.308). If your baby is breech in the last weeks of pregnancy, though, don't worry—he'll probably turn himself before labor actually begins:

- 30 percent of babies are breech at 30 weeks. More than half of these will turn spontaneously during the next two weeks

- 14 percent of babies are still breech at 32 weeks. There's a 60-percent chance that a baby who is bottom-down will turn of his own accord before labor starts

- Less than five percent of babies are still breech at 37 weeks. One-quarter of these will turn on their own, although this is less likely if the legs are extended or there isn't much room in the uterus for some reason—for example, if you're having more than one baby or a large baby

- A few babies will kick themselves around once labor starts, as long as there's room.

Are you overdue?

**If you go past your EDD, your
healthcare provider will keep a
close watch on your baby by a
number of different methods.**

Fetal movement recording
The most accurate sign that all is
well with your baby is if you can
feel regular movements. Since all
mothers, and babies, are different,
the amount of movement that's
normal differs from one pregnancy
to another. You are the best judge
of whether your unborn baby is
acting normally, and you may be
asked to monitor his activity using
a kick chart (see p.195).

Electronic fetal monitoring
This may be used to check your
baby's heartbeat by providing a
continuous sound or paper
recording (see p.275). If the
heartbeat is satisfactory, you're
unlikely to need other tests or
induction of labor.

Ultrasound You'll probably be
given an ultrasound scan to assess
the volume of amniotic fluid. If this
is becoming dangerously low, your
doctors will probably advise you to
have your labor induced.

Only about five percent of all babies arrive on the actual date that
they're expected. The expected date of delivery (EDD—see p.63)
is only a statistical average, and studies have shown that as many as
40 percent of babies are born more than a week after their EDD.
This 40 percent of babies that are "overdue" arrive as follows:
25 percent of babies are born in the forty-second week of
pregnancy, 12 percent in the forty-third week, and three percent of
babies are born in the forty-fourth week of pregnancy.

BEING OVERDUE

The exact date of conception in any particular pregnancy is
extremely difficult to pinpoint, and this makes it hard to decide
whether a baby is overdue. Even if you have a regular menstrual
cycle of 28 days (the standard on which the EDD chart is based), the
date of ovulation is only known approximately (see p.63).

As well as this uncertainty about the exact date of ovulation,
every baby is different, so it's unrealistic to expect them all to
mature in precisely the same number of days. Since labor is
initiated by your baby's producing certain hormones as he
reaches full maturity, it makes sense that the actual date of
delivery can vary fairly widely—even in "textbook" pregnancies.

Doctors do become worried, though, if a pregnancy continues
much beyond the estimated date of delivery. This is because post-
maturity and possible problems with the placenta (placental
insufficiency) pose some risks to the health of your unborn baby
(see **Postmaturity, Risks**, opposite). The longer your baby goes on
growing inside your womb, the larger he is likely to become,
which, in turn, will increase the chances of a difficult labor.
There's also the risk that the placenta will not be able to continue
to support your baby over an extended period (see **Your baby's
placenta**, opposite).

Doctors will also ask about your family history—have you or
your mother had longer-than-average pregnancies (lasting 43 or
44 weeks, for example)? If so, your doctor will probably be more
willing to let you to go more than two weeks overdue without
suggesting that you're induced—although you'll be closely
monitored in case any problems do develop. (In practice, most
women are desperate to have their babies by this stage of
pregnancy.) After 40–41 weeks, you will have antepartum testing,
either ultrasound or non-stress testing, to determine if you need
to be induced, or if you can safely continue your pregnancy.

Pelvic disproportion Your labor may be delayed if your baby's
head is too big to pass through your pelvis. This disproportion
may prevent your baby's head from becoming engaged. If this
is the case (see column, right) you may a cesarean section.

POSTMATURITY

An overdue baby is in danger of being postmature. A postmature baby will have lost fat from all over his body, particularly from his tummy. His skin will look red and wrinkled, as if it doesn't fit him, and it may have begun to peel. Very few babies are actually post-mature because postmaturity depends not only on the baby's condition, but also on his placenta (see below). It is difficult to predict which babies will be at risk.

Risks A postmature baby tends to be bigger than average, which can make your labor longer and more difficult. Also, the bones in his skull tend to be harder, which means that his descent through the birth canal is likely to be more traumatic, both for him and for you, and there's also an increased risk of stillbirth—the risk of stillbirth doubles by the forty-third week of pregnancy and triples by the forty-fourth week. Another risk is that a uterus that's slow to start labor may also be relatively inefficient during the labor itself.

YOUR BABY'S PLACENTA

At term, the placenta—the organ that links the blood supplies of the mother and baby—looks like a large piece of raw liver. It is about the size of a dinner plate, and measures about 1 inch (2.5 centimeters) thick. The maternal side is divided into wedge-shaped chunks called *cotyledons*.

The placenta has substantial reserves, readily adjusts to injury, repairs damages due to *ischemia* (lack of oxygen), and does not undergo aging. The widely-held view that the placenta ages progressively during your pregnancy is due to a misinterpretation of the appearance of different parts of the placenta over the duration of the pregnancy.

Unquestionably, though, there are changes in the character of the *villi* (small projections) around the placenta during the pregnancy, and by the thirty-sixth week there may be deposits of calcium within the walls of the small blood vessels, and a protein deposit may appear on the surface of many of the villi. Both of these changes can limit the flow of nutrients and waste across the placenta, but this is balanced by the fact that the fetal blood vessels and villi are close together, which makes the exchange of nutrients easier.

Risks If labor does not start at the right time (this varies from pregnancy to pregnancy, but is usually considered to be two weeks on either side of the EDD), the placenta may then start to become relatively inefficient. This happens slowly, and at 42 weeks the placenta should still be capable of supplying your baby with enough nutrients for his needs.

There can be problems when, occasionally, the placenta fails to nourish and support your baby adequately. This is known as placental insufficiency, and in these circumstances you'll be advised to have your labor induced.

LATE ENGAGEMENT

When engagement is late in a first pregnancy, doctors may suspect pelvic disproportion. This means that if your baby is very big, it might be difficult for him to pass through your pelvis.

To check whether your baby's head will actually engage in, and pass through, your pelvis, your doctor will perform this simple test:

Step 1

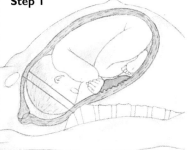

You'll be asked to lie on your back. When you're in this position, your doctor will be able to feel your baby's head resting just at the pelvic brim.

Step 2

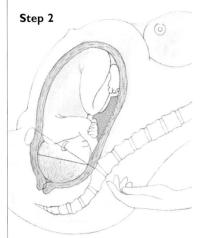

When you're propped up on your elbows, however, your baby's head slips easily into your pelvis, showing that you have no problem with pelvic disproportion.

CHAPTER 13

Managing your labor

Labor is the culmination of your pregnancy. Very few labors are pain-free, but you can choose the method of pain relief that suits you best. The help and support of your partner can be invaluable in making your labor a smoother, more comfortable experience.

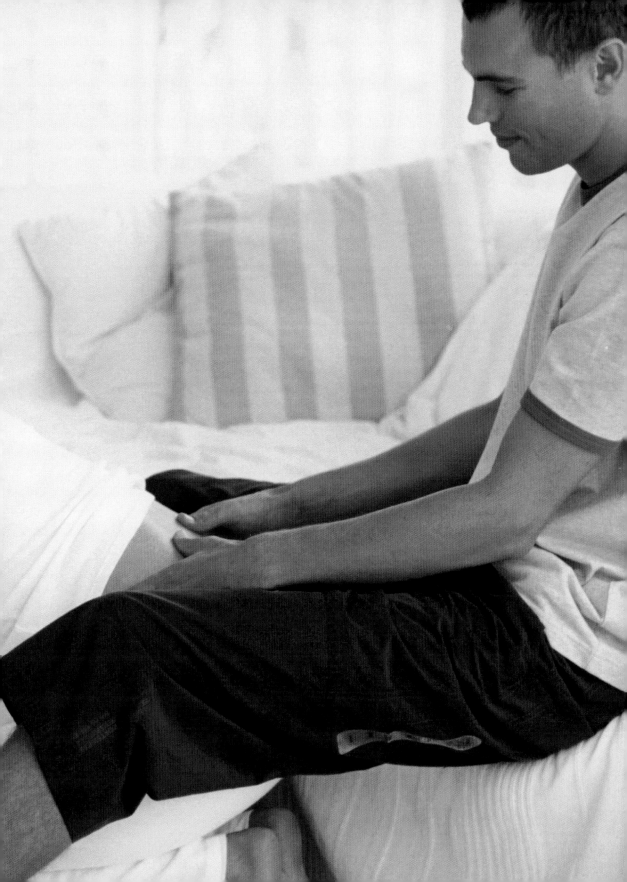

YOUR CHECKLIST

Most preparations can be made well in advance, but you'll still have a few things that you need to take care of at the last minute.

When you go into labor (see p.270), you should:

- call your midwife

- make contact with your partner or birth coach

- get in touch with whoever's going to care for your other children, if it's not your partner

- make sure your overnight bag is packed

- check that your labor aids are packed and ready to go

- make sure you have easy access to your health insurance card, ID, and any medical records you may need

- make yourself a hot, sweet drink

Getting ready for the birthing center

If you're planning to have your baby in a birthing center, your midwife will tell you what to bring and what to expect once you arrive. Do as much as you can a few weeks before your due date so that you don't have to rush around getting everything organized at the last minute, and you are at least partly prepared if your baby comes early.

WHAT TO TAKE

Whether you're having your baby in a freestanding birthing center or in a hospital that offers birthing rooms called LDRs – labor/delivery/recovery or LDRPs (labor/delivery/recovery/postpartum – you will need to bring the same things : clothing for yourself and the baby – including newborn diapers – your labor comfort aids, and your personal effects.

For you You will need a couple maternity bras, underpants, a nightgown that opens in the front or a pair of comfortable pajamas, breast pads, super-absorbent sanitary pads, a pair of warm socks, toiletries, (including soap, your toothbrush and toothpaste, your comb and brush, makeup and tissues); and, if you

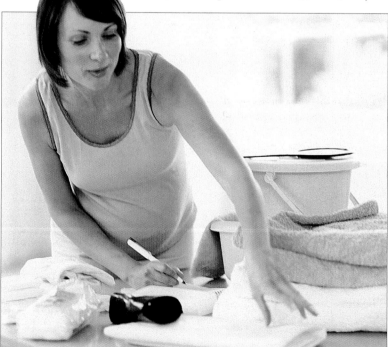

Advance preparations
Get as much as possible ready well in advance.

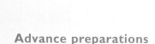

like, bring a towel, a washcloth, a pair of slippers, and a bathrobe. If you wear glasses or contact lenses be sure to bring them. You may also want to bring a camera, a CD player and some soothing music, your cell phone, and a list of important phone numbers. Double check to be sure you've brought your health insurance card, any registration forms that may be needed, and your ID.

For your baby A few newborn diapers and an infant car seat – for the ride home with your new baby – should be at the top of your list of things to bring to the birthing center or hospital, but you'll also need to bring some essential baby clothes, such as a couple pairs of footed pajamas, a soft hat, a couple baby nighties, and one or two receiving blankets.

IS IT TIME?

As it gets closer to your due date, your body will begin to give you signals that it is preparing for the birth. You may experience the symptoms of pre-labor (see p.270) and, in some cases, labor. Although you don't have to rush to the birthing center when any of the following occur, you should be prepared for them and ready to go to at a moment's notice. The show usually comes first, and either the waters breaking or contractions will follow, although contractions sometimes precede the first two. A fuller explanation of each one can be found on page 270.

The show A plug of blood-tinged mucus, which seals your cervix prior to birth, becomes dislodged during the first stage of labor, if not before. It can happen days or even weeks before labor.

The waters break Pressure due to contractions or the baby's head pressing on the membranes of the amniotic sac may cause it to rupture in advance of the start of labor. The amniotic fluid will then escape, either as a trickle or in a rush.

Regular contractions You will start to experience contractions in the form of severe cramp-like pains or a strong "tightening" sensations that come at regular intervals and last longer and longer. The time between contractions gets shorter.

WHEN TO GO

If, for over an hour, you notice that your contractions are coming every 5–15 minutes, and last for about one minute – and don't go away when you move around – call the birthing center and ask your midwife if you should come in. She'll probably tell you that there's no need to rush because the first stage of labor lasts at least eight hours for a first baby. You will also be more comfortable at home, rather than waiting anxiously at the center. Stay in close contact with your midwife, however, and let her know each time you feel there has been a significant change in your pre-labor. If you live a long way from the center or if you are worried about getting there in time, go as soon as you feel you have to.

HAVING YOUR BABY AT HOME

Fewer than I percent of all babies in the United states are born at home, due to a shift in thinking, over one hundred years ago, in which childbirth came to be viewed as a medical rather than a natural condition.

For some women, however, the idea of a home birth is appealing, because it allows for continuity of care, a homelike environment, and the ability to make their own decisions. If you are considering a home birth, you should, according to the American College of Nurse-Midwives, meet these guidelines:

- be in a low-risk category — no hypertension, diabetes, or other chronic medical problems, and no history of a previous difficult labor and/or delivery.

- be attended by a physician or a CNM (Certified Nurse-Midwife). If using a CNM, a consulting physician should be available, preferably one who has seen the mother during pregnancy and who has worked with the nurse-midwife.

- have transportation available and live within thirty miles of a hospital, if the roads are good and traffic negligible, or ten miles if these standards aren't met.

- for more information on home births, check www.home-birth. org

Going to the hospital

YOUR CHECKLIST

When your contractions begin, keep calm and don't rush: labor can last for as long as 12–14 hours for a first child and about seven hours for subsequent children.

When you go into labor, you should:

- notify the hospital

- call your insurance company if your policy requires advance notice of hospital admission, or else you may not be covered. (Many companies will make exceptions for emergencies if you or a representative notify them as soon as possible after you're admitted)

- call an ambulance if you aren't going to be driven to the hospital by your partner, birth assistant, or a friend. If someone drives you to the hospital or birthing center, make sure they drive safely

- contact your partner or birth coach

- advise whoever's going to take care of your other children, if it's not your partner

- double-check that your bag, your baby's bag, and your bag of labor aids are packed

- sit down and wait calmly for your transportation to arrive

- make yourself a hot, sweet drink.

Getting ready
Make sure you have everything ready and packed well in advance.

If you get everything ready in advance and pack the things you'll need to take with you to the hospital, you won't have to worry about being caught unprepared.

WHAT TO TAKE

The items you'll need with you in the hospital fall into three groups: clothes and other personal things for you; your comfort aids for labor (see p.268); and clothes and diapers for your baby.

For you You'll need maternity bras and front-opening cotton nightgowns, breast pads, a bathrobe and slippers, underpants, and super-absorbent, sanitary napkins (these may be supplied by the hospital). Pack an overnight bag with your hairbrush, shampoo, some towels and washcloths, a small mirror, makeup, face cream, hand cream, and tissues. If you've made a birth plan (see p.122), remember to take it with you, along with a photo ID, your insurance card, eyeglasses, a camera, and phone numbers of people you want to call.

For your baby Hospitals don't provide baby clothes, and most don't supply diapers, so you'll need to take some with you. You'll also need a nightgown or stretch suit, bonnet, footed pajamas, a blanket in which to wrap your baby when you leave the hospital, and a car seat.

IS IT TIME?

When your due date is near, your body will begin to give you signals that it's preparing for the birth. You may have some of the symptoms of prelabor (see p.270) and, in some cases, labor. Although you don't have to rush to the hospital when you have any of the following, you do need to be ready for them and make your final preparations. The show normally comes first, and either the water breaking or contractions will follow, although sometimes contractions precede the first two. For a fuller explanation of each one, see page 270.

The show This plug of blood-tinged mucus, which has been sealing your cervix prior to birth, becomes dislodged during the early first stage of labor, if not before. It can happen days or even weeks before labor. It's usually easily recognizable.

The water breaks Pressure caused by contractions or your baby's head pressing on the membranes of your amniotic sac may cause it to rupture before labor starts. The amniotic fluid will then escape, either as a trickle or in a rush.

Regular contractions Whether or not you've been aware of any contractions before, you start to experience them as severe cramplike pains or "tightening" sensations that come at regular intervals and last longer and longer. The interval between contractions gets shorter.

WHEN TO GO

If, over an hour, you notice your contractions are coming every five to 15 minutes, are about one minute long, and don't die away when you move around, or when you feel you can't cope without pain relief, call your labor ward or midwife, according to what you've arranged. At this time, your first level of breathing (see column, p.282) will probably no longer be enough, and you'll be getting ready to use other breathing patterns as prelabor eases into the first stage. There's still plenty of time to check that you have everything you need and to get to the hospital.

There's usually no need to rush into the hospital because the first stage normally lasts at least eight hours for a first baby. It may be more comfortable to stay at home. But if you live a long way from the hospital or you're particularly worried about getting there in time, go as soon as you feel you have to.

Transportation You'll probably travel to the hospital in an ambulance, by car, or by taxi. Never drive yourself. If you need to call an ambulance or taxi, be sure to give your full address and, if necessary, a clear description of how to get to your house so there's no unnecessary delay. If you plan to go by car, make sure that the car you're going to use has had a recent tuneup, and keep a check that there's always plenty of gas in the tank from about week 38 on.

YOUR TRIP TO THE HOSPITAL

If you're traveling to the hospital by car rather than by ambulance, try to make yourself as comfortable and safe as possible—and always wear your seat belt.

In the weeks leading up to the birth, make sure that both you and whoever's going to drive you to the hospital know the route really well. Find out how long the trip is likely to take at different times of day, and work out alternative routes in case there's exceptionally heavy traffic or other delays on the day. If you think you might have to park at a meter, make sure you have plenty of change ready. It's also a good idea to check all the entrances to the hospital—especially at night, and find out exactly how to get to the maternity ward.

The car The bigger the car you travel in, the more comfortable you're likely to be. You'll probably feel safer and more comfortable in the back seat with your seat belt on.

Sudden birth If your baby starts to arrive while you're still on your way to the hospital, stay as calm as you can. If you're close to the hospital, you have a good chance of getting there before your baby is actually born, but if you're farther away, stop the car at the nearest telephone, call for an ambulance, and then get ready for an emergency delivery (see also p.304).

DRINKS AND FOOD

It's important to save your energy during the first stage, in case you have a long and tiring labor.

Many hospitals suggest that you don't eat anything during labor in case there's an unexpected emergency and you need a general anesthetic. Take glucose candy to suck, and high-energy isotonic sports drinks to help you keep up your energy levels. Your partner will also need food, so he'll need to make himself a snack to take—perhaps sandwiches and fruit and a thermos of coffee.

Take something for you to have later as well—you'll probably be ravenous after the birth and you'll want something to eat right away.

You'll also need plenty to drink—a bottle or thermos filled with diluted, unsweetened fruit juice or cold water is ideal.

Comfort aids for labor

When you're gathering together all the things you'll need for the birth, think about any items that will make your labor a more comfortable experience. It's best to get your comfort aids ready in advance. That way you won't forget anything in the excitement when labor starts, and you won't be caught unprepared if your labor starts sooner than you expect.

ITEMS YOU'LL FIND HELPFUL

Your midwife or hospital attendants will suggest things you might find helpful during your labor. Pack all these items in a bag and put it next to your overnight bag. Make sure your partner or birth assistant knows where these things are and doesn't forget them at the last minute.

Distractions Many women find that being massaged soothes the discomfort of labor (see p.283). Your partner can provide counterpressure with his hands, a spinal roll, or even a tennis ball or rolling pin. Ask him to use a small amount of talcum powder or some vegetable-based massage oil on his hands to keep your skin from being dragged or pinched. A hot water bottle or a heating pad placed in the small of your back can act as a compress to soothe backaches.

In the early stages before labor really gets going, you might feel that nothing much happens for long periods. You might find it

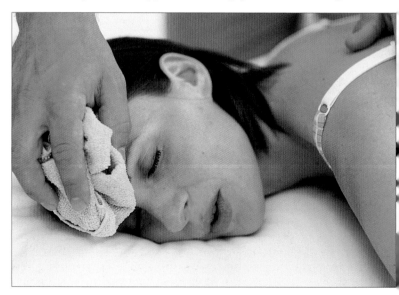

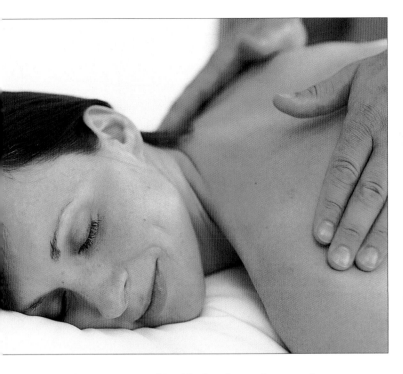

Your birth partner will need to take along some comfort aids, too, so that labor is a pleasurable experience. Here are some suggestions:

- a pack of wipes for freshening face and hands
- snacks and drinks
- change of clothing
- camera, or video camera if permitted
- coins and or calling card and numbers of family and friends.

helpful to distract yourself with books and magazines or even some playing cards and board games.

Keeping cool If you want something wet and cool in your mouth but you don't want a drink, try sucking an ice cube or crushed ice. Most hospitals now provide ice. Alternatively, moisten your lips and mouth by sucking on a small natural sponge that's been dipped in cold water. If you feel hot and sweaty, ask your partner to bathe your face with a cool washcloth and create a refreshing breeze with a handheld fan.

Keeping warm During the later stages of labor, and particularly immediately after the birth, some women begin to shake quite visibly with cold. Have some legwarmers or thick socks ready in case this happens to you.

General comfort If your hair is long or falls in your face, tie it back with clips or a hairband so it doesn't irritate you. Your lips are likely to become very dry because of breathing through your mouth, so include lip balm that you can rub on your lips to keep them from cracking.

If you feel nauseous and actually vomit, you'll feel much better if you can brush your teeth, so don't forget to take your toothbrush and toothpaste.

A box of tissues may come in handy, as may some scented wipes in single packs that can be opened when needed and used to cleanse your face, neck, and hands. For freshening up, you may want to spritz on a light cologne or body spray.

YOUR CHECKLIST

Use the following checklist when packing your bag of comfort aids:

- food and drink
- spinal roll, or tennis ball
- massage oil or talcum powder
- hot-water bottle
- books, magazines, cards, board games, etc
- small natural sponge
- washcloth and handheld fan
- leg warmers or thick socks
- hair clips or hairband
- lip balm
- toothbrush and toothpaste
- box of tissues or wet wipes
- cologne or body spray.

YOUR MOOD CHANGES

As you wait for signs that your baby is ready to be born, you may feel a number of emotions.

Contentment As your body changes in preparation for labor, you may find that you respond to the ripening of your womb in a sensual way. Particularly if this is your first baby, you might like to enjoy these last days on your own indulging your whims, sharing moments of intimacy with your partner, or spending the time just daydreaming. Pamper yourself, and allow your feelings to flow naturally and easily.

Elation You may feel a great sense of joy when your body alerts you to the moment that you've been waiting for with such excitement. Don't try to suppress this feeling; share it with the other people around you, since this may help to release any pangs of nervous tension.

Anxiety The signs of prelabor may also make you feel a little apprehensive. You may worry about the pain of labor and its effect on your baby, and you may wonder if you'll be able to cope. You may feel nervous about your water breaking in an embarrassing situation.

Impatience If your expected date of delivery comes and goes without any sign that your baby is about to be born, don't be depressed. Remember that it's only an approximate date and that most babies arrive either sooner or later than expected. This is particularly likely if you yourself were born sooner or later than expected.

Prelabor and labor

Medically, labor is divided into three stages. In the first stage, your cervix opens fully to allow your baby to pass through; in the second stage your baby is born; in the third stage the placenta is delivered. All these stages are discussed in detail over the following pages. In addition to these stages, most women experience prelabor. Your experience of labor will be much more colorful and exciting than the medical definition above. Go into it believing that very little can go wrong, and very little will go wrong.

PRELABOR

Before real labor begins, hormones from your uterus and your baby prepare your body for birth. During the last few weeks, you'll probably notice signs of your coming labor. But just as each woman's experience of labor and birth is unique, so these prelabor symptoms affect everyone in different ways. They do provide useful signals to warn you that labor is imminent.

Engagement To position himself for the journey through the birth canal, your baby will move lower down so that his presenting part, usually his head, settles into your bony pelvis (see opposite). This is known as engagement, and you'll experience it as a feeling of lightening. You may actually see your belly drop down. If this is your first pregnancy, your baby will probably engage two to three weeks before the labor starts. If you've had previous babies, your baby's head may remain higher until just before labor starts, because your uterine muscles may have stretched and so will exert less pressure on your baby. You'll know when your baby has engaged because there's less pressure on your diaphragm and breathing becomes easier. On the other hand, you'll probably find you have to pass urine more often, as your baby will now be pressing down on your bladder.

Braxton-Hicks contractions Your uterus practices for the strong contractions needed in labor with weak, irregular contractions, named after the doctor who first described them. Most women feel these during the last few months. If you place your hand on your abdomen, you may feel a hardening and tightening of your uterus, which lasts for approximately 25 seconds.

Unlike real labor contractions, these are usually painless, although some women find them uncomfortable. If you do feel any discomfort, sit down quietly until the feeling eases. You may find you get more and stronger Braxton-Hicks contractions as real labor approaches. This is your body's way of preparing the cervix to dilate and increasing the circulation of blood to the placenta. When you feel a run of Braxton-Hicks, practice the relaxation techniques you're going to use during labor; the tightening and relaxing of your uterus will give you a good idea of how a contraction feels as it waxes and wanes.

Some mothers misinterpret Braxton-Hicks as real labor pains and go to the hospital, only to be told they can go home again (see A false labor? p.272).

Nesting instinct You may suddenly feel like making final preparations for the arrival of your baby. If you want to rush around cleaning or decorating the house, or cooking large meals, try to restrain yourself. Save this extra energy for coping with labor and delivery.

The show An obvious sign that labor is coming soon is the appearance of the show—the plug of mucus that seals your cervix in pregnancy, providing protection against infection. Although the show often doesn't appear until labor is underway, the cervix may widen enough for the mucus plug to be dislodged up to twelve days before labor begins. This sticky substance may be slightly brown, pink, or blood-tinged from the capillaries that attached it to the cervix. The show signals dilation of the cervix.

Premenstrual feelings You may notice some physical and emotional changes similar to those you have before a menstrual period. You may also feel crampy, with some pressure in your rectum, and feel the need to empty your bowels and pass urine more often than usual.

Your baby's descent

Your doctor or midwife will check this by internal examination and measure it in "stations," lines measured in centimeters from –5 to +5 in relation to the level of your *ischial spines* and your baby's head. When his head first enters your pelvis, it is at station –5. When the top of his head is level with your ischial spines it is at station 0 (engaged). The remaining stations describe the head's position as it passes via the birth canal to the vaginal opening, station +5.

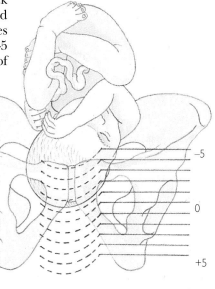

–5

0

+5

WHAT YOUR BABY'S DOING

While no one actually knows for certain why labor starts, there's increasing evidence to suggest that your baby plays a major role.

Hormones The start of labor is triggered by hormones—the levels of some pregnancy hormones drop, others rise. New hormones are secreted, one of which is produced by your baby.

Engagement Throughout your pregnancy, your baby will be floating in his amniotic sac above your pelvic brim. As his birth approaches, his head, or his bottom if he is in a breech position, will descend lower down into your pelvis and become engaged.

Kicking less You may notice that your baby becomes quieter than in previous months. From time to time you may feel a slight flurry of movement, but if his actions seem to decrease significantly, get in touch with your doctor or midwife immediately. While you are waiting for a call back, lie down and rest for an hour and count at least 10 kicks. If you can't count 10 kicks in an hour, go to the hospital.

The first stage

The months of preparing for your baby's birth have now reached their climax as labor begins. In medical terms, the first stage starts when your contractions bring about the opening (dilation) and thinning (effacement) of the cervix and ends when these are complete. At this point your midwife will confirm that you are fully dilated.

Although false labor is only a rehearsal, don't be disappointed— false labor means that real labor isn't too far off and you won't have much longer to wait.

WHAT HAPPENS IN LABOR

It's difficult to be sure about the onset of labor because it differs from woman to woman. Certain classic signs—intense contractions, dilation and thinning of the cervix, and rupturing of the membranes—are taken to mean that labor is underway.

There are some simple differences between the contractions of false and real labor.

Regularity False contractions never really settle down and become truly regular.

Contractions When true labor starts, the nature of your contractions changes. They become more rhythmic and more painful, and they come at regular intervals. These contractions are not within your control and, once they have begun, won't stop until your baby is born.

Frequency False contractions are sporadic. They may vary from 10 minutes to 20 minutes to 15 minutes, with no steady pattern.

You can time your contractions from the start of one contraction to the start of the next. In early labor, contractions are usually about 30–60 seconds long and come at intervals of about five to 20 minutes. This can vary; some women may not notice their first contractions until they are closer together—say, every five minutes. During the active phase, contractions usually last 60–90 seconds, at intervals of two to four minutes.

Effect of movement False contractions usually weaken or stop altogether if you get up and move around; real contractions increase.

As your uterine muscles tighten, you may feel something like menstrual cramps, spreading around your lower abdomen like a tight band. This is because the uterine muscle runs short of oxygen as its blood vessels are compressed. The uterus is a huge muscle and needs a lot of energy during contractions.

Strength False contractions do not get progressively stronger. They may even weaken from time to time and disappear altogether.

Every woman feels contraction pains differently, but in early labor they may be similar to menstrual cramps or a mild backache. Some women experience a persistent and severe backache (see p. 296). Very often a contraction feels like a wave of discomfort all the way across your abdomen that reaches a peak for a few seconds and then diminishes. At the same time, you can feel a hardening and tightening of the uterine muscle, which is held at the peak of its intensity for a few seconds before the muscle begins to relax.

Some women, especially if they are working and get overtired or overexcited, slip in and out of false labor for a few days before real labor begins.

Women assume that contractions will get steadily longer, more frequent, and stronger. This is not so; don't be disturbed if your contractions seem to vary. It's as normal for a strong contraction to be followed by a weaker one that doesn't last quite as long, as it is for contractions to follow one another relentlessly.

Tell your doctor or midwife about the contractions. If you can't get in touch with them, check with your hospital and go to hospital if you want to. If you stay at home, keep on the move and stay upright to help labor progress.

Your cervix dilates and thins The cervix is usually a thick-walled canal about three-fourths of an inch (two centimeters) long, and rmly closed. In the last few weeks, pregnancy hormones may often your cervix, but the intense contractions of first-stage bor are needed to dilate and thin it. Dilation is measured in entimeters from 0–10 (up to four inches). Your cervix will only ilate about four centimeters (or one-and-a-half inches) during he latent phase, then progress to 10 centimeters (four inches) in he active phase (see below). The pain increases as it becomes ully dilated during transition. Eventually, the whole cervix opens p and is made one with the body of the uterus, creating a ontinuous channel that your baby can pass through.

our water breaks The membranes of the amniotic sac may upture painlessly at any time during labor, although this usually appens toward the end of the first stage. Fluid may leak or gush ut; the flow depends on the size and site of the break and hether or not the baby's head is plugging the hole.

Usually, if the membranes rupture spontaneously near term, bor follows within a short time, although occasionally it's elayed—if your baby's presenting part is not engaged, or if your aby is presenting abnormally. Delay also occurs in normal cases. hen this happens, you'll be advised to have labor induced.

ow long does labor last?

abor times vary greatly, but an average labor lasts about 12–14 hours or first-time mothers, and about seven hours for subsequent bors. If your labor lasts longer than 12 hours the first time, or ine hours in subsequent labors, your doctor will want to find out hy progress is slow, and may intervene.

The first stage of labor can be further divided into three eparate phases. The latent phase is the longest, lasting about ght hours for first babies, and you'll feel contractions coming ith increasing frequency and length, but they won't be too istressing. Try to conserve your energy during this time as your ody will be warming up for the more demanding phases to ollow. The next, active phase, will be shorter, lasting about three o five hours, but this is when your contractions become more ainful, and you may want some pain relief (see p.280). The final, ansitional phase, is the shortest and most intense of all, usually usting just under an hour, and comes right before the delivery.

ransition This is the most intense phase of the first stage. Your ontractions will now last about 60–90 seconds, with intervals of nly 30–90 seconds. As the contractions become more forceful, ou may find it hard to relax and this is the time you may feel the nost discomfort. You may also feel a very strong urge to push, but hould not do so unless you're fully dilated. The intense pain may nake you feel extremely irritable, even bad-tempered with your irth partner. This is natural. Don't think you're failing if you ear you lack the energy to go on any more; you'll find hidden esources of energy to help you cope. Remind yourself that this hase means your baby's birth is now just minutes away.

WHAT HAPPENS TO YOUR CERVIX

During the first stage of labor, the cervix, which is normally tough, must be stretched thin and needs to open wide before your baby's head is able to pass through.

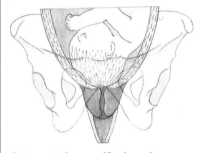

Latent phase (0–4 cm)
Your cervix remains about ¾ in (2 cm) long until contractions start thinning it out (effacing).

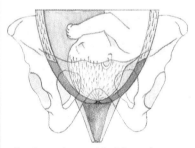

Active phase (4–10 cm)
When the cervical canal is thinned out, further contractions will widen (dilate) your cervix.

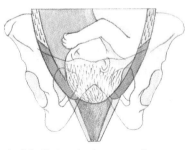

At full dilation the last part of your cervix at the front has opened to 10 cm (4 in).

GOING TO THE HOSPITAL

When you arrive at the hospital, your doctor will prepare you for the birth and give you a few routine checks.

- Your doctor will look at your records and ask you some questions about how your labor is going—whether your water has broken and how often you're having contractions.

- Then she'll examine you: she'll palpate your abdomen to feel what position your baby's in; she'll listen to your baby's heartbeat, take your blood pressure, pulse, and temperature, monitor your contractions, and give you an internal examination to see how far your cervix has dilated.

- You'll be asked to give a urine sample to test for the presence of protein and sugar.

- You'll be asked when you last had a bowel movement. You won't be given an enema or a suppository unless you ask.

- Then you'll take a shower or bath and settle in to your delivery room. If you have any questions or there's anything you want to tell the hospital staff about your preferences, now is the time.

Hospital procedures

Each hospital has its own set of routine procedures for labor. If you've visited beforehand, you'll probably have a good idea what the regulations are. Hospitals can be intimidating, but are much less so when you get to know them, so it's a good idea to take a look at the labor and delivery rooms, meet the staff who'll be caring for you, and get some idea about ward routines before your due date.

Admission to the hospital Once you've arrived at the hospital, you may be offered a wheelchair to transport you from the hospital entrance to the labor ward. If your labor is well advanced, you'll welcome the chair; if not, you'll be able to walk comfortably, so make sure you are allowed to do so.

You'll have outlined in your birth plan (see p.122) how you'd like your labor to proceed, and once you've met your midwife or doctor, this is the time to make sure they have a copy of your plan so that you can look over it with them. They'll also make some checks and ask you a few questions about your labor (see column, left, and p.116).

If there's anything you're not happy with—if equipment, lights, and needles frighten you, for example, or if you're upset by a staff member—do something about it right away. Don't wait, letting your fears and anxieties fester and grow. Your partner or birth coach can voice your feelings if you aren't feeling strong enough to be assertive.

Examinations Your baby's heart will be monitored regularly by Doppler or an electronic fetal monitor (see right). Your midwife will probably give you an internal check every two to four hours during the first stage to see how far your cervix has dilated, but there's no hard and fast rule.

Each time you have an internal check, ask how things are going. It's very comforting to know how far your cervix has dilated between examinations. If you're asked a question while you're having a contraction, concentrate on your relaxation techniques and answer the question when the contraction is over.

Pain relief Once you've been admitted, an anesthetist will visit you if you've asked for an epidural (see p.281), and the procedure will be set up. This usually takes 10–20 minutes. If a top-off is needed, this can usually be given by your midwife. If you've decided not to have any medical pain relief, you will be left with your birth coach and a midwife who'll stay with you throughout your labor.

Electronic fetal monitoring

This high-tech replacement for the stethoscope is used to track your baby's heartbeat. In all high-risk pregnancies, electronic fetal monitoring (EFM) will be used throughout labor for your own and especially your baby's safety. You'll have EFM if you are being induced or your labor is being accelerated for any reason, or if you're having epidural anesthesia. The main function of the monitoring is to give early warning if your baby is in any distress.

What it is   There are two kinds of electronic monitors, external and internal. An external monitor is used for routine short periods of monitoring, and it's sometimes used in pregnancy if it's necessary to monitor the baby's heartbeat over a period of time. Belts are strapped around your abdomen with sensors that record your baby's heartbeat and your uterine contractions, which are then printed out on a graph.

The internal monitor is slightly more accurate. You'll have belts strapped around your body and a tiny electrode will be clipped to your baby's scalp once your cervix is 2–3 cm dilated. The baby's heartbeat is printed out on a paper trace.

The latest type of EFM, known as *telemetry*, uses radio waves. The baby's monitor is attached to a transmitter that's strapped to your thigh, so in theory, at least, you're able to move around while being monitored. The older equipment confines you to a bed or chair.

How it works   During a contraction, the blood flow to your placenta is reduced for a few seconds, and your baby's heart rate may drop from its baseline. The heart rate should return to what it was before when the contraction passes. If it doesn't or the return is delayed, your baby may be distressed and your medical team may need to take action to protect his well-being.

How monitoring helps doctors   EFM provides medical staff with a second-by-second report on your baby's condition. It warns the doctors if your baby is in distress so they can intervene before anything untoward has happened. If your doctors decide that you and your baby would be better off with monitoring, try not to resent it and to see it as something that gives reassurance that your baby is doing fine.

Disadvantages   The use of monitoring means that there'll be more electronic equipment in the delivery room, making the atmosphere very clinical. You may also feel that the nursing staff might concentrate more on the machine than on you. As staff are aware of any tiny changes that may take place, they're more likely to intervene rather than letting labor take its natural course. However, many mothers do find it comforting to know that the doctors and midwives will know right away if there is a problem with the baby.

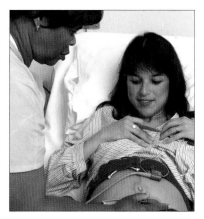

Monitoring in labor
Contractions are recorded by an external monitor strapped to your abdomen. An internal monitor is attached to your baby.

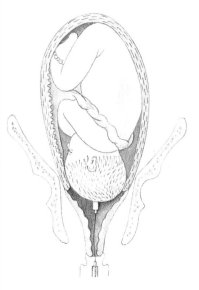

Monitoring your baby
The electrode is attached to his presenting part, usually his head, by piercing the skin and provides an electrical contact that picks up his heartbeat. Some babies' heads will be bruised or have a rash where the electrode was attached to them. Many mothers find EFM reassuring because they can watch their baby's heartbeat throughout labor.

Partner's role in labor

The more secure and relaxed a mother feels during labor, the better she'll be able to cope with pain. Her partner is the natural person to give this loving support, since he'll have been closely involved in the pregnancy, and eager to share his child's birth. Otherwise, ask a friend who's had children herself to be your birth coach. Most hospitals welcome fathers, friends, or relatives to support the mother.

UNDERSTANDING YOUR ROLE

It's normal to feel nervous about being a birth partner, so the best thing to do is prepare yourself. Find out as much as you can so you're able to help the mother meet the physical and emotional demands of labor. At prenatal classes there'll be demonstrations to describe labor's onset and the effect of contractions, and you'll be taught techniques to help her relax.

Visit the birthing center or the hospital's labor and delivery rooms and introduce yourself to the staff. Make sure you know the route to the hospital in case of an emergency, and find out all you'll need to do; trust will create a calmer atmosphere.

HOW TO HELP DURING LABOR

You may have a very active role throughout the labor and birth, but sometimes your presence is all the mother needs. Make sure you're very familiar with her birth plan and the alternative version (see p.122) and that you know all her wishes.

Use your intuition Judge the situation by observing your partner's moods. She may want to stay quiet, going through contractions alone without being touched. Or she may needs lots of encouragement or distractions.

Supporting your partner
If your partner leans back against you, you can support her weight and cuddle her at the same time.

Provide emotional support   Remain as close and intimate as you can, using loving words, and keep your movements slow, quiet, and steady. Be positive: praise her and don't criticize. If she wants to hear your voice, constantly tell her how well she's doing (how far dilated) and how she can relax herself. Tell her what the midwife is doing and what will soon happen. Also, help her to see how much she's achieved already—it's easy for her to be overwhelmed by how far she thinks she has to go. Massage and stroke her slowly, but if she just wants to hold your hand, you can encourage her by the expression on your face and lots of eye contact. Sometimes just the look of love in her partner's eyes can help a woman bear the pain of contractions.

Combat tiredness   Before labor, encourage her to rest as much as possible, particularly if she seems to want to rush around cleaning during the nesting period. If her labor is long and tiring, try to help her relax between contractions and save her energy for the second stage. If she's not feeling nauseous, provide her with any drinks or nourishment she wants (see also p.268).

Help her cope with pain   It's hard to see someone you care about in pain, but try not to show your anxiety—it could make her feel more worried. On the other hand, don't dismiss her suffering. Acknowledge it positively, telling her each contraction is bringing your baby's birth closer, and make different suggestions for relief. Help her not to be embarrassed about saying what hurts—encourage her to be as uninhibited as possible. A woman in labor should never be ashamed of needing pain relief.

  If she feels particularly anxious during a contraction, it might calm her fears to talk about how she felt before the next one starts. Don't take it personally if she's critical or aggressive toward you—this often happens when the pain is very intense.

Help with breathing   You'll probably have practiced your partner's preferred method in prenatal classes, but let her follow her own rhythm. If she seems to lose control, stay nearby and slowly guide her through the pattern until she's able to continue on her own. Be ready to adapt—very few people follow exactly what they practiced at prenatal classes.

Make her comfortable   You can be a great help here. Suggest different positions (see p.278) and support her with pillows or blankets, or let her lean against you while you cuddle, and rock together. Look for signs of tension in her neck, shoulders, or forehead, and gently stroke these areas. Massage may give some relief from pain. If she's using visualization techniques, gently talk her through them. She'll probably find having her face and hands wiped very soothing, or you can offer her ice cubes to suck. If she feels cold, help her put on socks or leg warmers. As labor progresses, she may want to talk less, but you can keep in touch by touching or caressing, or by using eye contact.

HOW YOUR PARTNER CAN HELP

A birth partner can do a lot to help you during labor, not only providing you with plenty of comfort and reassurance, but also dealing with staff for you. Try to remember that although the hospital uniforms and equipment may appear daunting, the medical team is there to support both of you and your baby.

Your birth partner can:

- answer questions for you (if allowed to by the staff), which saves you from having your concentration disturbed

- support you in the positions you choose for pain relief and/or to give birth

- stroke and massage you if you find it comforting

- change the atmosphere (dim the lights, change the music) for you

- ask people to leave if there are too many of them in your personal space, and ask any medical students present at a delivery to leave if they are inhibiting you or your partner

- be the one you can really rely on to deal with the medical staff on your behalf and to stand by your decisions on pain relief—whether to accept it or not, and if so, when and how much. If you decide to ask for relief, he should encourage you to have a breathing space of about 15 minutes before it's administered, since things can change very quickly and you may find you don't need it after all.

First stage positions

There are many different positions that you can take to ease your discomfort. Some women prefer to stand and move around during labor, as this helps to strengthen contractions, which then accelerates labor. If you do stand, try leaning forward against your partner or a wall. This will take the weight of your baby off your spine and make contractions more efficient. As your contractions get stronger, you may prefer to sit or kneel, using cushions or chairs for support.

Let your shoulders drop. You can rest against a cushion during contractions

Make sure your back is straight

Sitting

If you find it more comfortable to sit down, try leaning forward with your legs wide apart. You can sit facing the chair back, resting on a pillow or cushion. Or you may prefer to support yourself by leaning against your birth assistant, who can also rub your back.

Rock your pelvis backward and forward during contractions to relieve backaches

Make sure your back is straight and don't allow it to arch

Kneeling

As your contractions strengthen, you may find it less tiring to get down on your hands and knees. This helps to ease any backache. Keep your legs wide apart, and rock your pelvis. Between contractions, lean forward onto your folded arms or sit back on your heels.

During transition

If your cervix isn't fully dilated toward the end of the first stage, just before giving birth, use gravity to slow down your baby while the cervix continues to open. Lean on a pile of cushions with your legs wide apart, or kneel with your head down and your bottom raised.

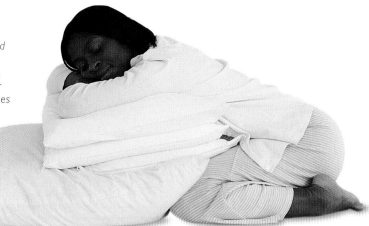

Take the pressure off your lower back by leaning forward with your head on a pillow

Kneeling on the floor with your bottom raised and your head on the floor may relieve backaches

Lying down

There may be times during labor when you just want to lie down. Try lying on your side, and place cushions under your head and upper thigh. Keep your legs wide apart.

Relax your shoulders, and concentrate on your breathing with your eyes closed

HOW DRUGS AFFECT YOU

Drugs give you relief from pain, but they can affect your experience of childbirth in other ways. Make sure you opt for the type that will help to improve, rather than detract from, the pleasure of your baby's birth.

Drowsiness This is a common side effect of gas, tranquilizers, and narcotics. Some women enjoy the feeling of drifting, but sometimes the sleepiness can make mothers feel they lack control. After using narcotics, a few women can become so lightheaded that they're unaware of what's happening around them.

Dizziness Pethidine and other narcotics can sometimes bring on a feeling of confusion or disorientation, and some mothers have even had hallucinations.

Nausea The sensation of nausea is usually quite slight with gas, but is common after using pethidine and other narcotics. A few mothers may have vomiting attacks. To counteract this, an antinausea medication (or antihistamine) can be given (it's safe for the baby).

Your state of mind can have a major influence on how much pain you feel during labor. If you feel very tense, your uterus may be affected, slowing down labor and adversely affecting your baby (see column, opposite), so if having some pain-relief drugs makes you feel less anxious, there's no point in depriving yourself.

Pain relief

Many women, particularly first-time mothers, find that the excitement about their baby's birth is overshadowed by worry about pain during labor. Labor invariably involves pain, but you can build up your confidence by preparing for the intensity of contractions, by understanding your own limits of pain tolerance, and by learning about different methods of pain relief. If you can, think of the pain in a positive way—each contraction brings the birth of your baby closer.

COPING WITH PAIN

The kind of pain you'll experience during contractions varies from woman to woman. Very often, it feels like a thick band being squeezed around your abdomen as the uterine muscles harden and tighten for a few seconds before relaxing. Some women describe it as being like severe menstrual cramps, others feel a backache, but there may be a combination of sensations as the contraction reaches its peak, culminating in a wave of discomfort, which then subsides.

Individual response You may prefer not to use drugs during labor because they can dim your awareness of what's happening and deprive you of the sensation of giving birth. It's difficult, though, to know your own pain threshold, particularly if this is your first baby. Some women are surprised by the overpowering intensity of their contractions; for others, the pain may be made worse by fear and anxiety.

Pain relief in childbirth can be complete, as in epidural anesthesia, or or it can reduce pain to bearable levels as with gas and air and narcotics. Many women choose to have no drugs in the early part of the first stage. Don't blame yourself if you want some pain relief with drugs—it isn't a sign of cowardice. Your labor isn't a test, and the use of drugs may even be essential for you to deliver your baby.

If you haven't made up your mind about the use of painkillers, you may want to go without drugs for as long as possible. If so, a useful tip is to wait 15 minutes after you feel you want pain relief before actually having it. During that time, your labor may progress well, and it gives you and your birth partner time to discuss whether or not you can get by with encouragement, or whether you really do feel the pain is increasing to the point where you need some relief.

If you want to participate fully in your baby's birth without dimming your consciousness of the feelings involved, there are alternatives to drugs for pain relief. Also, your body can provide its own brand of painkiller and relaxant, *endorphins*. The more natural your labor, the more quickly your own endorphins will be produced and your pain threshold increased.

A clear choice Find out as much as you can about the types of pain relief available. Talk to your doctor, midwife, and hospital staff, and outline your choices in your birth plan (see p.122). Have an alternative version ready in case any complications arise.

Many doctors and midwives want to make labor and delivery as pain-free as possible with the help of drugs, but you have the final say in whether or not to use pain relief, so do make your preferences clear. Don't hesitate to question the use of drugs, or ask your healthcare provider's advice.

PAIN-RELIEVING DRUGS

Some types of pain relief will only be available in large or teaching hospitals; others are available in all hospitals and birthing centers.

Regional anesthetics These remove feeling from part of your body by blocking the transmission of pain from nerve fibers. There are several different sorts. Caudal anesthesia is given by an injection into your spinal area around the sacrum, and numbs your vagina and perineum. This may be used for short-term relief if you need to have a vacuum extraction or forceps delivery.

For a pudendal block, anesthesia is injected straight into your vagina near the pelvic region, blocking the pudendal nerve. This numbs the lower part of your vagina, and may be given if you have an episiotomy, although it isn't used often.

Most widely used is the epidural block (see below). This prevents pain from spreading beyond your uterus by acting as a "nerve block" in your spine. A well-managed epidural removes all sensation from your waist to your knees, but you remain alert. Doctors may recommend an epidural if you have a difficult labor, preeclampsia, or severe asthma, if you have a forceps delivery, or if you have complications while delivering twins. Most mothers

HOW DRUGS AFFECT YOUR BABY

Once they're in your bloodstream, most drugs will cross the placenta to affect your baby. There'll be a higher concentration in your baby's blood than in your own.

Drowsiness Pethidine can make your baby drowsy after the birth, which may affect his ability to nurse and to respond to you after he's born.

Breathing difficulties Narcotics can depress your baby's respiration. If you take pethidine late in your labor, it will remain in your baby's bloodstream for longer.

Drugs used in epidural anesthesia cannot enter your baby's blood. A baby born after epidural anesthesia will be unaffected by the procedure and should be alert and breathe normally after delivery.

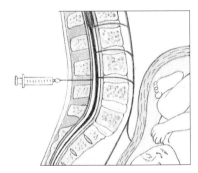

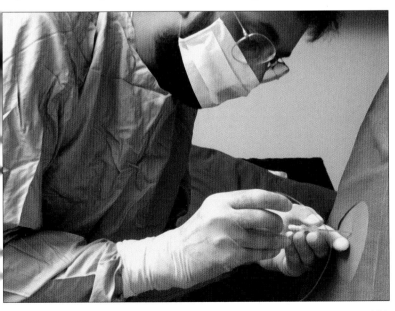

Epidural anesthetic
Once you've had an injection of local anesthetic in your back (to numb the skin), the anesthetist will ask you to lean forward (right) so he can insert a fine, hollow needle into the epidural space—the region around the spinal cord inside the spinal column (above).

WAYS YOU CAN BREATHE

Relaxing your body and focusing on your breathing will help to soothe your tension and anxiety and let you ride out your contractions. Practice breathing patterns beforehand with your partner or birth coach so they can help you during labor.

Slow breathing In the early stages, calmly and deliberately breathe out through your mouth as a contraction begins. Then slowly breathe in through your nose. Keep up the same steady pattern throughout the contraction, which may last about 45–60 seconds.

Light breathing As your contractions come more often and get more intense, you may find it easier to breathe above them. Take light, short breaths that seem to involve only the upper part of your body, and not your abdomen where the contraction takes place.

You'll probably find that you'll use different breathing techniques at different stages of your labor.

who have a cesarean now have an epidural instead of a general anesthetic so they're awake during the birth. First of all, you'll be given a local anesthetic in your back to numb the area for the injection. The anesthetist then inserts a fine, hollow needle into the epidural space (see previous page) and a thin tube known as a *catheter* is threaded down inside the hollow needle. The needle is removed, leaving the catheter in position. The catheter is then taped firmly in place. Anesthetic is syringed down the catheter, which is then sealed, although it can be topped off if necessary. If you do want to have an epidural, you need to let the hospital know in advance since it has to be given by a skilled anesthetist, and usually takes 10–20 minutes to be set up. The anesthetic takes effect within a few minutes.

Narcotics The most commonly used is meperidine, a morphine-like drug. It's given by injection in your thigh or buttock, or via intravenous drip if you have one in place, in varying dosages during the first stage, and it dulls the pain by acting on the nerve cells in your brain and spine. If you choose to take a narcotic, your doctor will start with a lower dose and raise it as needed. It is usually given with an antihistamine to reduce nausea. Narcotics usually take about 5–10 minutes to work and last 3–4 hours.

RELIEF WITHOUT DRUGS

Make sure you know as much as you can about your chosen pain-relief method, and you've shown your birth coach the technique, before you go into labor. If you need any special equipment, make sure it will be available in the hospital. One method on its own may not be enough—you may need a combination for more complete relief.

Positions Walking around, leaning against your partner or the wall, and rocking your pelvis will probably feel much more comfortable than lying on your back. There are some positions that may feel more comfortable than others, since they relieve the pressure on your back (see p.278).

Massage This is a wonderful way of relieving discomfort, whether you're lying, standing, or squatting, and it's greatly reassuring. It's particularly good if you have a backache in labor, as about 90 percent of women do (see column, right), or if you suffer from a backache labor (see p.296). Your partner will need to practice the technique beforehand.

Water Lying in warm water can be very relaxing and soothing. When in water, you're virtually weightless, and this brings relief between contractions. More and more mothers are using birthing pools under supervision (see p.107) and many hospitals are installing the facility. If you want to use a birthing pool, check early on in your pregnancy so that you can be sure one will be available.

Visualizing Creating images in your mind can be a very effective way of calming fear and reducing pain. As your contraction begins, imagine something that you find particularly soothing—for example warm, bright sunshine. Contractions in the first stage are opening your cervix and you may find the image of a bud of your favorite flower opening very slowly, petal by petal, helpful. Many women find thinking about ocean waves comforting, matching the flow of the waves with their own contractions.

Sounds You may find it helps to diffuse the pain and anxiety of labor if you make different sounds. Sighing, moaning, groaning, and grunting are all ways of releasing tension—don't feel inhibited about the noise you make, or worry too much about disturbing others.

Many women find that listening to music is helpful. Your partner can play different pieces on a portable player, according to how you're feeling. Light, uplifting music may help you rise above your contraction. When your contractions intensify, more dramatic music, building to a crescendo, may help you cope.

Hypnosis This isn't something to try on a whim, as you need to be able to respond to hypnosis very easily. Women who go into a deep trance have been able to have a forceps delivery, stitches, or even a cesarean without feeling pain. You'll need to have some practice sessions, and both you and your hypnotist should be completely familiar with what you'll have to do during your labor and delivery.

Acupuncture Only choose this method if you've already found that it can relieve pain in other situations. You'll also need an acupuncturist who's familiar with labor and delivery. Acupuncture treatment may not completely relieve pain, but it will certainly reduce it, and also helps to stop nausea.

TENS (Transcutaneous Electrical Nerve Stimulation.) In this technique, pain impulses conducted by nerves are blocked by an electric current, which also stimulates the production of the body's own endorphins. You have a battery-powered stimulator that's connected by wires to electrodes placed on either side of your spine. You'll be given a handset that regulates the amount of stimulation, allowing you to control the amount of pain-relief that you receive. If you're interested in this, ask your midwife or obstetric physiotherapist well in advance if the TENS method is available at your hospital.

RELIEVING BACKACHES

Many women have a backache during labor, sometimes because of the baby's head pressing against the sacrum. Your partner can help to soothe any back pain by gently rubbing and massaging your lower back during labor.

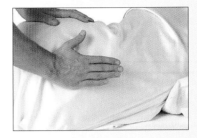

Rubbing the sacrum
Using the heel of your hand, rub all around the mother's sacrum and lower back.

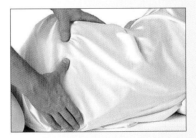

Circular pressure
Press your thumbs over the sacrum and move them gently in a circle. Rest your hands on the mother's hips for support.

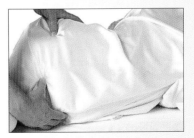

Deep pressure
Press your thumbs into the middle of each buttock. Make sure she is focusing on her breathing to help her relax.

BREATHING IN THE SECOND STAGE

You'll be shown breathing exercises in prenatal classes. I can't stress enough how important good breathing techniques are during the second stage of labor. They can make you feel in control of your own body and this is very empowering.

As you begin the second stage of labor, you may want to accelerate your breathing. This is the most shallow form of breathing you use in labor. Instead of using your chest and throat, focus on breathing only through your mouth. Breathe lightly in and out through your lips, starting slowly and gradually speeding up. Be careful not to breathe out too deeply or you'll start to hyperventilate. If you start to feel at all dizzy, place your hands lightly over your nose and mouth while you're breathing.

Into the second stage
At the end of the first stage of labor, your cervix will be fully dilated. The first sign that this has happened is that you'll feel a tremendous urge to push. Always ask your midwife to check your cervix. Don't hang on and fight the urge, even if it isn't long since you were checked—the last few centimeters of dilatation can be reached in seconds. Once you know you're fully dilated, you can push with force. Your mood will change and you'll feel reenergized and positive as you work hard toward the birth of your baby— now only a short time away.

The second stage: delivery

Delivery is the main event: it's what you've been getting ready for over the last nine months. Your expectations are realistic— a manageable labor, not necessarily painless but happy and relaxed, with your chosen birth partner and staff you know around you in familiar surroundings. One of the key factors in your feeling happy and relaxed is that everyone around you is a familiar friend.

CONTRACTIONS AND PUSHING

The second stage is the expulsive stage—you push your baby out. It lasts from the time your cervix is fully dilated until your baby is born and, for a first baby, generally takes less than two hours. The average second stage lasts about one hour, and it may be as little as 15–20 minutes for subsequent babies. At this time contractions are 60–90 seconds long and come at two- to four-minute intervals.

You'll almost certainly feel the urge to push, known as bearing down. The urge is caused by your baby's head pressing down on your pelvic floor and rectum, and is quite involuntary. Keep your pushing as smooth and continuous as you can; make the muscular effort smooth and slow so that your vaginal and perineal tissues and muscles have enough time to stretch and will be able to accommodate your baby's head.

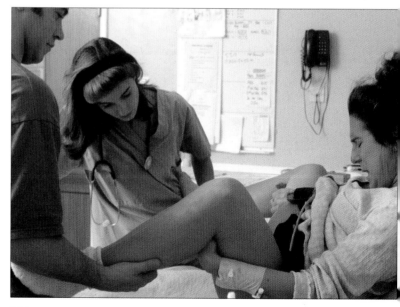

The most efficient position to be in when you're pushing is upright, whether you sit on a birthing stool, stand with your arms around your partner's neck, or squat. This means that the downward muscular force of your body and the downward force of gravity are working together to push your baby out.

If you're lying on your back, even if you're supported by pillows, you're pushing your baby out uphill against the force of gravity. This is much harder work, and so delivery is slower.

As you push, it helps if your pelvic floor and anal area are fully relaxed, so make a conscious effort to let go of this part of your body. Don't be embarrassed if you urinate or lose a little stool—lots of women do and your attendants have seen it all before. When you've finished a push, take two slow, deep breaths, but don't relax too quickly at the end of a contraction. Your baby will continue to maintain her forward progress if you relax slowly. If doctors think that your second stage is going on too long, they might suggest using forceps to assist the delivery of your baby (see p.306).

NORMAL DELIVERY

The first sign that your baby is coming is the bulging of your anus and perineum. With each contraction, more and more of your baby's head appears at your vaginal opening, until it doesn't slip back at all between contractions. This is known as crowning.

You'll probably feel a stinging or burning sensation as your baby stretches your vaginal opening. As soon as you feel this, try to stop bearing down, pant, and allow the contractions of your uterus to push your baby. This may be difficult since you'll probably still feel like pushing, but if you continue to push, you run a greater risk of tearing or needing an episiotomy. As you stop pushing, lean back and try to go limp. Make a conscious effort to relax the muscles of your perineal floor. The stinging or burning sensation only lasts for a short time and is followed by a numb feeling as your baby's head stretches your vaginal tissues so thin that the nerves are blocked, having a natural anesthetic effect. If the medical staff feel you are going to tear badly, this is the moment they may do an episiotomy (see p.110).

When her head has been delivered, your baby will be face down, but almost immediately she will twist her head so that she's facing your left or right thigh. Your doctor will wipe your baby's eyes, nose, and mouth, and clear any fluid from her nose and upper air passages. The doctor will also make sure the umbilical cord is not around your baby's neck—if it is, she will gently lift it over the head and make a loop through which the baby can be delivered. If the cord is very tight, she may clamp and cut it.

After delivery of your baby's head, your contractions will stop for a minute or so. When they start again, the first will usually deliver one shoulder and the next will deliver the other. Once both shoulders are delivered, the rest of your baby will slide out quickly and easily. Your attendants will hold her firmly because she'll be slippery with blood, amniotic fluid, and vernix.

WHAT YOUR BABY DOES

Her body goes through several twists and turns as she comes down through the birth canal, all of which are aimed toward having a smooth, safe birth.

Your baby has a pliable body but a fairly firm, oval head. Both these parts have to adapt themselves to passing through a curved lower birth canal. This is made up of the lower part of your uterus inside your pelvis, your dilated cervix, and stretched vagina. There are various adjustments that your baby makes as labor progresses.

- She'll bring her chin down on to her chest as she descends through your pelvis.

- She'll turn her head.

- She'll extend her head backward so that the back of her head touches her back as she emerges from the birth canal and vagina.

- She'll make a little sideways wriggle so that her head turns to one side or the other; the shoulder of that side can then be delivered through your vagina.

- She'll make another little wriggle to swing her head all the way around so that the other shoulder is delivered. (If you imagine this in quick succession, it's like a shrug of one shoulder after the other—it's so fast that you hardly notice it happening).

- Her trunk, buttocks, and legs follow her head out through your birth canal.

Giving birth

The urge to push your baby out is usually overwhelming and irresistible

Your baby's journey down the birth canal lasts about an hour on average. You'll probably feel swept along by an unbelievably strong, fundamental urge to bear down and push your baby out of your uterus. If you've had an epidural anesthetic your urge to bear down may be reduced.

Your caregivers will be there with you at all times to give you support and encouragement. They'll also be ready to act promptly if there are any complications

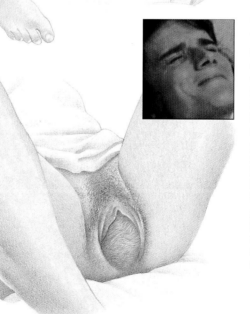

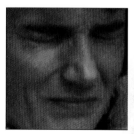

Pushing

As each contraction builds until it reaches its peak, you'll experience powerful urges to bear down and push out your baby as she descends. Bearing down is not something you decide to do; it's an instinctive reaction that you won't be able to resist.

The head crowns

There comes a point when your baby's head doesn't slip back between contractions, but remains visible at the vaginal outlet. This is when the baby's head is said to crown, and you'll feel a burning or stinging sensation as her head stretches your vagina. You'll need to stop pushing at this point so that you give the tissues of your perineum a chance to thin and stretch. This may be difficult since you may still want to bear down, but you must try to resist. If you continue to push at this stage, you'll put too much stress on your perineal area and you're more likely to tear or need an episiotomy. Panting is a good way to try to control your desire to bear down.

The head emerges

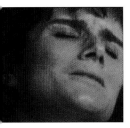

As her head is born, she'll immediately turn her head sideways. Your contractions will probably pause for a few moments at this point, and your caregivers will feel around your baby's neck to make sure that the cord's not there. If it is, hey'll either lift it up over her head or make a loop hrough which she can be born. Her shoulders will be lelivered in the next contraction.

With a couple of almost imperceptible shrugs, her shoulders emerge and she slithers out into the hands waiting to catch her

Once her head is born, she turns it immediately so that she's facing the inside of one of your thighs

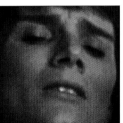

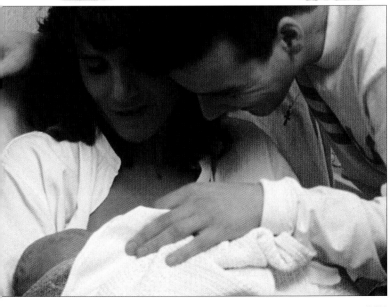

Your baby is born

As soon as her shoulders are free, the rest of her body will emerge right away. As she slithers out of your vagina, she'll usually be followed by a great gush of amniotic fluid. Your caregivers will hold her very carefully since she'll be slippery. She may be breathing and crying already.

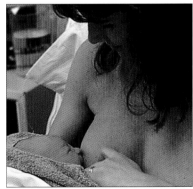

The first cuddle

If everything's gone well, your baby will be given straight to you to hold after her birth. She may start to suckle spontaneously.

RECORDING YOUR BABY'S BIRTH

Everyone wants to take photographs—or even video—of their baby's first moments, and all your family and friends will want to see pictures. There are a few points you need to bear in mind, though.

- Before labor begins, speak with your doctor or midwife to make sure it's okay to take pictures.

- If you want to take more than a few photos, or if you want to videotape the event, it may be better to ask a friend or relative to do it for you. Your partner will need you to be sensitive to her every need, not rushing around clicking the camera or focusing on the best image. You risk alienating yourself from her, and the doctor or midwife, if you're constantly behind a lens.

- Your partner will want soft, dim lighting in the delivery room to help her feel relaxed, so take this into account when assembling your camera equipment. Also, many hospitals don't like you to use direct flash since it can be irritating for the mother, distracting for the midwife, and may damage the baby's eyes.

Partner's role at the birth

By this second stage of labor, your role in providing loving support for your partner will be well established. You've now passed through the most painful phase and have reached the climactic stage of delivery.

SECOND STAGE JOBS

You'll need to continue doing many of the jobs you did during the first stage—making your partner comfortable, supporting her in different positions, providing drinks and food, and giving moral support. But you'll also now have to encourage her to push. All this will make the mother's job easier and help her feel emotionally secure and relaxed.

In the unlikely event of a medical emergency, staff have to move quickly and you might be in the way, so be sensitive to any situation that arises. You probably won't be asked to leave the delivery room, but be prepared to do so if necessary.

Helping with the delivery position Now that your partner has been through the first stage of labor, she'll probably know which position she finds most comfortable. Your support is very important to help her through the pushing stage, but always ask the midwife's advice if you're not certain what to do. If your partner doesn't want to be held, suggest other positions that she

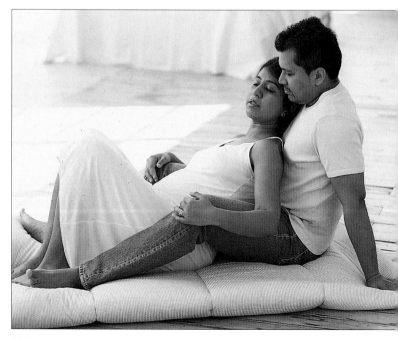

Semi-upright position
If your partner is happy for you to be as near as possible during labor, she can lean back against you for support. You'll be able to guide her through the contractions. Keeping close to her may help to make her feel more relaxed during the delivery.

might find comfortable, and place pillows or cushions under and behind her for support. It's a good idea to practice different ways of sitting or squatting before labor so that you're both familiar with them; if you feel unsure or uncomfortable about what you're doing, it can make your partner nervous.

If your partner is happy sitting on the bed or on the floor, she might like to try the knee–chest position, which many women find comfortable in the second stage. For this, she should drop her chin onto her chest while holding on to her knees. Between contractions, suggest that she relax against the pillow to conserve her energy.

Helping her with breathing and pushing To help her through these last few contractions, tap out a rhythm for the different kinds of breathing, using words like: "breathe, breathe, pant, pant, blow." As she's pushing, gently remind her to relax her pelvic floor.

At the peak of contractions, suggest that she take two or three deep breaths and push as hard as she can. She should push in a strong and steady way, and you can remind her that each push brings the birth of your baby a little closer.

Encouraging her to relax Between contractions, help your partner to relax—she needs to save her strength for pushing her baby through the birth canal. Massage her back (see p.283) if she has a backache or needs comforting and reassuring. If she is hot and flustered, mop her brow with a cool washcloth or mist her face with a water spray.

Standing by Once your baby's head has crowned, your role may become more passive for a while as you watch the doctor or midwife guiding your partner through this pushing stage. Don't be disappointed if your partner hardly seems to notice you during the birth and relies more on the hospital staff. She'll be fully preoccupied and involved with what's happening.

Showing her the baby When your baby's head is emerging, hold a mirror nearby so that your partner can see his head crowning and then his whole body slithering out. Help her to reach down and touch your baby's head as he is born.

Loving reception Ask the doctor or midwife if you can catch your baby in your arms as his body emerges. After you've greeted your baby for the first time, place him on your partner's stomach. You can then cuddle them both to help keep them warm and to let them know that you're there.

You and your partner will have a range of reactions—relief, tears, awed silence, exhausted collapse, whoops of joy. You may even feel squeamish at the sight of his bloodied, greasy, tiny body. Whatever your feelings, they're all perfectly understandable, and this moment marks a new phase in your family's history.

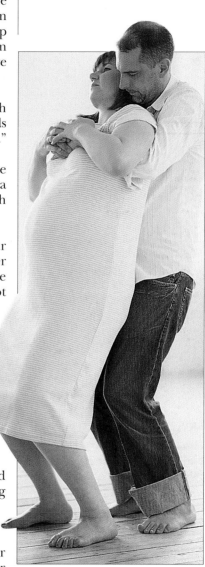

Supported squat
If your partner wants to deliver standing up, you can help support her by standing behind her and taking her weight on your arms. Supported in this way, her pelvis will be completely open and she'll be able to take full advantage of gravity. Her legs should be apart.

The third stage

Once your baby's been born, your uterus rests for about 15 minutes. But soon it starts to contract again to deliver the placenta. This is the third stage of labor, and it is comparatively painless—you'll be so absorbed in your baby that you'll probably hardly notice it.

THE THIRD STAGE

During the third stage of labor, the placenta becomes detached from the wall of your uterus and is delivered down the birth canal. The large blood vessels running to and from the placenta, which are about the thickness of a pencil, are simply torn across. Despite this, bleeding is rare because the muscle fibers of the uterus are arranged in a crisscross fashion so that when the uterus contracts down, the muscles tighten around the blood vessels and prevent them from bleeding. This is why it's absolutely essential that your uterus contracts down into a hard ball once the placenta has been expelled. Massaging every now and then for an hour or so after the third stage is complete can help keep your uterus tightly contracted. Normally the third stage lasts about 10–20 minutes.

DELIVERING THE PLACENTA

Usually your doctor or midwife won't try to deliver the placenta until there are clear signs that it's separating from the wall of your uterus and moving downward into your vagina. The signs your attendants will look for are contractions starting up again a few minutes after the birth of your baby, which shows that the placenta is about to separate, and your desire to bear down—this also shows that the placenta has separated from the wall of your uterus and is pressing down on your pelvic floor.

Once these signs have appeared, your doctor or midwife may encourage the delivery of the placenta by pulling gently on the cord, at the same time pressing above the rim of the pelvis to control descent. You may be asked to push. The placenta is expelled from your vagina, followed by the membranes. Rarely, a blood clot will also be expelled.

How you can help It may take up to half an hour before the placenta arrives. You can help speed things up by breastfeeding your baby because the sucking action stimulates your uterus to contract, thereby helping to expel the placenta. If your baby isn't ready to suck, stimulating your nipples with your fingers can have the same effect.

Delivery The placenta may pass through your vulva in two different ways. In the first, the center of the placenta comes out first, dragging the membranes behind it. In the second, an edge of the placenta presents first, then it slips out of the vulva

Most first-time mothers are eager to have a look at their baby's placenta.

The placenta measures about 8–10 in (20–25 cm) in diameter and weighs about 1 lb (0.5 kg). It's shaped like a disc and its surfaces look very different from each other.

The baby's side was continuous with the wall of your uterus and covered with membranes. It's flat and smooth, with blood vessels radiating out from the umbilical cord. Your side of the placenta was embedded in the wall of your uterus, and is made up of wedges (*cotyledons*) to make a larger surface area for the exchange of gases. This side is dark red and looks like several pieces of raw liver joined together.

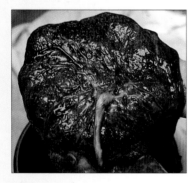

The baby's side
The side of the placenta that was facing toward your baby is flat and smooth. The umbilical cord emerges from its center, and there are prominent blood vessels.

290

sideways. Most women want to see the placenta—it's an amazing organ that's been the life-support system for your baby for nine months (see column, left).

After delivery Once the placenta is delivered, medical staff will check it carefully to make sure it's complete and none of it has been left behind. If any of the placenta has been left in the uterus it can cause hemorrhaging later on, so it must be removed as soon as possible. If there's any doubt, you may have an ultrasound scan to see whether the uterus is completely empty. The membranes should form a complete bag except for the hole through which your baby has passed. Your midwife will also check the cut end of the cord to make sure that the umbilical blood vessels are normal. After the placenta is delivered, the whole of your vulval outlet will be examined carefully for tears. Anything other than a minute one will be stitched immediately.

After the placenta is delivered

After the uterus is completely empty and the placenta is delivered, *Pitocin* is usually given by intravenous infusion. The *Pitocin* helps the uterus contract and reduce the amount of bleeding. Blood runs through sinuses in the uterus, and when the uterus contracts down to a small ball, these sinuses are closed off. If the uterus does not contract well, you will continue to bleed. At At this point your doctor will start an IV (if you don't have one already) and give you *Methergine* to control postpartum hemorrhage and help the uterus tone up. If you have high blood pressure, your doctor can give you a prostaglandin, which will have the same effect as *Methergine* to stop postpartum bleeding.

Oxytocin The hormone oxytocin is naturally produced by your body when you see and touch your baby and put her to your breast. This natural production of oxytocin helps control excessive bleeding and tone the uterus. At the same time, both you and your newborn benefit from close, skin-to-skin contact.

How you will feel

You may find yourself shivering and shaking after the placenta is delivered. After delivery of my second child, I was shivering and my teeth were chattering so much that I couldn't speak or breathe properly. My own explanation for this is that for nine months I had a little furnace inside me, producing quite a lot of heat, and my body had adjusted to take account of the extra heat by turning my own thermostat down slightly. When my baby left my body, I was deprived of that heat and my body temperature probably dropped a few degrees. The only way the body can raise its temperature is to generate heat through muscular work. That's exactly what shivering does—rapid contraction and relaxation of muscles produces body heat. The shivering usually stops in about half an hour, during which time your body temperature is back up to normal and your own thermostat is reset.

POSTPARTUM HEMORRHAGE

This is rare because your uterus has a self-protecting device to stop it from bleeding.

Once your uterus is completely empty, it contracts down to about the size of a tennis ball. The contraction of the uterine muscles nips the uterine arteries so they can't bleed. Under normal circumstances there's little bleeding after the delivery. What little bleeding there is appears as the lochia—the usual vaginal discharge after delivery. The lochia is red for two to three days, then turns brown, and disappears within two to six weeks.

If part of the placenta is retained in the uterus, it will bleed. a condition called called postpartum hemorrhage. This is why the placenta is checked— if any part is missing, it can be located and removed. The mother is given a general or regional anesthetic and the placental tissue is gently removed manually from inside the uterus.

If there's any bleeding more than 24 hours after delivery, your lochia may become bright red again. This can happen if you're too energetic. Check with your doctor, who'll probably suggest that you rest for several days. If the bleeding starts again or becomes heavy, it can be the sign of infection or that a small piece of placenta has been retained. Call your doctor immediately. If you pass clots of blood, or have a fever, call an ambulance and ask to be taken to the nearest emergency room.

THE APGAR SCORE

Within a minute of your baby's birth, five simple assessments of her condition are carried out to check that she is fit and healthy. These are scored on the Apgar scale (named after Dr. Virginia Apgar, who devised it). The Apgar score includes the following checks:

Pulse/heart rate This measures the strength and regularity of your baby's heartbeat: 100 beats per minute scores 2; below 100 scores 1; no pulse scores 0

Breathing This checks the maturity and health of your baby's lungs. Regular breathing scores 2, irregular 1, none 0

Movements Gives an indication of your baby's muscle tone. Active movements score 2; some movements 1; limp scores 0

Skin color This shows how well your baby's lungs are working to oxygenate her blood. Pink skin scores 2, bluish extremities 1, totally blue skin scores 0

Reflexes Crying and grimacing can show that your baby responds to stimuli. Crying scores 2, whimpering 1, silence 0.

Most babies score between seven and 10. A second test is done about five minutes later.

Baby's first hours

Once your baby is delivered, all the attention will be given to her, not to you, and rightly so. She may cry first when delivered and will be bawling robustly a few seconds after birth. She'll probably be a bluish-white color at first and may be covered with vernix—a white, cheesy substance that protects her skin in the womb. She'll have streaks of blood on her and, depending on your delivery, her head may look slightly pointed after her journey down the birth canal.

HER FIRST MOMENTS

If her breathing is normal, there's absolutely no reason why you shouldn't hold her immediately. If there's a danger of her being cold, you can be covered with a towel or blanket. Your gentle stroking movements and the sound of your heartbeat and voice will reassure your baby. Her eyes will almost certainly fasten on your face and she may scrabble as if trying to swim toward you.

Cutting the cord The first procedure after the delivery is the clamping of the cord. At the appropriate time, two clamps are applied to the cord, one a short distance from the navel, the other about an inch away. These clamps prevent the cord from bleeding, the one closest to your baby being the most important. At this point, your partner may be invited to cut the cord between the clamps. Some practitioners prefer to wait, however, until the

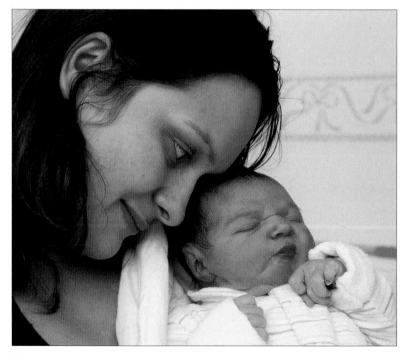

Your brand new baby
As you hold her, you'll feel the glow of motherhood—a mixture of love, pride, awe, and wonder, mixed with the all-encompassing tiredness that comes with a hard job well done.

placenta is delivered or the cord has stopped pulsating before cutting the cord. The cord may also be clamped and cut during delivery if it is looped tightly around your baby's neck.

Her general condition   The doctor or labor nurse will check your baby's general condition. She'll remove any fluid remaining in your baby's mouth, nose, or air passages by sucking it out with disposable plastic tubing or a bulb syringe. If your baby doesn't start to breathe immediately, the doctor will take her and give her oxygen, and the neonatologists will be called to the room.

WELCOMING YOUR BABY

Once the nursing and medical staff have checked that both you and your baby are well, by all means ask them to leave if you want to be left alone in the warmth of your birthing room with your partner and your baby.

If you've had an episiotomy, you may have to wait until after you've been stitched; your doctor will be able to make a much neater repair if you're stitched as soon as possible after the birth before the tissues swell. Once this is done, you can relax after your hard work and enjoy this amazing new experience together. It's a good idea to put your baby to your breast immediately because it stimulates delivery of the placenta, even if your baby isn't hungry at first.

Spend these first few moments concentrating on your baby, getting to know her, learning to recognize her face and cooing at her so that she can hear the sound of your voice. Ideally, hold her about 8–10 inches (20–25 centimeters) away from your face—at this distance she can make out your face quite clearly. Smile and talk gently in a sing-song voice, because newborn babies are attuned to high vocal pitches.

Let your partner hold his baby for the first time within half an hour of the birth. Men can bond as deeply and as quickly with their newborn children as women do.

After this initial bonding process, you'll be washed down and asked to pass urine to make sure that everything's in working order. You can then change, and the nurses will check your baby more thoroughly.

A MORE THOROUGH CHECK

Shortly after birth (in addition to the Apgar score, see column, left), the doctor or nurse will make some specific checks on your baby. The doctor will check that her facial features and her body proportions are normal. She'll be turned over to make sure that her back is normal and there are no indications of spina bifida. Her anus is checked, as are her fingers and toes. The number of blood vessels in the umbilical cord is recorded—there are usually two arteries and one vein. Your baby will then be weighed and her head circumference and possibly her body length measured. All this takes only a few seconds in the hands of an experienced doctor or midwife.

YOUR BABY'S IDENTIFICATION

Before your baby leaves the delivery room, she'll have some form of identification fastened to her, so that all the staff know she's yours.

Plastic bracelets will usually be sealed around both your baby's wrist and her ankle. The identifying bracelets must remain on your baby at all times while she is in the hospital. These bracelets are usually marked with:

- your last name (she'll be referred to by the staff as "baby Brown" for example)

- her date of birth

- an identification number (an identification number is used by most hospitals for both you and your baby).

In addition to the above:

- her footprints may be taken

- her crib may be marked with her name and number.

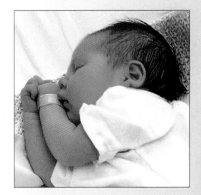

Keeping her bracelets
Like many parents, you may want to keep your baby's identity bracelets as souvenirs. As your baby grows day by day, it will soon seem astonishing that her wrists and ankles could ever have been quite so tiny.

CHAPTER 14

Special deliveries

Most babies are delivered without a hitch and are fit and healthy. Nonetheless, labors vary enormously. No two labors are alike, even for the same woman. From time to time, some need a special approach or even intervention. Don't worry—they can turn out just as well for mother and baby.

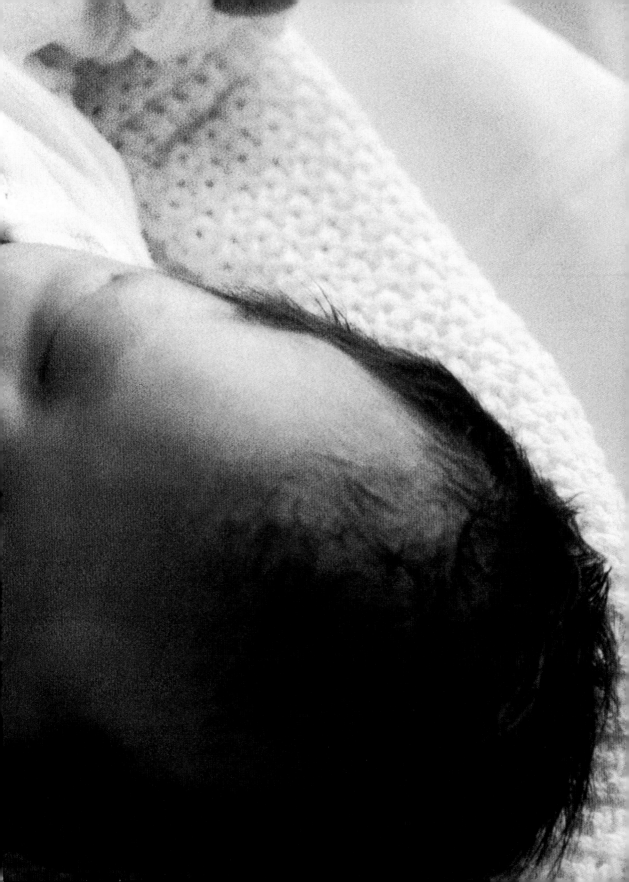

Special labors

Don't worry—most labors are quite straightforward, but just occasionally there may be a complication that needs a special approach. With good prenatal care, any potential difficulties are usually spotted well in advance and avoided. Now and then, though, the first stage is underway before a problem becomes apparent.

BACKACHE LABOR

Occasionally, a woman may feel the discomfort of uterine contractions mainly as low back pain. This is usually due to stretching of the cervix as it dilates. It may also happen if your baby lies in the posterior position with the back of his head up against your spine (this is not abnormal—one in 10 babies lies this way). In this position, your baby's neck may not be properly flexed and a larger proportion of the head than normal presents, which may mean that labor takes longer. Usually, your baby will rotate the 180 degrees into the anterior position and labor will go ahead smoothly. If, as sometimes happens, the baby fails to turn, there's still no cause for alarm, although your doctor may deliver him using forceps or, more rarely, vacuum extraction. This kind of labor may start slowly and take a while, so it can be tiring. There are various ways in which you and your birth assistant can relieve your backache.

Counterpressure This is the most effective way of relieving a backache (see p.283). But if you find being touched by someone else irritating—for example, during transition—you can apply counterpressure with your own knuckles by placing a hand underneath each buttock.

Change in position When you're lying flat on your back, your baby is pressing down hardest on your spine and its nerves. Try to stay upright and walk around as much as you can. You can also relieve the pressure of your baby on your spine by sitting tailor-style (see p.150), leaning forward, or rocking your pelvis. If you feel more comfortable lying down, lie on the side that your baby is turning toward (your midwife will be able to tell you which side that is).

Application of heat A heating pad or hot-water bottle placed against your lower back may help between contractions. A hot shower, directed onto your back, may also give some relief.

PROLONGED LABOR

Labor is said to be prolonged when contractions fail to bring about the expected delivery. This may be because the cervix hasn't dilated, or the baby hasn't descended through the birth

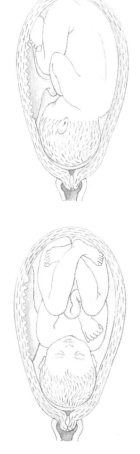

Your baby's presentation
The way your baby is presenting can affect your labor and birth. The usual presentation is when your baby's spine faces outward (top), but if your baby's head is facing outward (bottom), labor might be delayed. Most babies rotate to the correct position before passing down the birth canal.

canal. Doctors and midwives keep a very careful eye on the length of each stage of labor. If labor appears to be going more slowly than normal, your attendants may suspect obstruction and make an early decision to intervene—with a forceps delivery or vacuum extraction, if suitable, or a cesarean section.

No woman is allowed to go on with a difficult birth for much over the accepted times (see p.273) because this may lead to maternal exhaustion and fetal distress.

It's usually easier to detect obstruction in a mother who has had several children. But your midwife will be monitoring your general condition throughout labor, and she'll be alerted to possible obstruction if your condition appears to get worse and you look tired and anxious.

If your labor is very long and you're going without food and rest, you might become too tired or upset to push enough. Your midwife won't let this happen.

Failure to dilate When contractions are weak and infrequent and your cervix is dilating slowly, the uterus may be failing to coordinate muscular activity. One way in which your midwife will be able to see exactly how your labor is progressing is by plotting a partogram (see below). If failure of the uterus to contract efficiently is the only reason for the lack of progress, your attendants may suggest speeding up dilatation. The membranes may be artificially ruptured and then *Pitocin* may be administered intravenously with a drip or with a pump. The dosage will be

CAUSES OF FETAL OBSTRUCTION

There are certain conditions that cause obstructed labor. Fortunately, most problems are discovered beforehand so everybody is well prepared.

- Your baby is too large.

- Your baby is lying in a transverse or oblique position.

- Your baby is in a breech, face, or brow presentation.

- Your baby is lying in the posterior position.

- Your twin babies are entwined.

- Your baby has a congenital abnormality such as hydrocephalus.

- Your pelvis is particularly small or an unusual shape.

YOUR LABOR'S PROGRESS

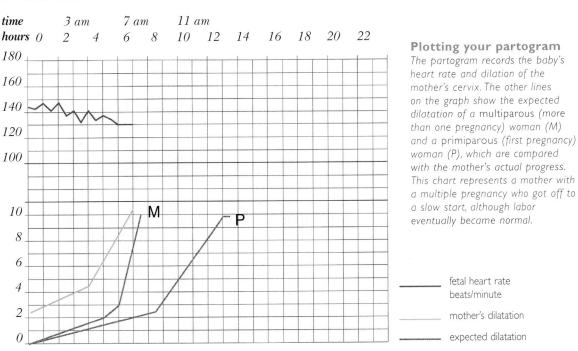

Plotting your partogram
The partogram records the baby's heart rate and dilation of the mother's cervix. The other lines on the graph show the expected dilatation of a multiparous (more than one pregnancy) woman (M) and a primiparous (first pregnancy) woman (P), which are compared with the mother's actual progress. This chart represents a mother with a multiple pregnancy who got off to a slow start, although labor eventually became normal.

———— fetal heart rate beats/minute

·········· mother's dilatation

▪▪▪▪▪▪ expected dilatation

MATERNAL CAUSES OF OBSTRUCTION

If your labor isn't progressing normally, there may be reasons why your pelvis or uterus is obstructing the descent of your baby.

- Deformity or disproportion of the bony pelvis.

- Pelvic tumors such as fibroids or an ovarian cyst.

- Abnormalities of the uterus, cervix, or vagina.

- A contraction ring of the uterus, which is when the uterus pulls in excessively and a band of tight muscle occurs. This can stop contractions from passing all the way down and may cause constriction of the uterus or cervix. Fortunately, this is very rare, unless the uterus has been overstimulated by oxytocin or prostaglandin, such as during induction (see p.300). A cesarean section is almost always needed.

carefully increased until strong contractions are coming regularly about every three minutes. Your midwife and doctor will keep a close watch throughout to make sure there are no unexpected increases in the strength or frequency of your contractions.

Failure to descend   I've mentioned breech and posterior presentation as causes of obstruction. One other reason for an obstructed labor is disproportion. This means that the size of your baby's head and the size of your pelvis don't match—for example, if your pelvis is too small relative to your baby's head. It's easy to understand how your baby might fail to descend in such circumstances (see also p.176).

If you're a first-time mother and your baby is still high and nonengaged during the last few weeks of your pregnancy (see column, p.261), your doctor may suspect disproportion. This will also be taken into account if your baby's head remains high during labor despite strong contractions.

If the disproportion is quite slight, your doctor may let you try having a normal labor (bear in mind that it's your uterus on trial, not you), provided there are no other irregularities, and the baby's head is felt to be descending. Once the baby's head enters the pelvic cavity, there can usually be a vaginal delivery. If the disproportion is major, which is rare, you'll need a cesarean section.

Don't worry—most of the abnormalities that cause obstruction and prolonged labor (see column, left, and p.297) will be picked up during your pregnancy so that early treatment is possible, and a plan of action can be laid out by the doctors and midwives before labor begins.

PREMATURE LABOR

A premature labor is one that starts at less than 37 weeks of gestation. The cause is a mystery in about 40 percent of cases, but it's known to happen in the following circumstances: premature rupture of the membranes; multiple pregnancy; preeclampsia; cervical incompetence; and uterine abnormalities. Overwork, stress, and some maternal diseases, such as anemia or malnutrition, may also have an effect.

Knowing whether you've actually gone into premature labor is almost as difficult for your doctors as it is for you (see column, right). The diagnosis is not easy, and criteria differ at different clinics—showing that often it's quite arbitrary. As a general rule, a premature labor begins without any warning; the first sign may be rupture of the membranes, the beginning of uterine contractions, or some vaginal bleeding. There's no stopping labor if your membranes have ruptured and labor has begun, but you or your doctor can take certain precautions while the membranes are intact or before labor really gets going.

What you can do   If your membranes have ruptured (see p.273) but labor hasn't started, go straight to the hospital. The risk of infection is great, and both you and your preterm baby will be vulnerable. The doctors will monitor you closely for signs of infection, such as a fever, and will give you antibiotics. Labor is unlikely to be suppressed once the membranes have ruptured spontaneously. Nonetheless, if labor doesn't start spontaneously, it won't usually be induced until after 34 weeks unless there are signs of infection.

What the hospital will do If labor starts between 24 and 34 weeks, the aim is to delay your labor with *ritodrine* or *magnesium sulfate* to allow time to mature the baby's lungs with steroids. A preterm baby (see also pp.344 & 345) has an increased risk of developing respiratory distress syndrome, and the shorter the gestation period, the greater the risk.

Being in hospital also allows your doctor to check for evidence of infection in cases of premature rupture of the membranes, and to monitor your baby's condition. It also means that your premature baby can be taken to intensive care immediately after delivery and cared for.

If your local hospital does not have a neonatal intensive care unit that can handle very premature babies, you may need to be moved to another hospital that has these facilities. This may be farther away, making it harder for your partner, friends, and family to visit you, but be comforted by the thought that the NICU will be able to give your tiny baby the best possible start in life after the birth (see p.344).

Drug treatments All of the drugs used cause some side effects, and for that reason they're only suitable in certain cases of premature labor. The main criteria for drug treatment are that you are healthy and have no heart disease, diabetes, high blood pressure, or an abnormally placed placenta. Another, of course, is that your baby is alive, with no evidence of a congenital defect.

If you are very anxious, a mild sedative may be given to help to calm you, but morphine and Demerol should not be given during labor unless your pain is extremely severe. These drugs may make your uterine muscles more irritable rather than calming them down, and they may also have a sedating effect on your premature baby.

Managing labor Once the membranes have ruptured, labor will go on as normal (see p.270). As a general rule, a premature labor tends to be shorter and easier than full-term, mainly because the baby's head is smaller and softer. However, an episiotomy is usually given to protect the baby's head from pressure changes within the birth canal.

You may prefer to have an epidural anesthetic instead of analgesic drugs, which can depress your baby's respiratory system. Doctors will take special care to avoid *hypoxia* (lack of oxygen to the tissues) throughout labor and delivery. Cesarean delivery is used to deliver some premature babies, particularly if there is fetal distress.

ARE YOU IN PREMATURE LABOR?

Here are some useful pointers for diagnosing whether or not you're in premature labor.

- You're less than 37 weeks into your pregnancy.

- You've had uterine contractions for at least an hour.

- You're having contractions every 5–10 minutes.

- The contractions last for 30 seconds and persist over the period of an hour.

- A vaginal examination by your doctor or midwife shows that your cervix is more than 2.5 cm (1 in) dilated and so more than three-fourths effaced.

According to these criteria, two-thirds of all patients who are thought to be in premature labor will actually be found not to be in real labor, and no treatment will be needed. This will be quickly confirmed if you go straight to the hospital so that staff can observe uterine activity very carefully.

IF YOU'RE OVERDUE

Toward the end of pregnancy, doctors are always on the look-out for any signs of placental insufficiency as the baby outgrows its food supply.

Whether to induce or not if you're overdue is a controversial issue, so it's worth talking about it at one of your prenatal checkups. Of course, induction isn't always necessary. A mother who reaches her estimated date of delivery, given that she and the baby are perfectly normal, should be allowed to go into spontaneous labor.

Once the EDD has been passed, though, I do think it's very important to have your own and your baby's condition monitored frequently. If there's any sign of fetal distress, I'd advise you to agree to medical intervention.

REASONS FOR INDUCTION

Anything that makes the uterine environment unhealthy is a reason for induction. Your labor may be induced if:

• you have hypertension, preeclampsia, heart disease, diabetes, or antepartum bleeding

• there are signs of placental insufficiency (the baby is in danger of not getting enough nutrients and oxygen from the placenta)

• your membranes have ruptured (see p.273) but labor hasn't started within 24–48 hours

• your pregnancy goes beyond 42 weeks.

Induction of labor

Induction is a way of starting labor artificially by rupturing the membranes and giving oxytocin or prostaglandins to stimulate uterine contractions. The same techniques are used to accelerate labor if your contractions are weak and progress is slow. If your induction is not done for the medical reasons below (see box) or as an emergency, you'll have an elective induction. An appointment will be made for you to go into the hospital at a certain time. Your partner will be able to be with you all the time. If you're in any doubt about why your doctor is suggesting induction of labor, ask for a detailed explanation—this should cover all of the alternatives. In the end, of course, the decision is up to you.

THE HISTORY OF INDUCTION

When induction was first available, it was often used for hospital or social convenience or so births could be arranged to happen during working hours. Such reasons are no longer acceptable.

When induction first became fashionable, doctors didn't have all the technological backup that we have today for checking fetal maturity, such as ultrasound and amniocentesis, and some babies were born too early and had respiratory problems. The rate of cesarean section also rose. Nowadays, fewer than one in five labors are induced.

Only five percent of babies actually come on their due date, and it can be hard for some doctors—and mothers—to remain calm when that magic date passes. They may worry that the placenta is becoming inadequate and that the baby is outgrowing its environment.

Don't worry if you have to be induced. Induction is fine, provided it's done strictly for medical reasons and either for your well-being or the baby's. And please don't feel angry with yourself if your birth doesn't turn out just the way that you'd planned.

HOW IT'S DONE

Most obstetric units will normally use a combination of three different methods to induce labor.

Prostaglandin suppositories One method of induction uses prostaglandin suppositories, which soften the cervix and start it dilating. They can be inserted at any time of day, although most units put them in at night, and they usually take full effect in six hours. This is a good method of induction since you are free to move around the labor room.

Artificial rupture of the membranes (ARM) This is also known as *amniotomy* and involves the use of an instrument not unlike a crochet hook. It is inserted through the cervix (when it is dilated) into the uterus to make a small opening in the membrane so that the water escapes. Amniotomy can be performed with or without contractions, but if there are no contractions, you'll need to have an oxytocin drip. If you have a drip, doctors usually advise fetal monitoring so they can check the effect of the induced contractions on the fetus. Labor usually reaches full intensity quickly after ARM because the baby's head is no longer cushioned and presses down hard against the cervix, encouraging the uterus to contract and the cervix to dilate. If left alone, the water doesn't usually break until late in the first stage.

Amniotomy is not just a method of induction. It will be performed if an electrode needs to be attached to the baby's scalp to monitor its heartbeat (see p.275). It will also be performed if the baby's heart rate goes down because of distress. In this case, traces of meconium, the baby's first bowel movement, may be seen in the amniotic fluid.

Oxytocin-induced labor Oxytocin is the natural hormone from the posterior pituitary gland in the brain that stimulates labor. The synthetic form is used for inducing labor.

Oxytocin used to be administered in tablet form, but it's now only given through a drip, which is easier to regulate. Ask for the drip to be inserted in your left arm if you are right-handed, and check that you can have a long tube connecting you to the drip. You'll then have more room to move around, even if this is just on the bed; some drip stands are on wheels so that you can still move around the room and change position if you wish, which will help you control the more intense labor pains. The oxytocin drip can be turned down if you go into strong labor quickly and the cervix becomes half dilated. The needle won't be removed from your arm until after the baby is born because the uterine contractions help to expel the placenta.

Contractions brought on by an oxytocin drip are often stronger, longer, and more painful than normal contractions, with shorter breaks between them, so there's an increased need for painkilling drugs. As the blood supply to the uterus is temporarily shut off during each strong contraction, it's thought that this may be detrimental to the fetus. Most obstetricians believe that only a small percentage of deliveries need an oxytocin-induced labor.

EXPECTATIONS OF INDUCED LABOR

If properly handled, induced labor needn't be more painful or difficult than natural labor and, using oxytocin, your doctor or midwife should be able to get you to the stage where you'll have a normal labor. You can still do all your breathing exercises and push the baby out at your own pace if you prefer to have a natural childbirth. If the induced labor does become too painful, you can ask for an epidural or other pain relief (see p.280).

AMNIOTOMY AND YOUR BABY

The membranes usually rupture naturally toward the end of the first stage of labor.

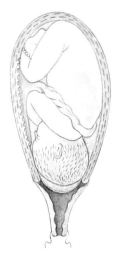

Intact membranes
The bag of water provides a cushion for your baby's head as it presses your cervix.

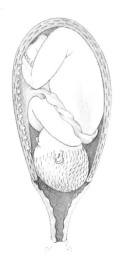

Ruptured membranes
Contractions get stronger, pressing your baby's head against your cervix and helping it to open.

An induced birth

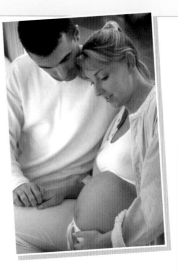

Case study

Name Rebecca Newland
Age 32 years
Past medical history Nothing abnormal
Obstetric history Normal pregnancy, baby born by vacuum extraction after an induced labor

Rebecca is married to David, age 40. This is their first baby, born in the hospital six days after term. The pregnancy went normally, and apart from feeling tired toward the end, Rebecca had no complications. Rebecca and David had decided that they wanted to have their baby in a birthing center, but things didn't go as planned and their baby was born in their local hospital after induction. The birth was induced because Rebecca's water had broken and after 48 hours there were still nos sign of labor.

Induction is a standard hospital procedure and is quite common (see pp. 300–301). Births are induced if labor hasn't begun 14 days after the woman's expected delivery date (known as post-maturity) or a maximum of 48 hours after the water breaks. Other reasons for induction include complications in late pregnancy such as maternal high blood pressure, preeclampsia, and suspected placental insufficiency, though in emergencies a cesarean is likely to be done. Induction is more common for older mothers.

WEDNESDAY AND THURSDAY

Rebecca's pregnancy passed by without anything unusual. Her water broke on a Wednesday morning about two days after her due date, before any signs of labor had appeared. It's quite normal for this to happen, and can be caused by pressure of the baby's head on the membranes of the amniotic sac. It's also quite normal not to go into labor immediately after the water breaks. However, once the water has broken, there's a small risk of infection for the baby, and most women are advised to have an induction within about 24 to 48 hours.

Rebecca and David went straight to the hospital. Their baby's heartbeat was monitored and all seemed to be going well, with no signs of distress. They were reassured that it was OK to wait for signs of labor to begin. But when there were no signs of labor by Thursday morning, the medical staff at the hospital recommended that if labor hadn't begun by Friday morning, 48 hours after Rebecca's water had broken, they should return to the hospital.

FRIDAY

Friday morning came without any signs of labor, so at 8 a.m. David and Rebecca went to the maternity unit at the hospital, where their doctor decided that Rebecca should have an induction immediately.

Rebecca was given a prostaglandin suppository at nine in the morning—a "vicious little pill," as the doctor described it. Prostaglandin can be very effective in inducing labor in some women, though many need to have more than one suppository. In Rebecca's case, the first one didn't work, so she was given another one a few hours later. That failed to have any effect, either, and so Rebecca had to spend the night in the hospital.

SATURDAY

On Saturday morning the hospital staff decided that a syntocinon drip was needed to start Rebecca's labor. Syntocinon is a synthetic form of oxytocin, and because it's given intravenously, it works very quickly. However, the hospital staff were very busy that day. Though the drip hadn't been given, Rebecca's labor finally began on its own at about 6 p.m.

LABOR

Rebecca's labor progressed very slowly. She had gas and asked for some Demerol after several hours, because her contractions were so painful. By midnight, David had to leave, since Rebecca's cervix still wasn't dilated enough for her to go to the delivery room. David went home and managed to get a little sleep. He was called back to the hospital at four o'clock on Sunday morning, where he found that Rebecca's labor had progressed enough for her to be taken to the delivery room.

Both of them were very relieved because it meant they had a room to themselves, so they were able to relax a little and doze in between the contractions. These were beginning to be very painful indeed, so a "walking" epidural was given to help Rebecca manage the pain, which meant that she could rest for a while in between each wave of pain. A "walking" epidural is so called because it numbs feeling from the chest to the knees, but still allows some movement, standing and even walking. A stronger, full epidural means that a woman can't move her legs much at all, and makes it harder to push.

The rest of Rebecca's labor was relatively straightforward. After several hours of contractions, a vacuum extraction was need at the end to deliver the baby's head. Rebecca finally gave birth to a beautiful baby boy at noon on Sunday. He weighed in at 9 lb 10 oz (4.3 kg) and was perfectly healthy.

AFTER THE BIRTH

Not surprisingly, Rebecca was absolutely exhausted after being on the verge of giving birth for so long, and David was also worn out by all the anxiety. Tiredness, though universal, is not the best start to parenthood, so I always recommend that parents-to-be try to stock up on their sleep in the weeks before their due date so they're able to cope with unexpected events like this. The two weeks or so before the birth is not the time to be making curtains—it's time to relax!

LOOKING BACK

Unforeseen eventualities can play havoc with the most carefully prepared birth plan, and induction is one of them. With the benefit of hindsight, Rebecca and David now feel that they'd have been better off letting nature take its course from the start. They've learned a lot from the experience, though, and feel that next time, if appropriate, they'd like to take a long, slow labor in stride, relaxing at home during the early stages. Then they might be able to have their baby at a birthing center, where they'd wanted to have their baby all along.

However, they also understand that the hospital was following standard procedures to ensure the safety of Rebecca and her baby son and that everyone was doing their best to help. And of course, they were completely thrilled with the new arrival, who's more than made up for all the trials of the past four days!

Why did Rebecca's labor take so long?

Induction is always done for good medical reasons, but it can affect your labor. Here are some of the reasons why Rebecca's labor went as it did.

- Rebecca's baby was a whopping big boy, and his very size made his passage through the birth canal very slow. Vacuum extraction was needed at the end because he was so big that he got stuck, even though Rebecca was fully dilated.

- The prostaglandin suppository, which softens the cervix, doesn't always "take." On average, two or three suppositories are given, with some women needing up to four, though this is unusual. It's necessary to wait for several hours between each one, which meant that Rebecca had to spend a long time in hospital rather than relaxing at home.

- Induced labor can be more painful than natural labor. The prostaglandin means that the onset of labor is speeded up, and the contractions are more severe and tend to be closer together. This makes it harder for the woman's partner to try "natural" forms of pain relief such as massage or breathing. Statistics show that women who have induction are also more likely to need pain relief such as epidurals.

Sudden birth

ON YOUR WAY TO THE HOSPITAL

If the urge to bear down comes as you're going to the hospital, use your breathing techniques to avoid pushing; do your best to stay calm.

If the urge becomes too strong for you to control, ask your partner to pull the car over and stop. Cover the back seat and car floor with a thick layer of newspapers or towels if you have them available, and get as comfortable as possible. You can then deliver your baby into his hands.

Follow the procedure for the birth in the main text. Once your baby is born, it's important that he's kept warm, so wrap him in a blanket or towel (or in your partner's shirt, sweater, or coat, if there's nothing else) and hold him close against your skin. If the placenta arrives before you reach the hospital, wrap it up with your baby, since this provides him with much-needed extra warmth. Do not cut the umbilical cord, but squeeze it in your fist so the baby doesn't lose blood.

Sometimes labor is so quick that the your baby is born before you can get medical assistance, whether at home or on the way to the hospital. If this should happen, the following information will help you and your partner deliver your baby safely. This is not intended to be used as a guide for an out-of-hospital birth without a professional attendant being present, because this can be very risky indeed. It's reassuring, though, that there are rarely any complications in emergency births of this kind.

WHAT TO DO

When you get the urge to push, try to pant or blow for as long as you can to delay your baby's birth. The contractions alone are usually enough to push your baby out when he's coming this fast, so this won't delay things for long, although it may be long enough for the ambulance to arrive. Never try to hold your legs together to delay delivery, or allow anyone else to do so: this may cause your baby to be injured. If you cannot comfortably delay your baby's birth, don't try to interfere. Deliver the head slowly. There's more chance that your vagina and perineum will tear if you push along with the force of your uterus, so pant lightly with each contraction.

Prolapsed cord   If a loop of the umbilical cord washes out when the membranes rupture and your partner can see a piece of gray-blue shiny cord bulging out of your vagina, this means that you have a prolapsed cord. You must get help as soon as possible because your baby's oxygen supply is in danger of being cut off. Don't panic; you have time. Get onto the floor on your knees, with your chest to your knees, your head on the floor, and your buttocks in the air. This will help to take the pressure of your baby's head off your cervix. If the cord is still protruding, your partner should cover it with a wet, warm, very clean towel after he calls the hospital or goes for help. Don't touch or put any pressure on the cord. Stay in the knee-chest position even on the way to the hospital, because it reduces pressure on the cord. A prolapsed cord means you'll have to have a cesarean delivery, unless the cervix is fully dilated, in which case forceps or vacuum extraction will be used.

WHAT THE BIRTH ASSISTANT SHOULD DO

If it looks as if your partner is going to give birth at home, call 911, then call the hospital, followed by your doctor or midwife. If you're not near a telephone, on no account leave the mother alone. However anxious and overwhelmed you feel, it's vital for you to stay calm and reassure your partner—she needs to feel confident and relaxed. Bear in mind that the vast majority of sudden births are uncomplicated. Encourage your partner to take up any position she finds comfortable (see p.278) and to eat and drink if she feels like it. Speak quietly and keep other people away. Between contractions, turn up the heat in the room. Wash your hands thoroughly in soap and water, then gather up as many clean bath towels as you have. Fold one and put it on the floor so that you have something soft on which your baby can be laid.

Then fill several bowls with lukewarm water, and collect as many clean hand towels, washcloths, and dish towels as you can. They can be soaked in the water and used as wipes for the baby and mother during and after delivery.

The birth   Your partner will know when her baby is coming because she'll feel a stinging or burning sensation as the baby stretches her vagina. Look to see if you can see the top of the baby's head in the vaginal outlet (known as crowning—see p.285). Remind your partner to pant or blow, so that her vagina and perineum have time to thin and stretch, which might help to avoid tearing.

Your baby's head will probably emerge in one contraction and the rest of his body in the next. When the head emerges, wipe each of your baby's eyes from inside to outside with separate pieces of moist cloth, and then feel around his neck to see if the cord is present. If it is, crook your little finger underneath it and pull it very gently over his head, or lift it so that his body can be born through the loop.

Do not interfere with the cord because it may go into a spasm and deprive your baby of oxygen. If the membranes are still present over your baby's face, gently tear them off with your fingernail so that your baby can breathe. Be careful to hold him firmly as he is born, since he'll be slippery with blood, mucus, and *vernix caseosa*. Never pull on his head, his body, or his cord.

Once he's born, he'll probably give a couple of gasps, a cry, and then start to wail. If he doesn't cry right away, place him across your partner's thigh or abdomen, with his head lower than his feet, and then gently rub his back while you dry him off. This helps any mucus to drain away and usually causes a change in blood pressure, which brings about his first breath. Talking to your baby lovingly will also help.

After the birth   Once your baby is breathing, pass him to your partner so she can put him to her breast, and keep him warm against her skin. If he's interested in feeding, the nipple stimulation will release oxytocin, which will encourage your partner's uterus to contract and expel the placenta.

Keep your partner and your baby warm with blankets or towels, especially your baby's head, since most heat is lost from here. Bear in mind that the normal color of a baby at birth is a bluish-white. He'll gradually become pink in the first minutes as oxygen enters his body; his hands and feet will take a little longer. Don't try to wash off the vernix, and never cut the umbilical cord.

THE DELIVERY OF THE PLACENTA

If the placenta is delivered before medical help arrives:

- never pull on the cord

- don't cut the cord

- after the placenta is delivered, firmly massage the mother's abdomen over her uterus, with a deep circular motion, gently pushing downward 2–3 in (5–7 cm) below the navel and rubbing. This is important to make sure the uterus contracts and stays hard after the birth so there's no hemorrhaging

- it's normal for a couple of cups of blood to be delivered when the placenta comes out

- getting your baby to start nursing immediately will help contract your uterus and minimize blood loss

- if your baby won't suck, encourage the mother gently to massage her nipples as a substitute way of releasing oxytocin into her system.

FORCEPS-ASSISTED DELIVERY

Forceps look like large tongs and are designed to fit snugly over the sides of a baby's head, covering the ears. They're rather like a cage that protects the head from any pressure as it passes through the birth canal.

The decision to use forceps is a medical judgment on the part of your attendants. Forceps are only applied when the first stage is complete, the cervix is fully dilated, and the head is in the birth canal.

Why forceps are used Forceps are applied when your baby's head has descended into your pelvis but fails to descend farther; when a baby presents in a posterior position; in a breech delivery (see main text); when the uterus fails to maintain contractions; and when you lack the strength to push. Occasionally, forceps may be used for a quick delivery early in the second stage if your baby shows signs of lacking oxygen, even if the birth is not imminent.

How it's done If you're going to have a forceps delivery, your legs will be put up in stirrups. A local anesthetic will be injected into your perineum. Then the forceps will be inserted into your vagina one at a time. A few gentle pulls on the forceps while you push, 30–40 seconds at a time, will bring your baby's head down onto your perineum. You should feel no pain. At this point you'll have an episiotomy (see p.110). Once your baby's head has been delivered, the forceps are removed and the rest of his body will be delivered as normal.

Complications at delivery

I've talked about the way delivery usually goes on the previous pages. Occasionally, though, there may be complications, and some special procedures may be needed. Something unforeseen may happen once labor has started, meaning that forceps or a vacuum extractor have to be used. Other special deliveries, such as multiple and breech births, are usually diagnosed well in advance.

ASSISTED DELIVERY

If, as sometimes happens, labor and delivery don't go quite as smoothly as expected, your obstetrician may need some help to complete a vaginal delivery. Forceps (see column, left) can be used to protect your baby's head, or, along with vacuum extraction, may be used to speed your baby's progress through the birth canal.

Vacuum extraction The vacuum extractor is a gentler alternative to forceps and is widely used. It's a cone-shaped cup of synthetic material that is placed over the baby's scalp. An attached pump is then used to create a vacuum that makes the cup hold fast to the baby's head. This instrument then becomes a "handle" that the obstetrician can use to rotate the baby's head and apply traction. Although the vacuum extractor leaves a bruise on the baby's head, it has many advantages (see column, right).

MULTIPLE DELIVERIES

If you're having twins, their delivery will always be treated as though you're having two single babies: if one has a vaginal delivery, it doesn't always follow that the other will. The risks of vaginal birth go up with the number of fetuses. As a result, women carrying more than two babies often have a cesarean delivery. Your doctor will probably suggest you have the babies in the hospital in case they aren't presenting properly. If all goes well, twins usually present head-down, the second one arriving eight to ten minutes after the first. Twin labors can be long, so an epidural anesthetic (see p.281) might help. Also, the second baby may have to be turned—this is done by rupturing the second baby's membrane and moving him by hand.

Twin deliveries are much safer than they used to be because the exact position of the second baby, and its condition, can be determined by ultrasound and fetal monitors. If you're carrying three or more babies, it's more likely that you'll have a cesarean section.

BREECH BIRTH

One out of twenty-five babies is born in the breech position, so this isn't all that unusual. However, most breech babies are delivered by cesarean section, especially babies lying sideways in the uterus rather than head-down. In these cases a cesarean birth is the only choice for delivery. Breech doesn't always mean a cesarean section, though, and if your attendants decide it's safe for your breech baby to be delivered normally, he'll usually be born buttocks first, followed by his legs and body.

Before your baby's head can be delivered, you'll almost certainly have to have an episiotomy. The head is the widest part and your baby's rump will not have stretched your birth canal enough for his head to pass through it unpressurized.

Once your baby's body is born, his weight will pull his head down to the vagina. His body is then lifted upwards and slightly backwards by the doctor, and one push is usually enough to deliver him. Forceps may be used to protect the baby's head. It's now fairly common practice to have an epidural if you're having a breech birth, which means that if you do need a cesarean section it can be done quickly and simply without further anaesthesia.

VACUUM EXTRACTOR

This device takes up less room in the vagina than forceps and is easier to apply. It has several other advantages over forceps.

- It can be applied to the lowest part of the baby's head.

- It doesn't affect the shape of the baby's head. It does, however, leave a bruise, but this will fade within a week or two of the birth.

- An episiotomy isn't always necessary.

DELIVERING A BREECH BABY VAGINALLY

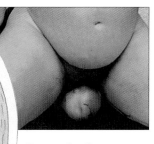

Buttocks first
In a breech birth, the baby's buttocks (here still covered by the amniotic membranes) are delivered first.

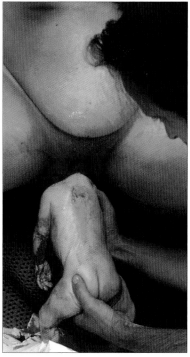

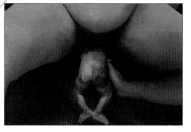

Breech position
Before labor begins, the baby's breech (buttocks) has not engaged within his mother's pelvis and her cervix is uneffaced.

Legs and body
Once the baby's buttocks are clear of the birth opening, the membranes rupture and the baby's legs and body are delivered.

Arms and head
In the final stages of a breech delivery, the baby's arms emerge. His body is gently supported as his head is guided out.

Cesarean section

A cesarean section operation usually takes 35–45 minutes, but the baby is delivered within the first 5–10 minutes. The rest of the time is spent stitching you up.

Preparation Before the operation begins, your pubic hair is shaved, you're given an epidural anesthetic or spinal block, and an intravenous drip is set up to supply you with fluids during the operation. Then a *catheter* (a thin, flexible tube) is inserted up your urethra and into your bladder to drain it of urine. A small screen is placed in front of your face so you don't have to watch the operation. Your abdomen is swabbed with antiseptic to prevent infection. If the operation is urgent—for instance, if your baby is in serious distress—you may need a general anesthetic, even if you already had an epidural in place.

The operation The obstetrician makes a short, horizontal incision along the "bikini line" at the base of your abdomen, then makes a similar incision in the lower segment of your uterus. The amniotic fluid is drained off by suction, and the baby is gently lifted out. Then the cord is cut, the placenta is removed, and your uterus and abdomen are stitched.

If a normal vaginal delivery could be dangerous or even impossible for you, your baby will be delivered by cesarean section (commonly called C-section). Small horizontal incisions are made in your abdomen and uterus, and your baby is delivered through them. The vertical cut is no longer used because there's a risk it may tear again if you have another child. The number of babies delivered by cesarean section has increased rapidly and is currently about one in four in the United States. One reason for this increase is that doctors are worried about being sued if a difficult birth causes complications that could have been avoided by a cesarean section. Another is that the operation is now so safe that it can be less risky than some other forms of delivery.

The need for a cesarean section may be apparent well before labor begins, so you, your partner, and your obstetrician have time to talk through what will happen—this is an elective cesarean. In emergencies, the need only becomes evident once labor is under way.

ELECTIVE CESAREAN SECTION

The most common reasons for choosing to have a cesarean include failure to progress in labor or dystocia (abnormally slow progress of labor), your baby being in a breech position (see p.307) or lying across your pelvis; placenta previa (see p.222); and certain medical conditions such as active herpes type II infection. A cesarean may also be necessary if you've had one for a previous baby—the worry used to be that the scar would open up again. Experience has shown that this does not happen with the horizontal or "bikini" cut, now generally used instead of the vertical cut, and so hospitals often allow a vaginal delivery to begin, and if there are no problems, labor goes on as normal— a "trial of labor."

Elective cesareans are often carried out under a spinal anesthetic (see p.281). This has several advantages over a general anesthetic: it's safer for your baby; you have no postoperative nausea or vomiting; and because you are conscious, you can hold your baby as soon as he's born. It's usually possible for your partner to be with you during the operation, just as he can be at a vaginal delivery.

When you've had a cesarean, you may feel deeply disappointed that you didn't have a vaginal delivery. It's natural to feel this way, and the best thing you can do is talk to your partner about it. If he describes the birth to you in detail it may help you to visualize and accept it. Also, remember that the way your child comes into the world isn't nearly as important as having a healthy baby.

It also helps, of course, to prepare yourself in advance for this type of birth. Go and see the obstetrician with your partner and find out what the operation involves, what procedures will be used, and whether your partner is allowed to be there. Ask if you can see a video so you'll know what's going to happen to you. If you can, talk to other women who've had cesarean sections. They'll be able to give you useful advice and reassurance.

EMERGENCY CESAREAN SECTION

An emergency C-section may be needed when something goes wrong during labor, such as a prolapsed umbilical cord, placental hemorrhage, fetal distress, or serious failure to progress in labor. Emergency cesarean sections may be carried out under epidural and the hospital may not allow your partner to be present at the operation.

AFTER A CESAREAN SECTION

As is the case with any major surgery, it takes time to recover from a cesarean, but even so you'll be encouraged to get up and walk around a few hours afterward to stimulate your circulation. You'll be given painkillers if you need them, and the dressings will be removed after three or four days. Your internal stitches will be made with absorbable sutures, which will dissolve away naturally. Skin stitches may also be absorbable, but if staples are used they should be removed within about a week.

THE EFFECTS ON YOUR BABY

Not having to pass through the birth canal is both a benefit and a drawback for the baby born by cesarean section.

Unlike a baby born by vaginal delivery, who has a rather squashed appearance at first after being squeezed through the birth canal, a C-section baby has smooth features and a rounded head. But often the cesarean baby needs more time to adjust to the outside world—first, because of his sudden entry into it, and second, because he's missed the journey through the birth canal that helps to clear amniotic fluid from a baby's lungs and stimulates his circulation.

CESAREAN UNDER EPIDURAL ANESTHETIC

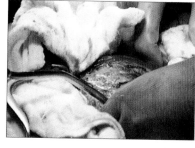

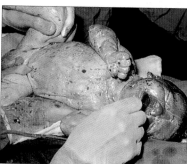

The delivery
Within 5–10 minutes of the incisions, the baby is delivered (above) and the cord clamped and cut. While the placenta is delivered and the incisions stitched up, you can hold your baby.

The operation
When the incisions have been made, the obstetrician begins to ease the baby out (left), sometimes using forceps.

If you've had an epidural you remain conscious

The screen hides the surgeon's activities from your direct vision

An emergency cesarean

Case study

Name Frances Ward
Age 27 years
Past medical history Nothing abnormal
Obstetric history One child aged three,pregnancy
and delivery both normal; second baby born by
cesarean

Fran's second pregnancy was uneventful. She and her baby were
both doing well. Three days before her expected date of delivery,
she went into labor, which went perfectly normally until the end of
the first stage, when Fran was suddenly told she would have to have
an emergency cesarean section.

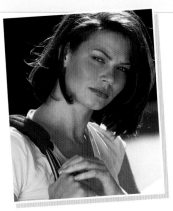

*About 25 percent of babies in the US are born
by cesarean section. A cesarean may be
planned, known as an "elective" cesarean, or it
may need to be carried out as an emergency
because the baby has to be delivered quickly.
Fran was glad she'd taken the time to learn
about cesarean sections in advance.*

WELL-INFORMED PARENTS

Fran had been surprised when I told her how many
mothers have cesarean sections. Her prenatal classes
didn't go into the subject in any depth, so she and her
husband, Jonathan, decided to find out as much as
possible themselves. They like to be well-informed about
anything they plan to do, whether it's visiting a foreign
country or having a baby. They questioned clinic staff,
read books, and watched videos on all types of birth,
including cesarean deliveries.

AN UNEXPECTED EMERGENCY

Fran's water broke halfway through the first stage of
labor, when her cervix was only four centimeters dilated.
Following the rule that every mother must have an
internal examination as soon as her membranes have
ruptured, the doctor examined Fran at once. She
discovered a prolapsed cord—a loop of the umbilical
cord coming through the cervix into the vagina in
advance of the baby. This is an extremely dangerous
situation because as the baby's head presses down on the
undilated cervix, the prolapsed section of the cord is

squeezed tighter and tighter, cutting off the baby's blood
and oxygen supply.

The doctor touched the cord and could feel that it
was pulsating. This was reassuring because it meant that
Fran's baby was still receiving enough blood. However,
within the next couple of minutes, the Doppler monitor
showed that the baby's heartbeat was starting to dip and
the baby was showing signs of considerable fetal distress.
Fran's obstetrician told her she need an emergency
cesarean section to protect her baby's well-being.

AVOIDING DISASTER

While the operating room was prepared, Fran was asked
to lie with her legs up in stirrups so that her baby would
slip backward, up into the pelvis, relieving the pressure
on the cord. Meanwhile, the doctor inserted three
fingers into Fran's vagina in order to keep the baby's
head pushed up away from the cervix.

Fortunately, Fran had chosen to have an epidural
anesthetic early in labor, so she didn't need to have a
general anesthetic or intragastric suction to prevent
inhalation of vomit. And there was the bonus that she'd
be awake during the birth.

THE OPERATION

Fran had chosen her particular hospital because it
encouraged fathers to be involved in their baby's
births. She was pleased that Jonathan was able to
watch the operation, because it meant that, even if
she couldn't see her baby being born, at least
Jonathan would see their child's entrance into the

world. The surgeon made a standard transverse incision (see column, p.308) through which Fran's baby was gently lifted out. As soon as the baby's head was delivered, the anesthetist gave Fran an infusion of Pitocin, which stimulates uterine contractions and reduces blood loss.

While Fran was being stitched up, Jonathan was able to hold their baby before taking her to Fran to see the baby for the first time. Although Fran was disappointed about not having a normal vaginal delivery, Fran and Jonathan had still shared the experience of Eleanor's birth, and Fran was able to hold and bond with Eleanor in the first few minutes after her birth.

After the operation was finished, Fran returned to the postnatal ward with Eleanor so that she could concentrate on nursing her new daughter and getting to know her better.

RECOVERING FROM THE CESAREAN

Fran found that getting back to normal after the cesarean was almost the hardest part. I suggested she join a self-help group for post-cesarean mothers, where she'd get useful advice on how to handle the postnatal period. Fran also worried that her next baby would have to be delivered by cesarean, too. I reassured her that most mothers can have normal deliveries following cesareans, although there may be good reasons for having another one.

REST AND HEALING

Fran had undergone abdominal surgery, so she needed plenty of rest and time for her scar to heal. When her stitches were removed, five days after the operation, she was told that the scar would heal in three weeks and would fade after six months. Fran was surprised to find herself losing blood from her vagina, just as she did after her first child, which was a vaginal delivery, but I explained that this is quite normal.

BREASTFEEDING

I told Fran that if she was going to breastfeed sitting up, she must sit up straight. Her abdominal wall was tender, so she used pillows to prop up Eleanor level with her breasts. She also found it comfortable to breastfeed lying on her side, resting on one elbow, with Eleanor on a pillow next to her.

MOVING AROUND

Fran found standing up quite difficult because her stomach hurt, but I encouraged her to try to stand up perfectly straight as soon as she got out of bed, and to place her hands over her wound, supporting it, whenever she wanted to laugh or cough. I told her that the more she managed to move around, the speedier her recovery would be. After her stitches were removed, she was allowed to go home but was told to rest and to be very careful when lifting anything, including picking up her other child for cuddles or carrying shopping bags. She had to avoid strenuous exercise and driving for at least six weeks.

Fran's baby

Some aspects of her birth were different from that of a baby who is pushed down the birth canal.

• Once the incision was made, the surgeon slipped a hand under her head

• Her head was gently pulled out by the surgeon's hand

• Her shoulders were maneuvered carefully through the incision

• Her body was gently pulled out—she was now delivered

• She was held with her head downward while her mouth and pharynx were cleansed of fluid with a soft catheter attached to suction apparatus

• She took her first breath

• Her cord was clamped and cut

• She was checked to make sure all her systems were functioning properly (see Apgar score, p.292)

• As soon as she was breathing normally, she was handed to her father for a cuddle

If a baby dies

The death of any child is always a tragic event, but the death of a baby before, during, or very soon after birth can be especially distressing. Today, in the Western world, the number of babies who are stillborn after 24 weeks or who die within the first few weeks of life has fallen to about one percent, largely thanks to improved obstetric and pediatric care.

WHY BABIES DIE

There are three main groups of perinatal deaths: stillbirths—babies who die before labor begins; intrapartum deaths—babies who die during labor; and neonatal deaths—babies who die within four weeks of their births.

Stillbirth About 45 percent of perinatal deaths are stillbirths, and in about one-third of these cases, the precise cause is not known. Of the rest, the most important causes are severe fetal defects (see also p.196) and a placenta that's not healthy. It could be that the placenta failed to develop adequately, became diseased in some way, or became unable to continue to support the baby (see p.260). Whatever the cause, the placenta was unable to provide adequate nutrition for the baby. It might even have begun to separate from the wall of the uterus before labor started. Less common causes of stillbirth include Rhesus incompatibility (see p.202), and maternal diabetes that is not carefully controlled.

The first thing that happens when a baby dies in the uterus is the almost complete disappearance from the mother's blood of pregnancy hormones—estrogen and progesterone. As a result, many of the signs and sensations of being pregnant fade quite quickly. Another early sign may be lack of fetal movement. If doctors or midwives suspect that a baby may have died, an ultrasound scan will be done to detect the baby's heartbeat.

Labor usually starts within two to three days of a baby's death, although many women want to have their babies removed as soon as they find out that they have died. If you find yourself in this unhappy situation, your wishes should be respected; usually doctors will suggest induction. It may seem very hard for a mother to have to go through this, but it is much less risky than a cesarean section—which puts the mother at great risk and is avoided at all costs—and less likely to affect any subsequent pregnancies.

When you go into labor, there will be no physical difference between this labor and a normal one. You'll need a great deal of sympathy and support, and will be given as much pain relief as you want. Everybody involved will recognize your feelings.

Babies who die in labor This is exceptionally rare, but the death of a baby during labor is usually caused by a lack of oxygen due to

A PARTNER'S REACTION

When a baby dies, both parents grieve. But a father may express his grief very differently from his partner, and this can lead to tension in the relationship.

If a father grieves in a different way from his partner, it doesn't mean his grief is any less intense. Some men try to hide their grief and throw themselves into work in order to find some relief from the pain they're feeling. Fortunately, all of us are learning that it's better for us to be open to feelings and express them. Hopefully, men will be more encouraged to let their true feelings show, especially to their partners.

Support groups for bereaved parents can put fathers in contact with other men who have lost their babies. Being with other men who've been through the same experiences may help a bereaved father express his grief, anger, and all the other possible emotions he may feel, in whatever way is best for him. What's important is that he's able to express his grief in his own way.

a problem with the placenta. Another possible cause is injury to the baby during labor and delivery. This is far less common than it was in the past, thanks to the high quality of modern care.

Neonatal death   Death of the newborn may be caused by breathing difficulties, especially in babies who are born preterm (see pp.344 & 348), are postmature, or are suffering from severe fetal defects. Fatal neonatal infections, once a significant cause of the deaths of newborn babies, are now very rare because of improved hygiene standards and modern antibiotics.

COPING WITH A DEATH

It's very important for both partners to come to terms with their grief, to be open about the death of their baby, to accept it, and to go through the grieving process.

It's absolutely normal for bereaved parents to feel isolated, angry with themselves, each other, the staff, or the unfairness of life, and often guilty about something they did or didn't do. However, accepting that everyone involved did everything possible and that nobody is to blame, while acknowledging how you feel, will help the healing process.

Parents are encouraged to hold their stillborn baby for a while after the birth, and most are very glad of this later. Having a photograph of the baby can also be a great comfort in the future. It helps to give the baby a name, to bury the baby formally, and to be present at the burial. Another important form of solace is to get in touch with other parents who have had stillbirths or neonatal deaths (see Addresses, p.370). Details of support groups are usually available from your hospital. Don't be afraid to ask for help from a counselor if you need it.

Emotional effects   The emotional and physical effects on the mother are due not only to the shock and grief of losing her baby but also to the sudden withdrawal of pregnancy hormones. This can affect her mood, bringing on tearfulness, depression, insomnia, appetite loss, and withdrawal, as well as loss of milk from the breasts. The milk can be suppressed with drugs. The comfort and support of her partner, family, and friends is vital.

It helps if both partners are open with each other and share their grief so that they can give each other support and comfort.

GETTING PREGNANT AGAIN

Grief over the death of a baby should have subsided before another pregnancy is contemplated. This usually takes at least six months and sometimes a year or more. Many women, however, find the key to normality and a return to happiness is through conceiving again. Once partners have decided to try to have another baby, they may find that worry about losing this baby will be hard to shake off. The risk of a recurrence is very slight, but where there has been predisposing cause, subsequent pregnancies are carefully managed.

LOSING A TWIN

The death of one twin or triplet is just as tragic for the parents as the death of a singleton, and carries additional problems.

The loss of a twin or triplet leaves parents with a complex emotional situation—they are mourning the death of the lost baby, while celebrating the life of the surviving twin or triplet(s). Faced with this impossible mix of emotions, many parents postpone their mourning. Others find they cannot attend to the needs of their living baby or babies properly because of the intensity of grief for the dead baby.

The loss of a twin or triplet may also cast a shadow over the life of the surviving twin or triplet(s), and birthdays may be particularly difficult for the first few years.

It must be stressed that a mother who's had a multiple pregnancy continues to think of herself as the mother of twins or triplets, regardless of whether any have died.

Parents who have lost a twin or a triplet may be told that they are "lucky" because they still have their other child(ren). This is not fair—no other parent is expected to find comfort for the death of a child in the survival of its siblings.

CHAPTER 15

Getting to know your newborn baby

Nurturing a relationship with your baby begins the second she's born. As you both learn how to care for her and meet her needs, your love will deepen and grow, and what she's able to do from the earliest days will amaze you.

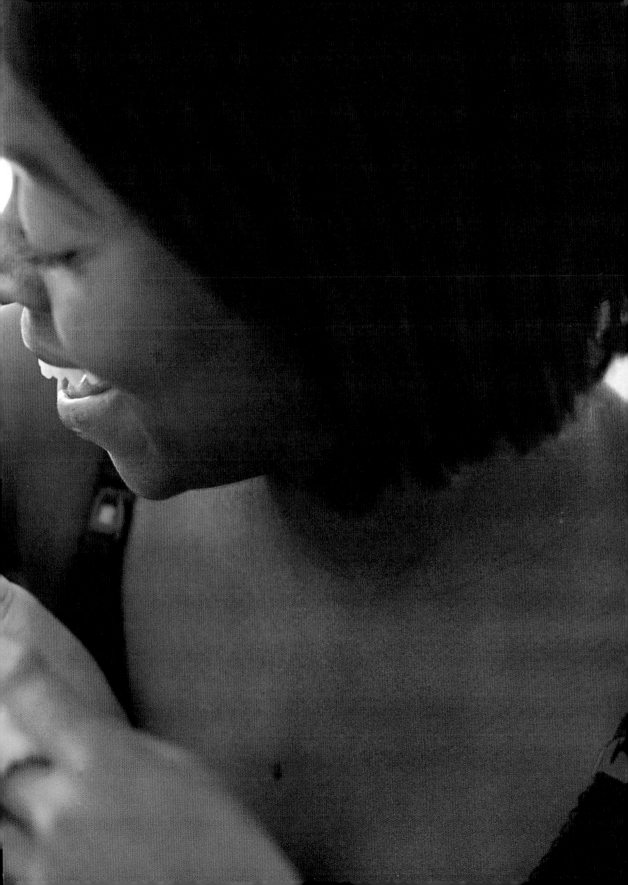

Your new baby

YOUR FIRST REACTION

Your newborn baby's appearance may surprise you when you first see him. He'll have wrinkly skin and you may think he looks more like an old man than a baby.

Some parents worry about how they feel when their baby actually arrives: he doesn't seem to be quite what they'd expected.

Unless you've had a cesarean, his head may be slightly squashed, with some bruising, and his eyelids may be puffy because of the pressure of passing through the birth canal.

He may look messy, since he'll be coated in a greasy substance (see right), possibly mixed with some of your blood, and he may have patches of body hair. His limbs may be a bluish color, and his genitals will look huge.

Don't be disappointed if you don't immediately feel love and tenderness when you first look at your baby. These feelings will develop as you get to know each other.

Genitals
Both boys' and girls' genitals often look swollen at birth. The swelling is caused by your pregnancy hormones and won't last long.

Take your baby in your arms and hold him as soon as possible after birth so that you can start to bond. Your baby will begin to learn about you and how much you love him as he hears your voice, smells and feels your skin, and is cuddled and nursed by you.

You're likely to feel many new emotions when you see your newborn baby's tiny, vulnerable body and realize his complete dependence on you. The way you react and what you do in these first moments are probably the most important interactions there'll ever be between you and your child.

Research shows that parents who can cuddle and be with their babies immediately after delivery tend to be more sympathetic to their children's needs later. Parents whose babies are taken away at birth may feel alienated for a while, but if this does happen to you, don't worry—just start bonding with your baby as soon as you're able to.

WHAT YOUR BABY WILL LOOK LIKE

Newborn babies vary greatly in weight and length. Average weights for a baby are generally 5 lb 8 oz to 9 lb 12 oz (2.5–4.5 kilograms), and average lengths are about 19–20 inches (48–51 centimeters).

Head Your newborn baby's head will be one-quarter of his length and it'll look large compared with the rest of his body. The younger the baby, the larger his head is in proportion to his body. On average a newborn baby's head measures about 14 in (35 cm) around. His head will be measured after birth, and this is an important check because the growth of his head is linked to the development of his brain.

A newborn baby's head usually looks pointed because it's been molded as it came through the birth canal. Molding is caused by the skull bones overriding each other. Sometimes this pressure also leaves one or both sides of the baby's head slightly swollen. This swelling doesn't affect your baby's brain and it goes down within a few weeks.

If your baby was delivered by forceps he may have some slight bruising. You'll feel a soft spot on the top, called a fontanelle, where the skull bones haven't yet joined together, and won't do so until your baby is 18 months old.

Skin Some babies are born completely covered in a greasy, white substance called *vernix caseosa*. Others only have vernix on their face and hands. Vernix makes it easier for your baby to slide through the birth canal and helps protect him against minor skin infections. In some hospitals the vernix is cleaned off right away, but others prefer to let it to rub off the skin naturally, which happens within two or three days.

Your baby's circulation takes a little while to settle down. While this is happening, the top half of his body may look paler than the bottom half, but this is nothing to worry about.

Your baby may have some downy hair on his body. This is called *lanugo* hair and it covered his body while he was in your womb (see p.80). Some babies only have lanugo hair on their head, but others may have hair on their shoulders. Both are normal, and the hair usually rubs off within a couple of weeks.

More permanent hair will appear later. Some babies are born with a full head of hair but others are completely bald. If your baby is born with hair, it might not be the color he eventually ends up with.

NEWBORN CHARACTERISTICS

Your baby's legs may look bowed because he's been curled up in your womb

His umbilical cord is clamped and cut right after delivery

A beating pulse can often be seen under the fontanelle. Although it's quite tough, it should never be pressed hard

His genitals may look swollen and large

His feet and hands may have dry, peeling skin because they've been immersed in liquid for so long

His eyes may look puffy

An identity bracelet will be attached to your baby's ankle

Your baby's stomach may look slightly bloated

His fingers are curled in toward his palms

Your baby's appearance
Your newborn baby may not look at all as you expected, and he'll have certain newborn characteristics that may surprise you.

Hands and feet These may have a slightly more bluish look than the rest of his body because his circulation hasn't gotten going. He may have dry patches with peeling skin, which will disappear in a few days. His fingernails may be long and sharp; gently nibble off the tips if he's scratching himself, but don't cut his nails.

Eyes Your newborn baby's eyes may be puffy because of pressure on his head during the birth, and he may not be able to open them at first. This pressure may also have broken some tiny blood vessels in his eyes, causing harmless small, red, triangular marks in the whites. These don't need any treatment and will disappear within a couple of weeks. Your baby may also have "sticky eye,"

YOUR BABY'S BIRTHMARKS

A group of small blood vessels under the surface of the skin may appear as a small blemish on your baby's body, but won't usually need any treatment.

Stork bites These are mild pink patches. They're very common and usually appear on the nose, the eyelids, and the neck under the hairline. They take about a year to disappear.

Strawberry birthmarks These first appear as tiny red dots and may get bigger up to the end of the first year. They almost always disappear by five years of age.

Mongolian spots These are blue and are found on the lower back of babies with dark skin tones (nearly all black and Asian babies, and some Mediterranean babies, have them). The spots look like bruises, but they're harmless and fade away naturally.

Port wine stains These are large, flat, red or purple marks on the baby's skin, usually on the face and neck. These marks are permanent, so if you're worried, talk to your doctor.

which is a yellow discharge around the eyelids. Sticky eye is quite common, and although it's not serious, it's best to take your baby to the doctor.

Your baby can see clearly to a distance of 8 in (20 cm) or so, but he cannot focus both eyes at the same time beyond that, so he may squint or look cross-eyed. Both problems should gradually clear up as his eye muscles grow stronger (usually within a month). Check with your doctor if your baby still squints at three months. If he doesn't seem to want to open his eyes at first, don't try to force them open. Instead, try holding his head above your head so that he opens his eyes naturally. All babies have blue eyes when they're born. Their adult eye color may not develop until about six months.

Umbilicus Your baby's umbilical cord will be clamped with forceps and then cut with scissors. A short length of cord is left; it dries up and becomes almost black within two to four hours after the birth. The cord doesn't come away from the navel until about ten days after the birth. Some babies have umbilical hernias (small swellings near the navel), but these usually clear up within a year. If the hernia goes on longer than this or gets bigger, check with your doctor.

Breasts Pregnancy hormones may cause both boy and girl babies to have slightly enlarged breasts and leak a little milk. This is normal, and will stop in a couple of days.

YOUR BABY'S CARE

Before you leave the hospital, your baby will be thoroughly examined by a pediatrician to make sure that everything's going well and there are no problems. Your doctor or midwife will also want to check that your baby is feeding well and that his stools are normal. He'll be given a blood test, usually by means of a tiny heel prick, to check for *phenylketonuria* (PKU), a rare metabolic disease, and for thyroid gland underactivity.

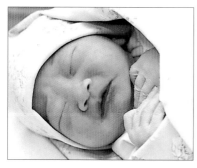

Puffy eyelids
Your baby's eyelids may be quite puffy because of pressure on the way through the birth canal. The swelling will go down in a couple of days.

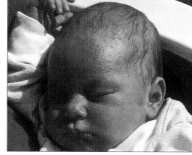

Pimply skin
Small white spots, called milia, are caused by blocked sebaceous glands that lubricate the skin. They're not serious and will soon disappear.

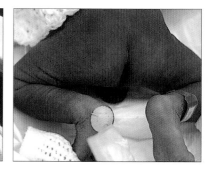

Blotchy skin tone
If your baby's circulation hasn't settled down, you may notice red and white blotches on his body, and his legs may be a different color.

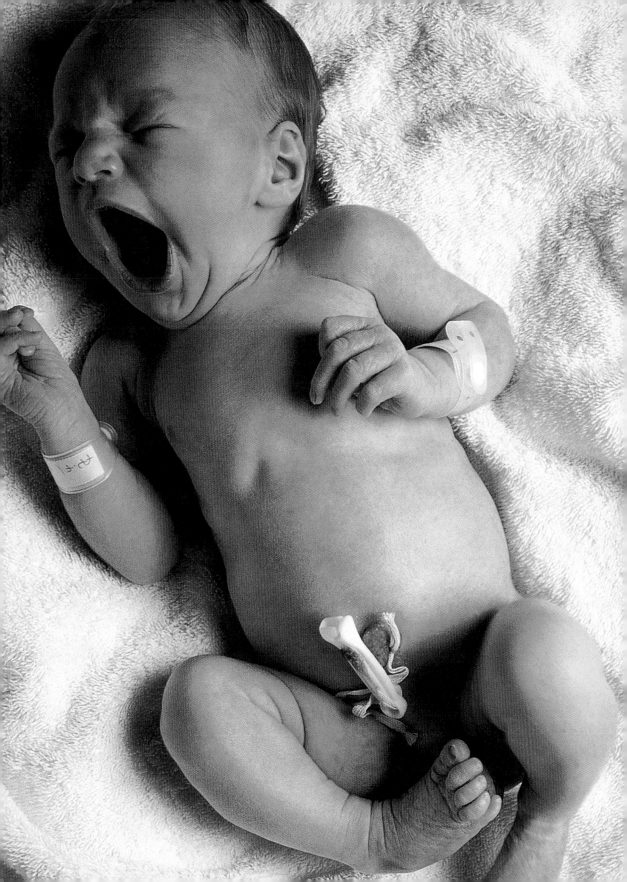

GET TO KNOW YOUR BABY

Spend as much time as you can playing with your baby— it's vital to her development.

Try to recognize her needs You'll soon start to understand her different expressions. When she's content, she'll look tranquil and quiet. When she's feeling miserable or uncomfortable, she'll look a little red and flustered.

Playing together Don't worry about looking silly when you're playing with your baby. Make funny faces and use a high-pitched voice to tell her how much you love her. She'll answer by nodding, moving her mouth, maybe sticking out her tongue, and jerking her body.

Step reflex
If you hold your baby under her arms and let her feet touch a firm surface, she'll make stepping movements.

What your new baby can do

Your newborn baby has her own very special personality, and she may surprise you with what she can do. Spend as much time as you can with her and you'll soon get to know every little expression and sound she makes.

POSTURE AND SENSES

At first, your baby's head is too heavy for her back and neck muscles to support. All her postures when not lying down are governed by her gradual development of the ability to control her head. If you put your baby on her back, she'll probably turn her head to one side, stretch out her arm on that side, and flex the opposite arm in toward her chest. By the time she's a week old, she'll raise her head in small jerks when she's supported on your shoulder. At six weeks she'll probably be able to hold up her head for more than a minute.

From birth, she has fairly good senses of hearing, smell, and taste. At first, she mainly touches things with her mouth. She'll soon recognize you by smell, and by sight, too, within a couple of weeks. When you hold your baby close to you for the first time, she'll focus on your face and look into your eyes. Babies like looking at faces more than anything else. Hearing high-pitched human voices gives her great pleasure, and she'll like yours, and your partner's deeper one, more than any others. She'll also respond to sounds with a change in her breathing, and she may be startled by loud noises.

REFLEX ACTIONS

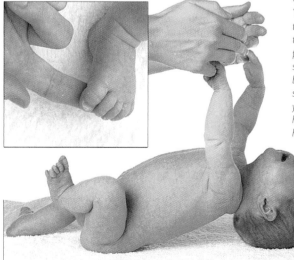

Grasp reflex
Your baby's fingers will tightly grasp anything that's placed in her palm. Her grasp is so strong that her whole body weight can be supported if she grabs your fingers with both her hands. The soles of her feet will also curl over if they're touched or tickled.

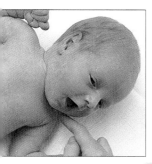

Rooting reflex
Your baby will search for your breast to nurse. Gently stroke her cheek and she'll turn in that direction and open her mouth.

Moro reflex
If your baby's startled, she'll throw out her arms and legs as if to catch hold of something. Her limbs will then slowly curl inward, with clenched fists.

All babies have certain automatic movements—reflexes—which help them protect themselves. They usually last until about three months and are then lost. For example, your baby will close her eyes if you touch her eyelids. All babies have a sucking reflex if you press the palate of the mouth. The sucking is more like chomping—it's very strong and lasts for some time. Babies are born with the swallowing reflex—they've had to use it when swallowing fluids in the womb—and so they can swallow colostrum or milk the instant they are born. If a baby swallows too much liquid, her gagging reflex will immediately act to clear her breathing passage.

WHY YOUR BABY CRIES

Crying is your baby's only way of speaking to you. You'll soon learn to recognize her different kinds of cries, and what to do in response.

- Your baby's first cry may sound more like a whimper, or splutter, before it turns into a full blown cry. She'll take a deep breath, her body will tense, her face will grimace and become bright red, and she'll open her mouth wide and literally scream. Distressing as you might find this, it does show that your baby's perfectly healthy.

- She'll cry when she's hungry, and usually won't stop until she's put to your breast or given a bottle. Some babies cry sooner than others when they're hungry.

- Tiredness, uncomfortable clothing, being too hot or too cold, or being undressed are all other reasons why babies cry.

- Loneliness is one of the main reasons babies get upset. Babies love being with you; if they feel abandoned, they'll cry until picked up and cuddled.

Sounds your baby will make

BREATHING	SNEEZES	HICCUPS
Your baby's breathing may seem much lighter than yours. At times it may be irregular or fast and noisy, and she may snuffle as she tries to draw air through her small nasal passages. You might not always hear her breathing at first, but it'll get stronger every day.	Light stimulates the nerves to your baby's nose as well as her eyes, and bright lights may make her sneeze. A sneeze will clear out her nasal passages and keep dust from getting into her lungs. Don't worry when your baby sneezes—it's very common and it doesn't mean she has a cold.	Your baby may hiccup often, and this is perfectly normal. Hiccups can be caused when the diaphragm makes sudden, irregular contractions. They're a sign that the muscles used in breathing are getting stronger and are trying to work together.

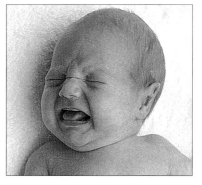

A cry for attention
Sudden movements, very bright lights, loud noises, or feeling too hot or too cold—all these things may make your baby start to cry.

GOING HOME

The routine for checking out varies from mother to mother, depending on how you're doing after delivery. If everything has gone well after a vaginal delivery, you can go home after 48 hours; if you've had a cesarean section, you can go home after three to five days. The usual stay is between two and five days. Before you're discharged from the hospital:

- a midwife or doctor will examine you. They'll check that your uterus is returning to its prepregnant size, that your stitches (if you've had any) are healing, and that your breasts are okay. They'll check your flow of lochia for color and amount, and to see if you've passed any clots. Clotting with persistent bleeding may be a sign that there's still some placental tissue inside you

- if you've had a cesarean, the doctor will check your incision and remove any nonabsorbable sutures

- your doctor will ask about your contraception plans, and give you a prescription for the pill if necessary

- if you weren't immune to rubella (German measles) during your pregnancy, you'll be immunized

- you'll be shown how to clean your baby's umbilical cord

- you'll be given a date for your postnatal checkup, and advised to take your baby to the clinic for a 6-week check-up

- when you leave, dress your baby warmly as he's not yet able to regulate his temperature very well.

Your stay in the hospital

What happens in the hospital after your baby's is born will vary, depending on whether you've had a vaginal or cesarean delivery (see p.306), which hospital you're in, how long you stay, and the health of both you and your newborn baby.

YOUR CARE

Immediately after the birth, your healthcare provider will take your temperature and note your pulse rate and blood pressure. These will be checked every four hours for the first day or so, then twice daily during the rest of your stay in the hospital. Your pulse rate may change slightly, but this is perfectly normal, so nothing to worry about.

Medical staff will also check that any stitches or tears you have are healing properly and that you don't have an infection. They may suggest that you apply ice packs to the area to prevent swelling and ease the pain, and you may be offered painkillers during the first few days for afterpains.

They'll also keep a close eye on the amount and appearance of your lochia in case there are any abnormal blood clots or excessive bleeding. Your uterus will be checked to make sure that it's starting to return to its prepregnant state, and your legs will be examined for any signs of thrombosis (blood clots). Your healthcare provider may also ask a few questions to get an idea of your general emotional state and make sure you're recovering from the birth.

Up and around Start moving around as much as you can soon after delivery. This will help you get your strength back, get your bowel and bladder working normally again (see also p.354), and prevent blood clots from forming in your legs.

Unless you're very tired and simply want to sleep, you can get up to go to the bathroom, take a shower, or walk around any time after the birth. It's a good idea to have someone to help you at first in case you feel faint or weak. You'll probably have a blood test on about the fourth or fifth day after delivery to make sure your hemoglobin is returning to normal.

Cesarean births About 26 percent of women in the United States have cesarean births. Many have epidural anesthesia, but if you do have a general, you may feel sick and wobbly. Your incision will be painful and the stitches will be covered by a soft dressing. You'll probably have an intravenous drip in your arm and may be given analgesics to help you sleep. If your baby is healthy and well, there's no reason why he can't be with you all the time. If your stitches aren't self-absorbing, they'll be taken out about five days after delivery, which is only mildly uncomfortable. After a cesarean, expect to stay in the hospital for three to five days if everything's normal (see also pp.306 & 308).

HOSPITAL PROCEDURES

You may find hospital routines a little annoying, especially if you're woken for meals or routine checks by the staff when you'd rather be asleep. But where breastfeeding is concerned, think about your own and your baby's needs above all else. Take the time you need to nurse your baby and ask for help if you're finding it difficult. Start slowly, with short periods of two to three minutes on each breast so that your nipples have a chance to harden up. That way they won't get sore and crack. Your baby may not seem very interested in nursing at first—he may be tired, too—but after the first day, try putting him to your breast whenever he seems to want it.

It's really important to eat properly yourself so you keep your strength up for breastfeeding. Hospital food can sometimes be bland and unappetizing—and it's not always very nourishing or plentiful—so ask your partner and family to bring in some treats such as fresh fruit for you. Better still, get friends to visit you around mealtime and bring in food you enjoy.

Visitors It's nice to see your family and friends, but you'll find that visitors will tire you out more than you'd expect, so try to limit each visit to half an hour at the most. Ask everyone except your partner and your other children to stick to hospital visiting times so you can rest when you need to. Partners are usually allowed to come and see you whenever you want, but this policy does vary from hospital to hospital.

Social contact Being in the hospital can be quite enjoyable. You'll have a chance to get to know the other mothers and to talk about your feelings and worries with them. You're all going through the same things, and by sharing your experiences and working out plans together, you may find that you make friendships that last well after your stay in the hospital.

Feeling unhappy Even the minimum stay of 48 hours in the hospital can seem like a very long time if you're feeling homesick and anxious. You can always talk to one of the hospital staff or to another, more experienced mother about your feelings. And, as eager as you may be to get home, don't forget that this is the ideal time to get help from the nursing staff, who will be glad to give expert advice on breastfeeding and caring for your newborn. You can also ask for additional assistance from a lactation specialist if your baby is having a hard time latching on, if you have any other problems with breastfeeding. Before you know it, you, your baby, and your partner will all be home together as a family.

REGISTERING YOUR BABY'S BIRTH

Birth certificates
Birth certificates are mandatory for all children born in the United States. Your baby's birth cerificate will serve as the official proof of her citizenship and date of birth.

Fortunately, when applying for a birth certificate, the hopsital staff will do most of the work for you. After your baby has been born and you and your partner have filled out a brief questionnaire, the staff will complete the certificate and send it to your state's department of health.

The process of obtaining a copy of your baby's birth certificate varies from county to county. Ask the hospital staff about the procedure in your area. Many hospitals will provide you with a souvenir birth certificate upon discharge, but keep in mind that this is not an official document.

Social security numbers
You are not legally required to apply for a social security number for your baby immediately after birth, but it is a good idea to do so, since she will almost certainly need one eventually. A number is mandatory for any child older than one year who is listed as a dependent on a tax return, and is also needed to open a bank account, buy savings bonds, or apply for government services on behalf of your child.

Upon request, most hospitals will apply for your baby's social security number at the same time that they send in the birth certificate. Usually, there will simply be a box to check on the questionnaire. Once a request has been submitted, a card should be mailed to you within a few weeks.

Holding and handling

From the moment your baby is born, you can develop a special feeling of intimacy by holding him close to your bare skin.

Skin-to-skin contact enables you to become intimate with your baby. You will enjoy "skin bathing" with your baby—the feel of his soft, warm skin against yours, and the wonderful smell of newborn baby.

When you're feeding your baby, whether by breast or bottle, don't let a barrier of clothing always come between you. You'll both benefit from his being held close against your bare skin (see column, right)—not least because he'll begin to recognize your smell (an important step in the bonding process, especially if you're not breastfeeding).

A newborn baby can appear very fragile and at first, many parents are scared to pick up and handle their baby because of the feeling that he's so breakable. Your baby is actually very resilient, and as long as you support him firmly, there's no need to be afraid.

FIRM SUPPORT

Even if he's crying to be picked up, don't use jerky or quick movements when lifting him—do it as slowly, as gently, and as quietly as you can. Most babies like to be handled in a firm way; it makes them feel more secure. He won't be able to support his head for several weeks, so you'll have to support it so that it doesn't loll. Always hold your baby close, keeping your arms close to your body, and bending over the place you're lifting from or putting down. To put him down, reverse the process of picking him up, always supporting his neck. When you lay your baby down, it's safest to put him on his back, or his side, if propped.

Loving support A mother often feels prime responsibility for her newborn baby, but most partners are eager to be fully involved as

PICKING UP YOUR BABY

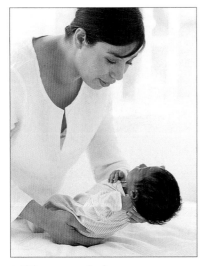

Lifting your baby
Slide one hand underneath his neck and head, and slide the other behind his lower back (above). Lift him gently so that his head doesn't fall back.

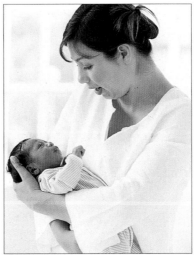

Support his head
Always be sure to support his head in the crook of your arm (above) so that it doesn't loll around.

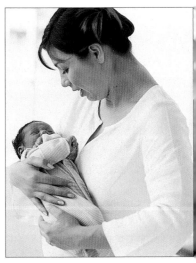

Cradle him in your arms
Your baby will feel secure cradled in the crook of your elbow, with his head and limbs well supported.

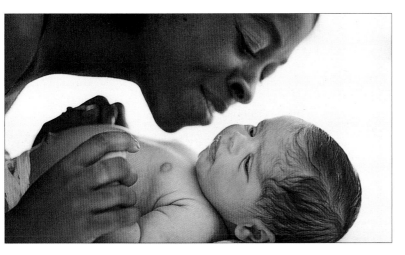

BENEFITS FOR YOUR BABY

Recent research has shown that the more physical contact babies have, the healthier and happier they become.

You can appeal to your baby's sense of rhythm by rocking and swaying him. Skin-to-skin contact stimulates his senses of touch and smell, and even helps him to grow. Human skin sends and receives warmth that has a positive effect on other human skin. Snuggling together will evoke a feeling of sensuous contentment.

early as possible. Both your baby and his father will develop a better understanding of each other through cuddling, handling, and carrying, and the more tactile their relationship, the more loving it will be.

All through the day, especially when changing him, you can discover ways to gently explore and caress his body. The best way to cuddle together is by lying naked in bed. In this way he can smell your skin, feel its touch and warmth, and hear your heart beating clearly.

Your baby will be comforted by the familiar beat of your heart

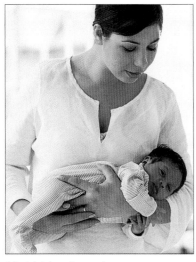

Hold him face down
Your baby may like being held face down in your arms, his cheek resting on your forearm.

Hold him against your shoulder
Held upright like this, your baby feels secure. Put one hand under his bottom, and support his head with your other hand.

PRODUCING MILK

Your breasts change during pregnancy to prepare them for producing milk. Your milk will being to come in a few days after you've given birth.

A female breast has 15–20 groups of milk-producing glands, connected to the nipple by the milk ducts. When you're pregnant, the placenta and ovaries make high levels of the hormones estrogen and progesterone, which stimulate the glands to make *colostrum*. Colostrum gives your baby water, protein, sugar, vitamins, minerals, and antibodies to protect him against infection. Your body stops making colostrum and starts making milk three to five days after your baby is born.

Stimulating milk
Your baby's sucking stimulates nerve endings in your areolae. *These send messages to your brain to produce* prolactin *and* oxytocin.

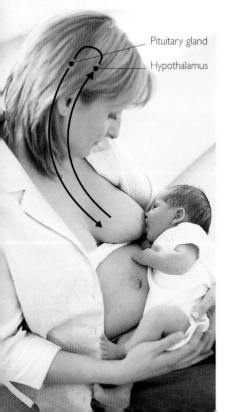

Pituitary gland

Hypothalamus

Beginning to breastfeed

If you're planning to breastfeed for the first time, you might be worried that you won't be able to produce enough milk or that your milk won't be nourishing enough. Don't be anxious—you're not likely to have any problems. All women are equipped to feed a baby. No breast is too small, and in most cases, your supply of milk will automatically adjust to meet your baby's needs.

FEEDING ON DEMAND

A baby can digest a full feeding of breast milk in an hour and a half to two hours (half the time it takes for a bottlefed baby to digest a full feeding of formula). So breastfeeding on demand means frequent feeding, but this doesn't mean your milk supplies will run out. Research shows that mothers who breastfeed their babies on demand produce more milk than mothers who feed their babies at regular but less frequent intervals.

One study compared babies breastfed on demand with those fed only every three or four hours. The babies fed on demand got an average of nearly 10 feedings a day, compared to an average for the others of just over seven. The more frequent feeding didn't mean that a daily amount of milk was being divided into more but smaller feedings—in fact, it was the opposite.

Better fed The fed-on-demand babies got an average of just over 73 milliliters at each feeding (725 milliliters a day), while those fed at fixed intervals got only 68.8 milliliters at each feeding (502 milliliters a day). As a result, after two weeks, the fed-on-demand babies had gained more weight than the others—an average of 561 grams compared to 347 grams.

KEEPING UP YOUR MILK SUPPLY

Milk production can be affected by many things, including how you're feeling, how healthy you are, and what you eat.

Producing milk The change from colostrum to breast milk is triggered by changes in your hormones after the birth, but continuing supplies of milk depend on the sucking action of your baby. When he sucks, nerve endings in your areolae are stimulated, sending signals to a part of your brain called the *hypothalamus.* The hypothalamus in turn sends signals to your pituitary gland telling it to release *prolactin*, the hormone that stimulates milk production—this response to your baby's sucking is known as the prolactin reflex. Your *pituitary* gland also releases oxytocin, a hormone that causes the muscle fibers around the milk glands to contract, squeezing the milk from the glands into your milk ducts. This is called the milk ejection or "letdown" reflex. When your breasts are full, it can be triggered not only by sucking but also by your baby's hunger cries or even simply when he's near to you.

A good milk supply   The best way to keep up your milk supply is to feed your baby often, so that the prolactin reflex and the milk ejection reflex are triggered frequently. This will also prevent en-gorgement—swelling of your milk-producing glands with milk.

If the glands do swell, they won't be able to make milk efficiently. And you won't feel like nursing because it'll be painful. For these reasons, the reflex that promotes the release of prolactin diminishes and so your milk production slows down. If this does happen, you can relieve engorged breasts by expressing milk (see column, right), and keep it from happening again by nursing your baby often.

It's also important to wait until your baby empties the first breast you give him before switching him to the other. This way he'll be sure to get not only the thirst-quenching, low-fat foremilk that comes from your breast first, but also the highly nourishing, fat-rich hindmilk that follows.

You'll need to eat well at this time, since your body has an even greater need for good nourishment than during pregnancy. You don't need to eat any special foods for breastfeeding, but it's best to have a balanced diet with plenty of protein, iron, and calcium, and lots of fluids, fresh fruit, and vegetables. Three good meals, with light snacks of fruit, cheese, or milky drinks in between, will give you energy and keep you from getting too tired. It's a good idea to keep taking an iron supplement daily. Caring for a baby can be exhausting, so relax or nap during the day whenever you get the chance. If you're diabetic, your doctor will keep a close eye on your diet, and your glucose and insulin levels. When you start making love again, don't use oral contraceptives until you stop breastfeeding (see p.364).

REFUSAL TO TAKE A FEEDING

Occasionally, your baby won't want to breastfeed. This is most likely to happen during the early days, when he may be too sleepy to be interested in nursing. If your baby refuses the breast, don't give up—express the milk your baby would have suckled and wait for him to want food. Babies take the breast much more enthusiastically when they're hungry.

If you find that your baby tends to fall asleep soon after you've started nursing, try lying on your side, with him lying beside you. This way he'll find breastfeeding less tiring.

Your baby may also refuse to nurse because he has difficulty latching on (see p.329). Your breasts may become engorged, as a consequence—and the swelling makes it almost impossible for your baby to latch on. If you express some milk from your swollen breasts before nursing, he'll be able to latch on more easily.

EXPRESSING YOUR MILK

You may sometimes need to express milk from your breasts, perhaps so that your baby can be fed from a bottle if you have to go out for a while, or you're returning to work, or if your breasts have become engorged (see p.356).

You can express milk by hand, but it's quicker to use a pump. When you've expressed your milk, put the cap tightly on the bottle. Refrigerate the milk until needed; it will keep for up to 48 hours in a refrigerator, or can be stored for up to six months in the freezer.

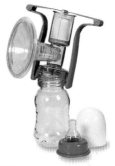

Using a manual pump
Fit the funnel of the pump over your areola to form an airtight seal, then operate the lever or plunger to express the milk.

Using a electric pump
Electric pumps are more expensive but quicker and easier to use. They also imitate a baby's natural sucking cycle more closely. An electric pump is best if you need to express often—for example, if you're going back to work before weaning.

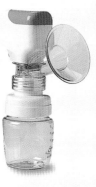

Breastfeeding your baby

Breastfeeding your baby is a loving, nurturing experience that strengthens the bond between you. It carries on the physiological relationship that began when your baby was developing in your womb. Your baby knows your milk will be there when he needs it and trusts it to be pure and good. Because of this, some people say that breastfeeding is the first way to tell the truth to a baby and to keep a promise.

Getting started
Hold your baby close to your own body, with his head a little higher than his body. If you're sitting, keep your back straight. You may find it more comfortable to rest your baby on a pillow on your lap so that you're not holding all his weight. Until your baby learns to seek out or "root" for the nipple, stimulate his rooting reflex by gently touching the cheek closest to you. He'll instinctively turn his head toward your touch, and so toward your nipple.

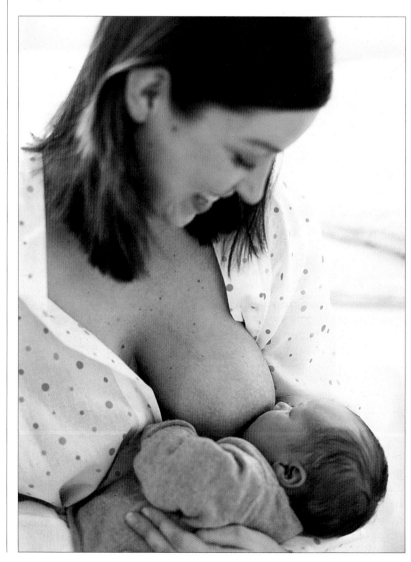

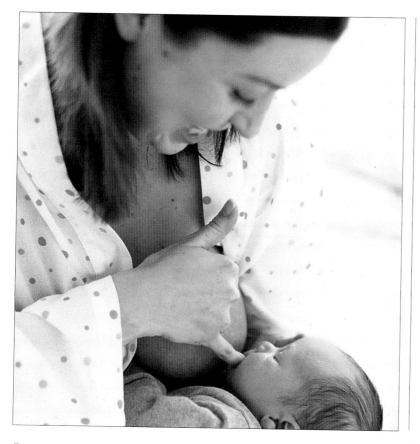

Releasing the breast

When he's nursing correctly, his mouth will be wide open and, as his tongue and jaw muscles work to suck milk from your breast, you'll see his ears and temples moving. When he's finished nursing, or when all the milk is gone from the breast and you want to switch him to the other, slip your little finger gently between his jaws.

LATCHING ON

The key to happy, trouble-free breastfeeding is knowing how to get your baby's mouth correctly fixed or latched on to your breast. If your baby's latched on properly, he'll get enough milk and you'll avoid breast and lactation problems. When your baby is nursing correctly, his jaws will be clamped on your breast tissue rather than just onto your nipple, which will be completely inside his mouth.

To encourage your baby to latch on as easily as possible, give yourself plenty of time to nurse and make sure you're comfortable and relaxed. Hold your baby high enough so he can reach your nipple without effort. Cradle his head in the crook of your arm, and support his back and bottom with your lower arm and hand. Express a little milk to soften the areola, and make sure that his mouth contains the entire nipple.

Correct latching on is important to both you and your baby for two reasons. First, it prevents your baby from sucking on the nipple itself, which can cause soreness and cracking. Second, it allows him to stimulate a good flow of milk and makes sure that he gets the rich hindmilk as well as the less nourishing but thirst-quenching foremilk (see p.327). A good flow of milk also prevents your breast from becoming engorged (see p.356) because it hasn't been emptied.

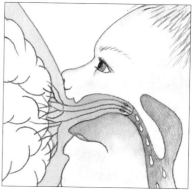

The sucking effect

A baby first stimulates milk to flow into your nipple by pressing the tip of his tongue against the areola at the base of your nipple. Then he presses the back of his tongue up toward his palate to squeeze the milk from your nipple into his throat.

329

BREASTFEEDING TIPS

Breastfeeding is simple—if it weren't, many millions of infants and mothers wouldn't have managed it successfully. Lots of new mothers have problems getting started, though, so don't hesitate to ask for help from friends, nurses, midwives, or the La Leche League if you need assistance.

- Establishing breastfeeding is always easier if you're able to put your baby to your breast within a few minutes of delivery. Once you've achieved successful suckling in the celebratory atmosphere that surrounds birth, you'll feel confident about future feeding.

- If your nipple is soft and small and your baby has trouble finding it, put a cold, wet cloth on it for a moment—your nipple will firm up and protrude.

- Milk flows in both breasts at every nursing and it's better to use both at each feeding. Start with the heavier breast.

- Once breastfeeding is going well and your nipples have toughened up, let your baby suck for as long as she likes on the first side so she gets both the foremilk and the hindmilk. (Foremilk is the dilute, thirst-quenching part; the hindmilk is the richer, creamier part.) Then switch to the other breast and let her stay there as long as she likes.

PREPARING YOUR NIPPLES FOR BREASTFEEDING

When you first start breastfeeding, your nipples will feel delicate. They need time to toughen up, so increase the length of time on each breast gradually. Two minutes on each breast will give your baby sufficient colostrum at first. Build up the time on each breast to ten minutes on each side by the time the milk has come in on about the third or fourth day.

All babies suck most strongly in the first five minutes, and during this time they take about 80 percent of the feeding. When she's had enough, she'll lose interest and play with your breast or fall asleep. Alternate the breast you begin nursing with each time.

TAKING CARE OF YOUR BREASTS

Your breasts need special care when you start breastfeeding. Buy at least two maternity bras—the best you can afford (see p.163)—and be very careful about the daily hygiene of your breasts and nipples. Bathe them every day with water; don't use soap because it defats the skin and can encourage a sore or cracked nipple to develop. Always handle your breasts with care. Never rub them dry—always pat them.

If you can, leave your nipples open to the air for a short time when you've finished nursing. Wear pads inside your bra to soak up any milk that may leak, and change these pads often. Don't leave a wet pad in contact with your breast for any length of time. To avoid cracked nipples, apply a drop of olive oil or hypericum and calendula cream to the pad.

BREAST CARE

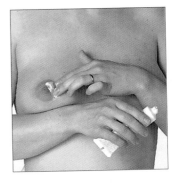

Sore nipples
Use lotion to relieve cracked or sore nipples. Apply often, especially after each feeding.

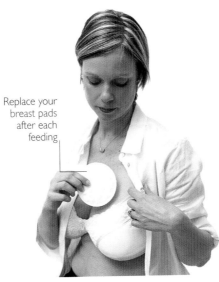

Replace your breast pads after each feeding

Breast pads
Leaking breasts can be embarrassing and uncomfortable, causing cracked nipples and staining your clothes. Breast pads are easy to use, so tuck them into the cups of your bra to soak up the leaking milk. Both washable and disposable pads are available, but avoid any that are backed with plastic.

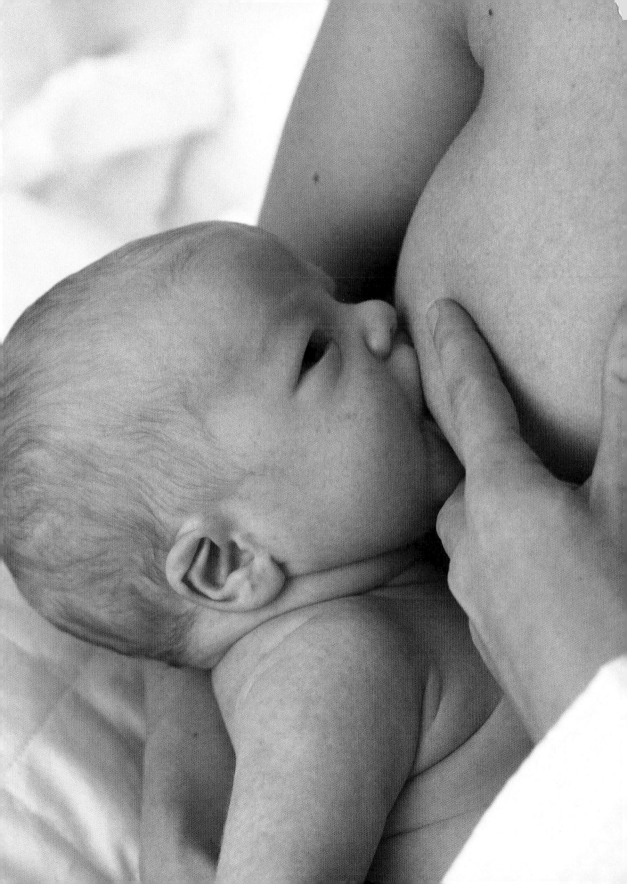

TAKE CARE

To reduce the risk of your baby's contracting a gastrointestinal infection, make sure that everything that comes in contact with your baby's food is thoroughly cleaned or sterilized before use. Use a pot of boiling water or a dishwasher (see opposite) and wash your hands before handling any formula or equipment. You'll also need to give pacifiers and teething rings a thorough cleaning each time they're used.

Always store prepared bottles of formula in the refrigerator, and never keep them longer than 24 hours. It's best to make up formula when you need it, not in advance. If your baby doesn't finish a bottle or if you warm up a bottle for him but he doesn't want it, throw it away—reheated formula is a prime source of infection.

Bottlefeeding

It's perfectly safe and healthy to bottlefeed your baby with an infant formula, instead of breastfeeding, but you must follow the manufacturer's instructions very carefully. When you feed your baby, give him plenty of warm, loving attention and eye contact.

PREPARING FORMULAS

Infant formula products range from relatively inexpensive dried-milk-based powders to ready-to-use but expensive liquid milk products. Infant formulas are enriched with vitamins and iron, and are carefully formulated to make them as close as possible to human milk. They're usually based on cow's milk, but there are soy-based formulas for babies who cannot digest, or who have an allergy to, ordinary milk. If you're unsure which product to choose, ask your healthcare provider to recommend one. Whichever formula you use, it's essential to keep all the bottles, spoons, measuring cups, and nipples absolutely clean, because a newborn baby is very vulnerable to infection. It's also very important always to wash your hands thoroughly before making up formula or bottlefeeding your baby.

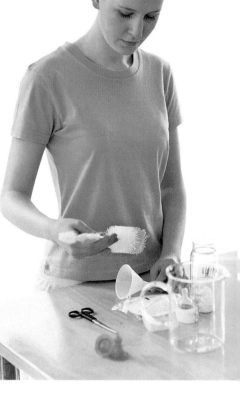

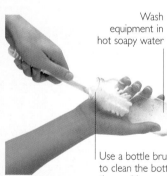

Wash equipment in hot soapy water

Use a bottle brush to clean the bottle thoroughly

Washing bottles and nipples
Wash all equipment in hot, soapy water. Scrub the insides of bottles with a bottle brush, and rub the nipples thoroughly to remove any traces of milk. Rinse bottles and nipples thoroughly under warm, running water to remove any soap.

EQUIPMENT

If you're going to bottlefeed your baby, you'll need to have the following items ready.

- bottles, with nipples, rings, and caps
- bottle brush
- measuring cup
- plastic knife and spoon
- plastic funnel
- a means of sterilizing bottles and nipples, whether it's a pot of boiling water or the dishwasher.

332

KEEPING EVERYTHING CLEAN

You'll quickly develop your own routine for cleaning bottles and nipples. For sterilizing, you can use the hot cycle on your dishwasher, but be aware that rubber nipples will deteriorate quickly in the heat of a dishwasher. You can also sterilize equipment if you put it in a large pot, cover it with water, and boil for 10 minutes. All items must be fully submerged during the boiling period. Use tongs to remove the hot bottles and allow them to cool before filling. Sterilize all feeding equipment until your baby is 12 months old.

Before sterilizing, wash the feeding equipment in hot, soapy water or, if you have one, in a dishwasher. Scrub inside the bottles with a bottle brush. Clean nipples carefully, and rinse everything thoroughly (see column, far left).

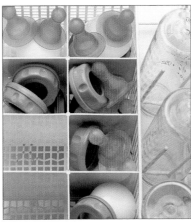

Cleaning in a dishwasher

If you have a dishwasher, you can put the bottles, measuring cup, and knife straight in it once your baby is 12 months old. Clean nipples separately before they go in (see column, left). Run the dishwasher on the normal cycle.

Make sure bottles are submerged when boiling

Boiling

Boil the bottles for ten minutes. Then take them out and leave them to cool down before using.

MEASURING AND MIXING

Follow the instructions on the can or package exactly when preparing a feeding. Never make the formula "more nourishing" by adding more powder than specified — your baby will get too much fat and protein and too little water. And if you always add extra water to the powder, because you want to make the formula more thirst-quenching, you run the risk of undernourishing your baby.

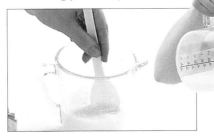

Measuring

Using the scoop provided, measure the quantities accurately. Use a sterilized knife blade to level off the powder in the scoop. Don't heap the powder in the scoop, or pack it down tightly.

Mixing

Use only freshly boiled water that has been allowed to cool down slightly, and measure it after it has cooled. If you measure it before you boil it, the made-up formula will be too strong because of the water lost by evaporation.

BREAST TO BOTTLE

If you've been breastfeeding your baby and for any reason you want to change over to bottlefeeding with formula, it's best to do it gradually.

Make the switch from breast to bottle very slowly so that your baby has time to get used to bottlefeeding and to the taste of formula. Your milk supply will then slowly reduce as your baby's demand for it lessens.

Before starting the change to bottlefeeding, ask your healthcare provider for detailed advice.

Giving the bottle

When you feed your baby with a bottle, whether its filled with formula or with expressed breast milk, be just as patient and loving as you would be if you were breastfeeding. Allow her to take a break if she feels like it and to decide when she's had enough.

GETTING COMFORTABLE

When you or your partner give your baby a feeding, it's important to look at her, cuddle her close, and talk to her. Find a quiet

Warming the formula
The best way to heat a bottle of formula is to stand it up in a bowl of warm water. Don't use a microwave to heat a bottle—it can cause "hot spots" in the formula that might burn your baby's mouth. Splash a few drops of milk on your wrist to check the temperature before giving the bottle— the milk should feel tepid on your skin.

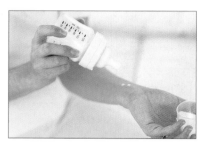

BOTTLEFEEDING

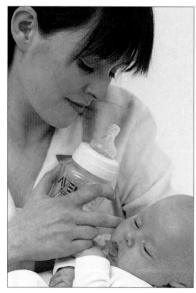

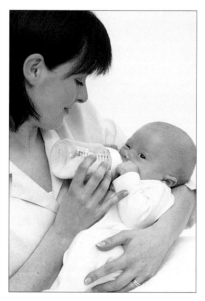

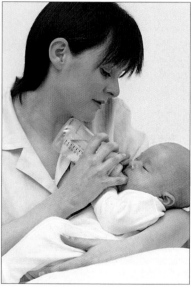

Preparing for a feeding
Hold your baby with her head slightly raised so she can breathe and swallow safely and there's no risk of choking. Until she's about 10 days old, you may need to trigger her sucking reflex by gently stroking the cheek closest to you.

Giving the bottle
When you gently put the nipple into her mouth, be careful not to push it too far back. When she begins to suck, hold the bottle at an angle to keep the nipple full of formula or milk and free of air.

Releasing the nipple
Sometimes your baby will want to keep sucking away at a bottle even though it's empty. If you want her to let go, gently slide your little finger between her gums.

comfortable place to feed your baby. You may like to sit on the floor or in a low chair so you can support her on your lap. Rest her head in the crook of your elbow, with her back supported on your forearm, and hold her securely.

Before feeding, unscrew the nipple ring a little so that air can get into the bottle when your baby sucks out the formula. This will prevent the nipple from closing up. Always hold the bottle at an angle so the nipple is full of milk or your baby will swallow air with the feeding. If your baby falls asleep during a feeding, she may have gas that is making her feel full. Sit her up and burp her.

BURPING YOUR BABY

The point of burping is to help your baby bring up any air she's swallowed during feeding, or when crying before feeding, so it doesn't cause her any discomfort. If your baby has gas, one of the best ways to burp her is to hold her against your shoulder and gently stroke or pat her back (below). Put a clean cloth over your shoulder first because your baby might dribble or spit up a little milk as she burps.

Another way to help your baby to clear any gas is to sit her on your lap and lean her forward, without bending her over at the waist. As you do this, support her head with your hand so it does not flop forward.

GAS AND BURPING

Babies vary a great deal in how they react to gas. In my experience, most babies aren't noticeably more contented for having been burped.

Babies differ in the amount of air that they swallow during feeding. Some, including most breastfed babies, swallow very little. Once a baby is clamped on to the breast, it's virtually an airtight seal, so it's almost impossible for a baby to swallow air while on the breast.

Swallowing air is much more common in bottlefed babies, but even then it doesn't really seem to be a problem.

One thing in favor of burping is that it makes you relax, take things slowly, hold your baby gently, and stroke her in a firm and reassuring way, which can help both of you. My feeling about burping is, by all means do it, but don't become fanatical.

Don't rub or pat your baby too hard—you may jerk her and she'll bring up some of her feeding. A gentle upward, stroking movement is better.

You don't need to stop halfway through a feeding to burp your baby. Wait until she pauses naturally, and then put her on your shoulder. If she doesn't burp, don't worry; it's because she doesn't need to.

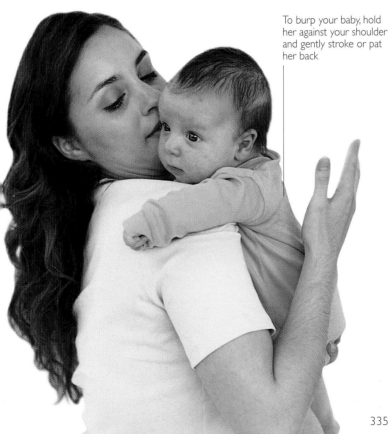

To burp your baby, hold her against your shoulder and gently stroke or pat her back

Choosing diapers

TYPES OF DIAPERS

There are range of different diapers available. Choose what's best for you and your baby.

Disposable

- disposable diapers, available in different sizes and sometimes in boy and girl styles

Reusable

- traditional cloth diaper for use with pins, plastic pants, and diaper liner

- shaped cloth diaper

- shaped cloth diaper with built-in waterproof covering

Sore bottom
Diaper rash is common. Don't wash his skin with soap and water: use baby lotion, and avoid plastic pants. You can treat rashes by using special cream bought from a pharmacy.

Your baby will need to wear diapers day and night for the next two to three years, until he's able to start using a potty. There are lots of different types of diapers available, so choose whatever's best for your lifestyle and budget.

TYPES OF DIAPERS

The basic choice is between disposable and fabric diapers. Think about which type will be comfortable for your baby as well as cost-effective and manageable for you.

Disposable diapers These are convenient and easy to use. They come ready-shaped with elasticated legs to prevent leakage, and there's no need for pins or plastic pants. Sizes range from newborn to toddler, and some come in boy and girl styles. However, disposables are expensive, and because millions are thrown away every day, they are creating a huge waste problem.

Reusable diapers Reusable cloth diapers may seem more expensive at first because you need to buy at least 24 of good quality. But they can be less expensive over the long term since you can use them over and over again, and for more than one child. Some parents also find that cloth diapers are better for older babies at night because they're more absorbent.

Reusables are more work, since they need to be washed and dried after every use, but in some areas there are diaper laundering services that will pick up dirty diapers from your home and return them clean and dry. Use reusable diapers with liners that allow urine to pass through and away from the baby's skin and lessen the risk of a sore bottom. You'll also need a supply of plastic pants to stop leakage.

Choose ones with that fit snugly, and never put them in the dryer. Traditional cloth diapers are a litttle trickier to put on, but the latest cloth diapers are shaped like disposables so they fit around your baby without having to be folded. They fasten with Velcro tabs and don't require pins. Some of these diapers come with a built-in plastic outer layer; others need to be worn with plastic pants.

Benefits of types of diapers

DISPOSABLE	REUSABLE
Advantages No washing, drying, pins, or plastic pants. No risk of hurting your baby with a pin. More practical when traveling because you need fewer accessories and you don't have to carry a bag of dirty diapers home	**Advantages** Only one set needed, so you don't need to keep buying new supplies. Work out cheaper in the long run and can be used for another child
Disadvantages Can only be used once. More expensive in the long run. Create mountains of garbage. Must never be flushed down the toilet	**Disadvantages** Washing and drying is a lot of work. More difficult to put on, unless you use shaped reusables. May prick baby with pin

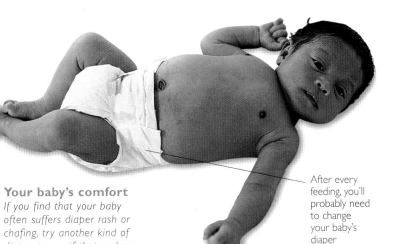

Your baby's comfort
If you find that your baby often suffers diaper rash or chafing, try another kind of diaper to see if that makes a difference.

After every feeding, you'll probably need to change your baby's diaper

DIAPER CONTENTS

After your baby is born, you'll notice some changes in the color and consistency of his stools. During the first couple of days, your baby will pass *meconium*, a sticky, greenish-black substance. This contains bile and mucus and comes from the amniotic fluid he swallowed in your uterus. Once he starts nursing, the stools will become greenish brown, with a looser consistency, and then a yellowish brown. The color, smell, and consistency of the stools varies, depending on whether you're breastfeeding or bottlefeeding your baby. The stools of breastfed babies are looser and bright yellow. Bottlefed babies pass a firmer, pale brown stool, with a more pungent smell. The number of movements also varies. Some babies fill their diapers after every meal, while others are less frequent. Sometimes, a couple of days may pass without a bowel movement—unless there are other problems (see column, right), this is nothing to worry about.

DIAPER CONTENTS

As long as your baby is healthy, don't worry too much about the contents of his diaper.

A baby's bowel movements may vary, but there are a few signs to look out for (see Newborn health, p.342). For example, streaks of blood in stools aren't normal, so if you spot these, call your doctor right away.

Immediately after birth, your baby's urine contains substances called urates that may stain his diaper a dark pink or red, but this is normal, so don't be alarmed. He'll urinate often, maybe every half hour, because his bladder can't hold urine for even a few minutes. Don't worry unless he stops urinating for several hours. If this happens, check with your doctor in case there is an abnormality in his urinary tract or he's dehydrated.

DIAPER WASHING

Remove all traces of urine and feces from cloth diapers, otherwise your baby's skin will become red and sore.

Each morning, fill two pails with cold water and sterilizing solution. Put wet diapers into one pail, and soiled diapers into the other one—flush as much of the feces down the toilet as you can first. The next day, rinse urine-soaked diapers in hot water before drying. Wash soiled diapers on the hot setting of a washing machine, then dry. Always put diapers used during the night into a fresh batch of solution.

Changing a diaper

DIAPER RASH

Bacteria on the skin break down urine to form ammonia, which is toxic and burns.

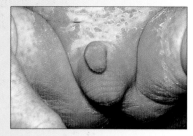

Sore bottom
Diaper rash is common. Don't wash your baby's skin with soap and water: use baby lotion. Avoid plastic pants. You can also treat it using special cream bought from the pharmacy.

You'll need to change your baby's diaper when it's wet or dirty, which will be very often—especially with a new baby. To prevent your baby from getting diaper rash, change her diaper when she wakes up in the morning, after every feeding, and when she goes to bed at night. Make sure you have somewhere safe to change your baby, with all the equipment you'll need close at hand. As often as you can, leave her diaper off for a while to air her bottom.

CLEANING YOUR BABY

Clean her leg creases
Wipe off any feces with a tissue. Lift up her legs and, using one cotton ball or pad at a time, moistened with water or lotion, clean inside all the creases at the tops of her legs, wiping downward and away from her body.

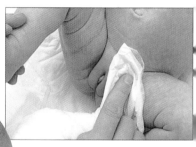

Airing her bottom helps prevent it getting sore

Clean her diaper area
Holding both her ankles in one hand, clean her genital area. Always wipe from her vagina back toward her rectum to prevent soiling her vulva. Never pull back the labia to clean inside. Wipe her thighs and buttocks inward toward the rectum. Remove the dirty diaper.

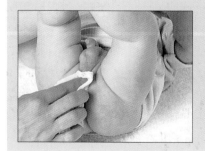

Cleaning a boy
Using some baby lotion on a cotton pad, gently clean under his testicles. Wipe all over his testicles and under his penis. Don't pull the foreskin back. Holding his ankles with one hand and lifting him up, clean his bottom; use petroleum jelly, not barrier cream, to protect his penis.

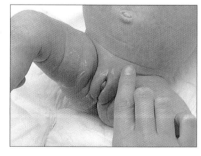

Dry her bottom
If you've used water, dry the area with a tissue, then let her kick her legs for a while so that air reaches her bottom. Apply barrier cream gently to prevent diaper rash.

PUTTING ON A DISPOSABLE DIAPER

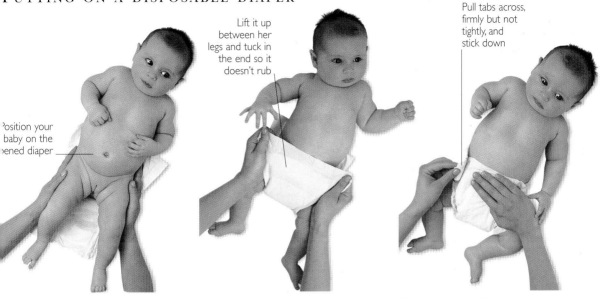

Lift it up between her legs and tuck in the end so it doesn't rub

Pull tabs across, firmly but not tightly, and stick down

Position your baby on the opened diaper

1 Open out the diaper with the adhesive tabs at the top. Then lift her legs, slide the diaper underneath, and align the top with her waist.

2 Bring the front panel up between her legs, smoothing the sides around her tummy so they tuck neatly underneath.

3 Peel the tabs. Pull one side over and across to the front flap and stick down the tab. Repeat with the other side, keeping the diaper taut.

PUTTING ON A TRADITIONAL CLOTH DIAPER

1 Fold the diaper into a triangle by lifting the bottom right-hand corner to the top left, and then the bottom left to the top right.

3 Bring the diaper up between her legs (with a boy, tuck down his penis first). Holding it in place, fold one side over the central panel and pull slightly to keep it firm. Then fold up the other side.

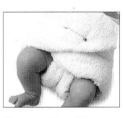

2 Raise your baby's legs and slide the diaper under her, aligning the top edge with her waist.

Secure the diaper
For a small baby, secure the diaper with a pin in the middle; for a bigger baby, use a pin at both sides.

Thumb on outer diaper; use fingers as a shield against the safety pin

Fold over, making sure other hand has other corners secured, then pin

Bathing baby

You might feel a little nervous the first time you give your baby a bath. But once you get used to it, you'll both relax and enjoy this chance to be extra close.

- Keep the room warm—at least 68°F (20°C)—and don't leave your baby undressed for too long.

- Make sure the bath is a at comfortable height for you. Wear a waterproof apron with a towel tied around your waist so you can dry your baby on your lap.

- Make sure everything you need for washing, drying, and dressing is within easy reach.

- Always test the water first, and don't add hot water while your baby is in the bath. Add baby bath liquid to the water; it's easier to use than soap.

- Talk and smile at your baby all the time while you're bathing him, and take the chance to have lots of body contact.

You don't need to give your newborn baby a bath every day—once a week on a regular day is often enough. You can bathe him more often if you both enjoy it—lots of babies like a splash in the bath once they get used to it. You can bathe him in any room in the house as long as it is warm enough. Always check the temperature of the water first to make sure it's not too hot by dipping in your elbow or the inside of your wrist.

TOPPING AND TAILING

This is a quick way of cleaning his face, neck, hands, and bottom without bathing him or taking off all his clothes. Instead of a washcloth, use cotton balls or pads dipped in cooled, boiled water and squeezed dry. Using a new cotton ball each time, wipe from the inside of his eyes outward. Clean behind his ears, over his face and chin, and around his neck. Dry him off carefully with a soft towel.

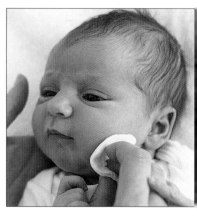

Clean his cheek and neck
Wipe his face, chin, and the creases in his neck with moist cotton ball or pad to remove any traces of milk or spittle.

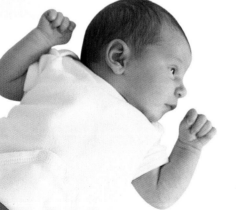

Wipe inside skin creases downward and away from his body

Clean his bottom
Undo any lower garments and remove his diaper. Using a new cotton ball or pad, wipe around his genital area (see p.338). If he's soiled, moisten the cotton ball with some baby lotion.

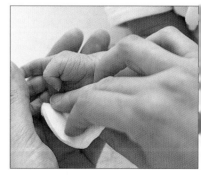

Clean his hands
Gently uncurl his fingers. Using a moistened cotton ball, wipe over the fronts and backs of his hands, and in between his fingers. Take a new cotton ball and wipe over his arms. Dry with a soft towel.

BATHING

Undress your baby down to his T-shirt and diaper. Before you put him in the bathtub, wipe his eyes and face with a moist cotton ball. Then undress him completely and wrap him in a soft, clean towel.

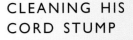

Fan out your fingers to cradle his head

Wash his head
Hold him just above the bathtub in a football hold, so that he lies along your arm and his head is supported by your hand. With your other hand, carefully wash his hair with the bath water. Then gently dry his hair with a soft towel.

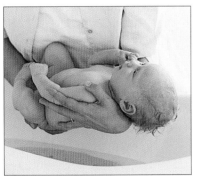

Put him into the bath
Support his shoulders and neck on your forearm, hooking your hand around his far shoulder. Cradle his bottom with your other hand.

Wash him all over
Keep him semi-upright and slowly splash water over his body with your free hand. Talk and smile at him all the time. When you're finished, lift him out, with your free hand held firmly under his bottom, and wrap him gently in the towel.

Always hold him securely

CLEANING HIS CORD STUMP

Your baby's umbilical cord stump dries and drops off within a week after the birth. Clean this area daily to avoid infection.

Gently wipe the skin creases around the stump with a surgical baby wipe containing pure alcohol. Ask your healthcare provider for these. Keep cleaning in the same way after the stump has separated so it heals quickly. If you notice any redness, discharge, or other signs of infection, ask your doctor what to do.

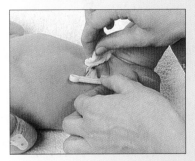

Avoid infection
Dry the area carefully every time you bathe your baby. Leave the area open to the air as often as you can in order to avoid infection.

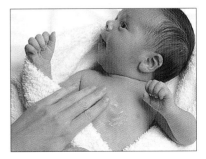

Dry and powder
Pat him dry—be particularly careful to dry his skin creases. Put some baby powder on his skin if you like, but don't use any in his diaper area because powder will cake when wet.

Newborn health

Newborn babies, especially breastfed babies, are generally healthy during their first weeks of life. But their immune systems and internal organs are not yet fully developed, so there are some ailments that can affect them at this early age.

WHEN TO CALL THE DOCTOR

As your baby gets older, you'll learn how to deal with common minor ailments, but there are times when you'll need to call the doctor.

Sometimes when your baby is ill you'll be torn between not wanting to bother the doctor unnecessarily and feeling more and more worried about your baby's well-being. If this happens, don't take any chances with your baby's health—call the doctor promptly, especially if your baby is showing one or more of the symptoms listed below or if you have any other reason to worry about his health.

Call your doctor sooner rather than later if your baby:

- is having convulsions

- is hard to wake up

- is having trouble breathing, is wheezing, and has a loud, dry cough

- has a very high temperature, or an abnormally low one

- has stools that are frequent, loose, green, and watery

- is vomiting a significant amount (not just the usual after-feeding spit-ups)

- has refused several of his feedings in a row

- is showing the symptoms of dehydration (see right)

- is listless and crying for no apparent reason

- seems to be bothered by his ears, head, or neck

- has an unusual rash.

JAUNDICE OF THE NEWBORN

Quite a few babies suffer from jaundice. This is a yellowish discoloration of the skin and whites of the eyes caused by too much bilirubin in the blood. Bilirubin is a yellow pigment that's produced when primitive red blood cells are destroyed—something that often happens after birth.

Infant jaundice usually appears by the second or third day after birth, and lasts for about seven to 10 days. By this time the surplus red blood cells have died off and the baby's liver has matured enough to mop up the excess *bilirubin* in the body. The jaundice usually clears up by itself, but if the bilirubin levels are particularly high, a baby may need phototherapy. In this treatment a baby is exposed to carefully controlled amounts of ultraviolet light, which breaks down the bilirubin pigment in his skin.

Hemolytic disease of the newborn   This is a more serious condition caused by too much bile in a baby's blood. It can result from the breakdown of large numbers of red blood cells due to the action of antibodies from a Rhesus-incompatible mother (see p.202). The main symptoms are jaundice, pallor, enlargement of the liver and spleen, and blood abnormalities. It's usually treated by blood transfusion.

DIARRHEA AND VOMITING

Mild cases of upset stomach or diarrhea will soon pass, but a young baby's digestive system is extremely vulnerable. Breastfed babies are less prone to these gastrointestinal infections than are bottlefed babies, because of the protective antibodies that are contained in breast milk, but all babies may suffer from them from time to time.

Contact your doctor immediately if your baby vomits up all his feedings over a six-hour period or is passing frequent, loose, green, watery stools.

Dehydration   The major danger to babies who are suffering from vomiting and diarrhea is dehydration because of the loss of fluids. Symptoms of dehydration include a dry mouth, sunken eyes, the fontanelle looking or feeling unusually low, irritability, lethargy, lack of wet diapers, and refusal to feed. Never ignore these symptoms, and seek medical help at once.

CONSTIPATION

Breastfed babies don't get constipated—the ideal composition and digestibility of breast milk keeps everything moving. Bottlefed babies can get constipated, usually because they're not getting enough fluid. If your bottlefed baby passes no stools for a day or two, then produces a hard one, give him drinks of water between feedings to increase his fluid intake. If this doesn't make his stools softer and more frequent, give him a little drink of diluted fruit juice twice a day, which should help to loosen his stools. If that fails, ask your healthcare provider for advice.

Urinary problems   Constipation is easy to treat and usually nothing to worry about. But if your baby starts to urinate infrequently, it might be a sign of a fever, a blockage, or an infection in his urinary system. If he goes for a couple of hours without wetting his diaper, give him plenty of water to drink. If his diaper is still dry two hours after that, call your doctor.

If your baby's urine becomes strong-smelling and deepens in color, he may not be getting enough to drink. This makes the urine more concentrated. The remedy is to increase his liquid intake by giving him several drinks of water between feedings. If this doesn't make any difference, he could have a urinary infection and might need medical treatment, so call your doctor.

FEVERS

When your baby has a fever, it's a sign that his body is fighting an infection—the rise in body temperature acts to make the body's own defense system work harder. If you think your baby may have a fever, take his temperature. Check it again in 20 minutes to see if it's changed, and note each reading. If your baby's temperature rises slightly but he seems like his usual self and shows no other signs of illness, it's probably a minor infection and will usually pass within a day or two, but tell your doctor just in case. Call your doctor right away if your baby's temperature rises by a degree or more, he gets hot and distressed, or he shows other signs of illness such as lethargy, vomiting, or diarrhea.

EAR INFECTIONS

Babies often get colds, and these can lead to an ear infection called *otitis media*. This happens when the bacteria travel along one, or both, of the eustachian tubes (which link the middle ear to the back of the throat and equalize pressure in the ears) into the middle ear. Babies spend most of their time lying down, which allows the bacteria to pass along more easily. When the mucus membrane of the eustachian tube gets inflamed, bacteria are trapped in the middle ear, where they multiply.

Symptoms include a high temperature, diarrhea, crying for no apparent reason, and any kind of discharge from the ear. Call your doctor right away. Your baby will need to be seen to confirm the diagnosis and to rule out meningitis, which has similar symptoms. Ear infections are easily cured by antibiotics.

COLICKY BABY

Colic is more common in male babies. The exact causes of this exasperating blend of indigestion and inconsolable crying are still not known.

Some medical researchers looking into the cause of colic suspect that it happens because the baby's digestive system is immature. Other research suggests that babies whose mothers have been particularly anxious while pregnant are more prone to being colicky (see p.193).

In a typical colicky baby, the problem begins at about two weeks and disappears at about three months. The colic attacks usually happen in the evening. The baby draws up his legs to his stomach or sticks them out straight in an attempt to relieve the stomach cramps and gas, and cries loudly from distress and pain.

There's really not much you can do about colic, except wait for him to grow out of it. Stomach massage can often ease the discomfort, as does laying him face down across your lap with a warm towel, or a hot-water bottle half-filled with warm water, placed under his belly. Other ways of helping include taking your baby for a ride in a car, putting him face down across your knees and stroking his back, and giving him a pacifier to suck on.

Colic doesn't damage your baby's health (although it can be very frustrating for you), but when it first starts to happen, check with your doctor to make sure that it's nothing more serious.

Special care baby

HOW TO HELP YOUR BABY

Your baby will receive lots of care and attention from neonatal specialists, but there are things you and your partner can do to help him thrive.

- Spend as much time with him as you can; he needs the same love and attention as a full-term baby.

- Touch and fondle your baby, both in and out of the incubator, whenever and as soon as you can. Cuddling, stroking, and gentle caressing all help him to grow and thrive.

- Express your breast milk at regular feeding times for your baby. You'll be giving him the best possible food and at the same time you'll build up your milk supply for when he's able to suck on his own.

- Research shows that the colostrum and milk of a mother whose child is preterm contain more of certain nutrients than those of mothers whose babies are born at term. This makes up for a preterm baby's missing out on nutrients he would have received in the uterus. A preterm baby fed on his mother's breast milk develops at almost exactly the same rate as he would if he were still in her uterus.

- Get involved with your baby's care. Ask the nurses to show you how to help with feeding, washing, and changing him. This will help you bond with your baby and give you confidence in caring for him.

- Don't struggle with feelings of anxiety, ignorance, or worry—ask the medical team for information and support.

About one in 10 of all newborn babies needs to spend some time, even if only a very short time, in a special care baby unit. Most have been born too soon or have not grown as much as they should have before birth. A small number may be ill. The aim of the special care baby unit is to protect your baby from any risks to his health and to nurture him until he has outgrown them.

LOW BIRTHWEIGHT BABIES

In general, any baby weighing less than 4½ lb (2 kg) at birth is probably smaller than he should be and may need special care. About four to eight percent of all babies have low birthweights. Of these, two-thirds are preterm—born before their due date—and one-third small-for-dates.

Preterm babies The pace of an unborn baby's development is geared to his being born at full term (40 weeks from your LMP). If for any reason he is born a few weeks or more before full term, he may not yet be ready for life in the outside world. A baby born before week 35 is said to be preterm or premature. Depending on how premature he is, he'll need the help of a special care baby unit or a neonatal intensive care unit (NICU).

Small-for-dates babies A baby is "small-for-dates" if he weighs less than expected for the number of weeks that have passed since he was conceived. A small-for-dates baby is usually a full-term baby who's very small at birth. A small-for-dates baby may present different problems of care after the birth from a premature baby. Babies who are only three or four weeks premature and low-birthweight full-term babies, who are otherwise healthy and taking feedings, can usually stay in the postnatal ward with their mothers, or in a special care area where their progress will be more closely monitored than normal.

Health risks A premature baby born before 35 weeks faces a number of health risks that don't usually affect a full-term infant, as well as more common ones such as jaundice. If his internal organs are underdeveloped, for example, he may have difficulty breathing, regulating his body temperature, and feeding; he'll also be very vulnerable to infection. He may also have a low blood sugar level (*hypoglycemia*), which can cause brain damage if untreated, and he may need iron or calcium supplements if he lacks these essential minerals.

CARING FOR BABIES WITH SPECIAL NEEDS

Today, a baby who's born preterm or small-for-dates, or with an illness or disability, has a far better chance than he would have had 20 or even 10 years ago. This is because so much more is known about how to care for newborn babies and this knowledge is applied in neonatal intensive care units (NICUs).

If a baby is simply too weak or young to be able to suck, and needs tube feeding, or has jaundice and needs phototherapy treatment, he'll be taken care of in the NICU. If he's very premature or sick, he'll also need the specialized, high-tech care that's available in a neonatal intensive care unit.

A neonatal intensive care unit is dedicated to caring for babies who need highly specialized nursing attention. In modern NICUs, the tiniest premature babies—even ones born at only 24 or 25 weeks' gestation and weighing barely 1 lb (450 g)—can be helped to thrive while they catch up on their growing. Neonatal intensive care units tend to be in major regional hospitals rather than community hospitals.

If you go into labor very prematurely, you may be taken to a hospital with an NICU, even if it's not the hospital with which you were registered, or your baby may be taken there by ambulance in a special incubator immediately after the birth. This can be upsetting for parents if the new hospital is some distance from home, but the NICU will be designed to be as welcoming and friendly as possible. If this should happen to you, ask the staff in charge to explain all about your baby's particular needs and how you can help.

Most NICUs encourage parents to play an active part in their baby's everyday care by helping with tasks such as feeding, washing, and diaper-changing. Many provide facilities so parents can stay at the hospital with their babies as much as possible. Parents are encouraged to cuddle their babies skin to skin, since this helps them develop more quickly (see also p.349). But with a very premature baby, it may be some time before he's strong enough to be handled outside the incubator, and parents may have to steel themselves for an anxious wait until their baby's condition has improved.

BABIES THAT NEED SPECIAL CARE

Every baby born prematurely or small-for-dates is assessed individually, but your baby will definitely be taken to a neonatal intensive care unit (NICU) if any of the following applies:

- birthweight less than 3 lb (1.5 kg)

- less than 34 weeks in the womb

- severe respiratory problems (*hyaline membrane disease*, sometimes known as respiratory distress syndrome)

- severe birth asphyxia (lack of oxygen or fetal distress)

- severe infection

- convulsions

- jaundice that requires an exchange transfusion

- drug withdrawal, in cases where the mother has been addicted to narcotics such as heroin.

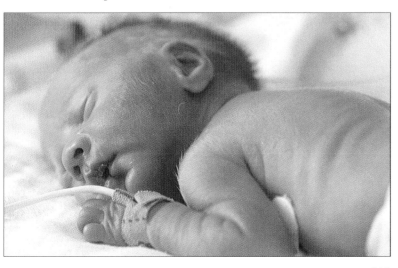

A special care baby
Most special care babies, like this premature baby, spend some time in an incubator. This keeps their temperature steady and monitors their breathing.

Neonatal Intensive Care Unit (NICU)

In the neonatal intensive care unit (NICU) your baby is cared for 24 hours a day by specially trained staff with a wide range of technology to help them. The main concerns for a baby in intensive care are temperature control, breathing, brain and immune system, and feeding. There'll be a lot of tubes, electrodes, monitors, and drips, but they're there to help your baby, so try not to be alarmed.

WHY YOUR BABY NEEDS CARE

Your baby needs intensive care to help him to grow and thrive independently. The following key areas are closely monitored.

Temperature control All babies are at risk of getting cold, but a premature or small-for-dates baby is even more at risk because he has so little fat for insulation. A premature baby is placed in an incubator, an enclosed cabinet in which he can be kept warm and supplied with warmed, humidified air (or oxygen, if he needs it).

YOUR EXPERIENCE

If your baby needs intensive care, you'll probably be concerned about the bonding process. Don't worry— the staff will encourage you both to be as involved as possible with your baby and his care.

- You'll be encouraged to watch the nurses care for your baby and to help with the practical care and nursing.

- Don't be afraid to touch and talk to your baby as often as possible. As well as helping you feel closer to him, this loving attention also has huge benefits for your baby, helping him thrive and grow.

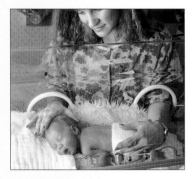

Physical contact
An incubator has circular doors in the plastic top so the nurses can attend to your baby and attach any monitor leads, feeding tubes, or intravenous drips he might need. The doors also allow you to reach in and touch your baby, helping you to bond with him and feel close.

YOUR BABY'S ENVIRONMENT

A preterm or small-for-dates baby's internal organs may not be completely developed, and he'll need help so he can breathe and grow. Inside the incubator (see right), the temperature, oxygen levels, and humidity are all carefully controlled to provide the best possible conditions for your baby to develop and thrive.

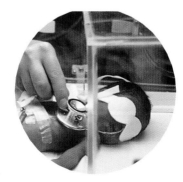

Checking heart rate
A stethoscope is used to monitor and record a premature baby's heart rate.

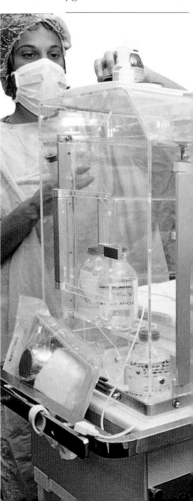

Breathing Under 30 weeks, and certainly before 27 weeks, a baby's lungs are not mature enough to allow the transfer of oxygen to the bloodstream. If you go into premature labor, you'll probably be given an injection to help mature your baby's lungs. Because the nervous system is immature, this can affect a baby's breathing mechanism, and may cause pauses in breathing, known as *apnea*, sometimes accompanied by a slowing of the heart rate, known as *bradycardia*.

Feeding Initially, your baby will have small feedings once an hour, progressing to one every three hours. A very premature or sick baby may be unable to digest milk and will be given a special solution of sugar, salts, and potassium. When he's able to take milk, he'll have a special infant formula or your own expressed milk. Breast milk is the ideal food for a baby in intensive care, just as it is for any other baby.

YOUR BABY'S NEEDS

A baby in intensive care needs his mother and father as well as expert medical care.

Although a baby in intensive care receives 24-hour medical attention, he also needs to feel his parents' love. Physical contact with you and your partner will reassure and comfort him, and help you to develop a warm, close, and loving relationship.

He needs to hear both your voices, so talk and sing to him all the time. Hold him close whenever you can so that he gets to know your smells and can feel close to you.

Central nervous system
This needs careful monitoring with electrodes that feed information into a visual display unit.

Feeding
Most premature babies have to be fed through a soft, thin tube which is inserted through the nose.

Assisted breathing
A premature baby's lungs are likely to be under-developed, so he may need help with his breathing through a special ventilator.

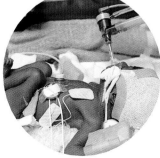

Detecting the heartbeat
Electrodes placed on the baby's chest monitor his heartbeat.

Premature baby

Case study

Name Carol Scott
Age 24 years
Past medical history Nothing abnormal
Obstetric history This was Carol's first pregnancy

At 28 weeks of pregnancy, Carol noticed that her hands and feet were swollen, and that she couldn't take off her wedding ring. Two weeks later she was found to have raised blood pressure, so she went to her doctor's office so that her blood pressure, blood, and urine could be monitored and checked. The well-being of her baby was checked too, with regular electronic fetal monitoring (see p.275) and ultrasound scans. There was albumin in Carol's urine, which is a symptom of preeclampsia, along with high blood pressure and swelling.

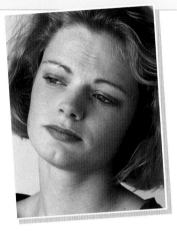

Carol's baby was born prematurely. Premature babies can have a difficult start in life, but most of them do well and grow up to be healthy, normal children, thanks to dedicated staff and high-tech neonatal intensive care units. Premature babies can look frighteningly small, but most have great fighting spirit.

BABY AT RISK

After a week of careful monitoring, Carol's blood pressure hadn't gone back to normal and there was still albumin in her urine. At the beginning of the thirty-second week there were signs of fetal distress. Her obstetrician decided that labor would have to be induced. After a straightforward induced labor, Carol delivered her baby, Alice, who weighed 3 lb (1.4 kg).

FAILING PLACENTA

Carol's obstetrician thought that her placenta had begun to fail at the beginning of the third trimester and so her baby's nutrition had been inadequate for some time. When this happens late in pregnancy, the baby's head is disproportionally large because of the relatively normal growth of the brain at the expense of the rest of the body.

KEEP BABY WARM

He explained that low-birthweight premature babies like Alice are born with insufficient energy stores and don't

have enough fat to maintain their body temperature. Premature babies are more likely to suffer from hypothermia, hypoxia (lack of oxygen to the tissues), and hypoglycemia (abnormally low blood sugar) so it's crucial that they are kept warm. Alice was put straight into an incubator and her immature lungs were helped by a ventilator. Carol was given a room next door so she could be with Alice as much as possible.

POSTNATAL REACTIONS

Carol and Mark were quite taken aback by the first sight of Alice (see box, right), even though they'd had time to get used to the idea that she would be premature. Throughout her pregnancy, Carol had dreamed of a curly-haired cherub. Instead, Alice was red and wrinkled, and her head looked very large in proportion to the rest of her body, which was very thin. When they looked at Alice inside the incubator, attached to a ventilator and taped with wires and tubes for monitoring and feeding, she seemed very far away and isolated.

SEEKING REASSURANCE

Carol found herself bursting into tears at the sight of her tiny daughter, so alone and shut away. At the same time, she realized she was having considerable difficulty relating to her baby in the incubator even though she knew she was her longed-for child. Mark encouraged Carol to explain her difficulties to the senior nurse in the unit who comforted Carol and said that her feelings were common and normal. The staff of the neonatal

ICU were understanding; they encouraged Carol and Mark to make contact with Alice by touching and stroking her through the portholes of the incubator. Research show that this helps a premature baby to establish breathing more readily. The staff explained to Carol that her love was more important for the baby's survival than all the technology they could offer.

GETTING INVOLVED

As Carol became involved in caring for Alice, she realized that she loved her and desperately wanted her to survive. The nurses showed her how to express her colostrum (see p.327) so that it could be fed to Alice via the tube. The colostrum of the mothers of premature babies is extra-rich in trace minerals—those minerals the baby would be getting if she were still in the uterus—and their milk contains extra protein to help their babies grow.

Meanwhile, Mark became very interested in the machines in the ICU. He wanted to know what each one was doing for his daughter. Busy though they were, the staff found time to answer his questions.

SKIN-TO-SKIN CONTACT

Once Alice had gained weight and her breathing had improved, she was taken off the ventilator and feeding tube. The staff of the ICU then encouraged Carol to tuck Alice under her blouse and hold her in an upright position between her breasts. Alice was naked except for a diaper, and this meant that mother and baby were in skin-to-skin contact for long periods of time.

Premature babies thrive on this treatment. A mother's body is better than an incubator for keeping a baby warm because her temperature rises automatically if her baby is cold, then falls again once the baby has warmed up. The nurses called it kangaroo care, because it is similar to the way in which kangaroos keep their infants in a warm, protective pouch. This skin-to-skin contact also strengthens the mother-and-baby bond that is so important for survival. Alice began to suckle spontaneously. The staff were delighted with her progress, and Carol and Mark were now eager to take Alice home. The obstetrician explained that it wasn't a question of Alice reaching any target weight; each baby was considered as an individual case and allowed to go home when her weight and general health were satisfactory, given her circumstances. Generally, premature babies are kept in the hospital until they reach 5 lb (2.5 kg).

BACK AT HOME

At home Carol and Mark were faced with new problems. Newborn baby clothes were too big for Alice, but Carol's mother found a special mail order catalog, and Mark found one or two large department stores that had a stock of tiny clothes.

Ordinary diapers were far too big, so Carol cut some disposables down to fit Alice and fastened them with tape. Alice thrived at home and soon began to catch up with full-term babies of the same age.

Carol's baby

Born eight weeks early, Alice had none of the fat that a baby normally puts on in the last few weeks, so she looked much too small for her skin, which was wrinkled and red. She was a sorry sight.

- Her head looked very large in comparison to her body, which was thin and tiny.

- Her skin was loose-fitting and dry.

- She had lanugo (fine downy hair) on her back and the sides of her face.

- Her chest looked small, with prominent ribs.

- As she breathed, her chest rose and fell dramatically.

- Her bottom looked bony and pointed due to lack of fat.

- Her movements tended to be jerky because of her immature nervous system.

- She seemed to have to make a huge effort to take every breath. Sometimes her breathing would stop for a few seconds, but this is not abnormal in a preterm baby.

CHAPTER 16

Adjusting to parenthood

You may find that the responsibilities of parenthood take some getting used to, particularly if they mean dramatic changes in your lifestyle. But you'll soon find that watching your baby grow and develop will bring you great joy as you start to experience the closeness that only a family can bring.

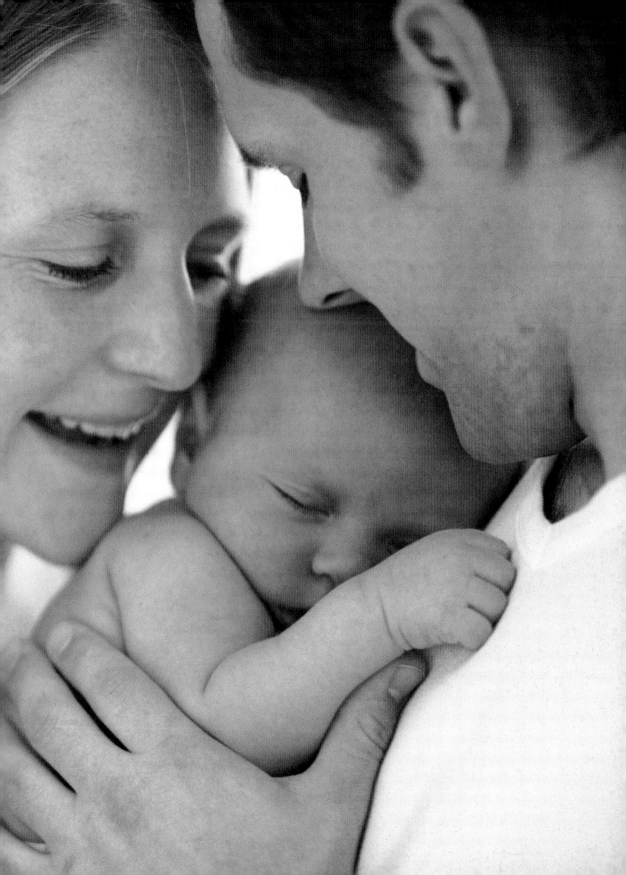

The first weeks

Plan to take some time out immediately following the birth of your baby. Don't feel you have to get back to normal right away—if you try, you'll become overtired and miss out on enjoying your new baby.

Provisions Before the birth, stock up as much as possible with things you'll need—favorite nutritious foods, drinks (you'll need plenty of fluid if you're breastfeeding), clothes, sanitary napkins, cotton balls, diapers.

Nurturing You and your partner will nurture your newborn baby, and your partner will nurture you. Spoil yourselves!

Bonding Give yourselves both time and space to get to know and bond with your baby.

Nesting Make your bed the center of the household—talk, entertain, cuddle, and picnic there.

Visitors Limit visitors. Don't feel you have to play hostess, and put a card on the front door saying you're resting if you don't feel like seeing anyone just then—they can always come back another time.

Callers If you have an answering machine, you could alter the message to include a birth announcement, and perhaps explain that you are resting at present, but that you would love to talk to the caller in a few days.

At one time, women weren't expected to appear in public for some time after giving birth. They spent this time getting their strength back. A period of peace and relaxation in the days immediately following the birth of a baby is vital. It gives both partners a chance to celebrate the birth, welcome and bond with their new baby, and adjust to their new roles as parents.

BECOMING PARENTS

It usually takes a while for new parents to adjust to their situation. Many feel a degree of panic when they realize the overwhelming responsibility they have to take on for this tiny, dependent human being. As with all major changes, it can take time for you to accept and feel comfortable in your new roles, and at the beginning, you may catch yourself hoping that someone else is going to come and take over.

The solution is to give yourselves time and space to get to know and feel comfortable with your baby. The first few weeks are also important for establishing breastfeeding, so it's best to stay as rested and relaxed as possible, and to continue to eat well.

Welcoming your baby Every mother daydreams about her unborn child. But fitting the image of this "dream child" to the reality of the newborn baby you're holding in your arms is not always easy— especially if your baby is the opposite sex from the one you expected, or isn't quite "perfect," or is simply different from what you expected.

It takes time to fall in love with your baby and to learn how to be a mother—or a father. Time spent together will give you the space you need to become adjusted, and to allow you both to get used to being parents.

You may prefer to keep your baby with you in your bedroom at the very beginning, even if you have already made a room ready for her. If she's close by, feeding her will be easier and your nights may be more restful.

RESTING AND RELAXING

The first few weeks can seem like a never-ending round of feeding and changing, with snatches of time for catching up or resting when your baby is asleep. If you're exhausted all the time, you won't enjoy taking care of your baby so much, and you may end up feeling resentful and irritable.

To prevent this, keep the first weeks after your baby's birth for you and your family to be together. Nurture each other, marvel at the new life you're entrusted with, and nest and picnic in your bed. All this will ease you into parenthood and help you regain your strength before you get back to real life.

Friends and family Close friends and relatives always want to help, so perhaps a couple of them could make this an extra-special time for you by taking on the household chores, food preparation, and so on. Your helpers might also be invaluable sources of support, particularly if they've had children themselves and know about baby care and behavior. On the other hand, some new parents find that everyone wants to give them advice, which can be confusing or different from your own ideas. If this happens, try talking things through with your healthcare provider, who'll be able to clear up any confusion.

Lots of people will call you and want to come and see you and your baby. Talk to your partner about this and decide together how best to deal with visitors. Don't feel that you have to entertain—you need to save your strength for your baby and breastfeeding. Being a good hostess every day is tiring, so please don't feel guilty about restricting visiting hours. Put a note on the front door saying "We're sleeping now, but we'd love to see you another time" if you want to rest. You could also add an announcement, such as "Matthew was born at 11:35 p.m., July 20. He was 7 lb 2 oz and we're all doing well." If you have an answering machine, you could also add the birth details to your message.

OTHER CHILDREN

If you already have a child or children, you'll need to include them in this family time after the birth. When you come home from the hospital, your other children will want their share of your attention now that you're back. They'll enjoy cuddling up with you, talking or reading to the baby, and playing on the bed. Just being together can help to fend off any feelings of jealousy. But they probably won't want to sit still for long, and it will help all of you if a friend or relative they love and trust can give them some extra individual attention during these first weeks.

YOUR BABY'S EXPERIENCE

Your baby has arrived in a brand-new world and into a warm, intimate, and loving environment.

Daily routine At first he won't have a recognizable pattern of behavior. He'll begin to settle down into an established routine of feeding and sleeping by the time he's 3–6 weeks old.

Sensations He'd rather look at your face than at unfamiliar people and things, and he'll be reassured by the smell of your skin and his father's. He'll look toward new sounds, and will be startled if they're loud or unexpected. He'll enjoy the taste of your milk, and he'll love being cuddled, touched, and massaged.

Communicating Crying is his main way of communicating. He'll cry if he's hungry, tired, upset, bored, or lonely. He'll also cry if he senses that you or his father are tense or tired.

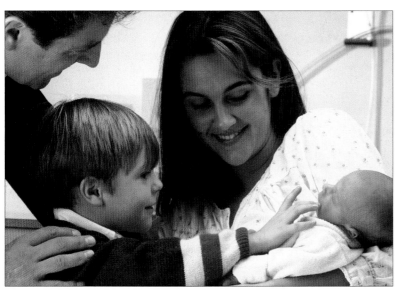

Family togetherness
Time spent cuddling, talking, and being together without everyday demands will give you a chance to adjust to the changes in your family.

Postnatal health

LOCHIA

While your uterus is contracting and getting back to its normal size and condition after delivery, you'll have a vaginal discharge known as lochia.

Lochia is the normal vaginal discharge from a healing uterus. The time it lasts varies from woman to woman—it can be anything from 14 days to six weeks, but the average is about 21 days. If you're breastfeeding, the lochia will end sooner, because the *oxytocin* that triggers the letdown reflex (see p.326) also causes uterine contractions; these help the uterus to shrink back to its normal size, cutting down on bleeding.

However long it lasts, lochia goes through three stages. For the first three or four days, the discharge is bright red. It then gradually reduces in quantity and changes to pink or brown as the uterine lining is shed, and by about the tenth day it becomes yellowish-white or colorless.

Lochia should have a fresh, blood-like odor. If it starts to smell bad, tell your doctor immediately because such a change is a sign of infection. Another warning sign is the flow becoming bright red again. This usually means that the placental site is not healing properly, perhaps because you're doing too much. Talk to your doctor, who'll probably suggest that you rest for a couple of days and generally take things easier.

Because there's a risk of infection, don't use tampons until about six weeks after delivery. Use sanitary napkins until the lochia flow ceases.

After your baby's been born, your body begins to reverse the changes it went through during pregnancy and labor. The withdrawal of the huge amounts of pregnancy hormones is like the withdrawal of a life force, and the time immediately after labor and delivery—known as the postnatal or *postpartum* period—can be very tiring for you. Take care of yourself—try to get as much rest and relaxation as you can and eat well. Make sure you have lots of healthy, fresh foods and plenty of liquid (at least two cups of milk a day and half a gallon of other liquids such as water or fruit juice). If you're breastfeeding, take good care of your breasts and nipples.

PELVIC AREA

After delivery, your uterus, cervix, vagina, and abdomen begin to shrink back to something like their prepregnancy and prelabor sizes. As your uterus shrinks, you'll have a vaginal discharge known as lochia (see column, left) and you'll feel some contractions or spasms called afterpains or afterbirth cramps.

Afterpains All women feel uterine contractions throughout their fertile lives. During a period these are known as menstrual cramps, during pregnancy as Braxton-Hicks contractions, and following delivery as afterpains. After delivery, uterine contractions are stronger and more painful than usual because your uterus is contracting down to its nonpregnant size. And the faster and harder it contracts down, the less likelihood there is of any bleeding. You usually notice afterpains more if you've had a child before, because the muscles of your uterus will have been stretched by your previous pregnancy and so have to work harder to help get your uterus down to its nonpregnant size. You may also feel these muscular spasms when you breastfeed, as the hormone oxytocin involved in the milk letdown reflex (see p.327) also causes uterine contractions. They usually disappear after three or four days.

Bowels and bladder It's best to get out of bed to use the toilet as soon as you possibly can after your baby's been born. But if you've emptied your bowels before delivery, you may not want to move them for 24 hours or more, and this is fine. When you do move your bowels, you may feel you want to bear down, and any pressure in the perineal region will stretch your tissues and be painful if you have a episiotomy wound (see column, right). To prevent stretching, hold a clean pad firmly against your stitches and press upward while you bear down. Do everything you can to avoid constipation and the need to strain. Eat lots of roughage, vegetables, and fruit, especially prunes and figs, and drink lots of water (see column, p.357).

Drinking plenty of water, as well as getting up and walking around, will help to get both your bowels and your bladder working normally. You may feel some hesitancy before your urine starts to flow for the first time after the birth. This is probably because your perineum and the tissues that surround your bladder and urethral opening are swollen, and it's nothing to worry about. A good way to start to pass urine is to sit in some water and try out the pelvic floor exercises (see p.148), passing urine into the water. This isn't unhygienic because urine is sterile—just wash yourself down afterward. You may find that turning on the bath faucet and letting it run while you sit on the toilet helps to trigger your flow of urine.

Cervix and vagina   These will have been stretched considerably during labor, and they'll be soft and slack for a while. It takes about a week for your cervix to narrow and firm up again, which it will do by itself, but you can help your vagina to recover by contracting and relaxing its muscles (pelvic floor exercises). It's a good idea to start these exercises within about 24 hours of giving birth. Begin with five contractions three times a day and gradually work up to five contractions 10 times a day if you can.

Exercise will also help to tone up your abdominal muscles again (see p.358), but don't start doing these until your flow of lochia has stopped.

Cesarean wound   If you've had a cesarean section, don't do any abdominal exercises until your wound has completely healed. Also, it's best to avoid lifting heavy weights; try not to climb stairs more than once a day; be careful how you move when you're getting up from a lying or sitting position; and generally try not to put too much strain or pressure on your abdominal muscles.

Hemorrhoids   *Hemorrhoids* or piles are quite common after childbirth. They appear as lumpy swellings just inside your anus, and they're caused by the great strain put on the veins in the pelvic floor during labor and delivery. Hemorrhoids will eventually shrink away with proper care—ask your healthcare provider what you should do to relieve any discomfort.

MENSTRUATION AND OVULATION

The dramatic fall in the levels of pregnancy hormones after the birth of your baby brings about the return of your periods and ovulation, as well as sometimes causing cold and hot flashes—you can even get both at once, which can be disconcerting.

Your periods will probably start again some time between the eighth and the sixteenth week after the delivery, but both menstruation and ovulation may be delayed much longer if you're breastfeeding your baby. If you want to begin making love again (see p.364) before your periods have started, remember that you'll ovulate before you get a period so it's important to use some form of contraception.

EPISIOTOMY WOUND

Unfortunately, the pain from an episiotomy wound gets worse before it gets better. The position of the wound means that fluid can collect in the cut edges. The skin then swells and the stitches become tighter and tighter, biting into the tender skin around the wound.

If you're bruised or if your stitches are really painful, you might find it helps to sit on an inflatable rubber ring, so try to keep one with you. Good hygiene is really important while the wound is healing, so make sure you keep it clean. Most stitches dissolve after five or six days.

Warm baths and showers, and special perineal pads that fit between your sanitary napkin and the wound, are soothing and help the healing process—so do pelvic floor exercises. Ice packs or local anesthetic creams can be helpful; your healthcare provider can advise you about these.

Don't use antiseptics in your bathwater—they can cause irritation. After you've had a bath, dry the wound area thoroughly with a hairdryer instead of using a towel, which would be uncomfortable.

If you sit down as usual when you use the toilet, urine, which is very acidic, will run over your episiotomy wound and make your raw skin sting. Standing up will probably help. You could also try standing in the bathtub or shower and pouring warm water over yourself as you're passing urine—this will dilute the acid and reduce the sting.

TIREDNESS

The first few weeks of caring for your newborn baby are very tiring, so it really helps to get as much rest and sleep as you can.

Rest whenever you get the chance, especially during the first week or so when you're still recovering from the exhaustion of labor. When your baby sleeps during the day, go for a rest or nap yourself—try not to waste these valuable opportunities for rest by using them to catch up on chores. Take advantage of any offers of help.

At night, go to bed half an hour or so before you plan on going to sleep, and unwind by sipping a warm, milky drink and listening to some music or the radio, or doing a little light reading to relax you physically and mentally before you sleep. If you're breastfeeding, express milk into bottles (see p.327) so that your partner can share the nighttime feeding duties just as he can if you're bottlefeeding.

Avoid climbing stairs and heavy lifting as much as possible, and encourage your partner to share in the care of your baby as well as household tasks. Eating well is important in keeping tiredness at bay, but don't eat too much late at night in case digesting your food interferes with your sleep pattern.

BREASTS AND NIPPLES

Your breasts will be bigger and heavier than usual, so you'll find a good quality, well-fitting cotton maternity bra both convenient and comfortable. Have several so you can wear a clean one every day. If you're using breast pads to prevent leaking milk from staining your clothes, avoid those that are lined or backed with plastic. Change pads after each feeding and whenever they're wet.

Cleaning and washing Clean your breasts and nipples every day with cotton balls and baby lotion or water. It's best not to use soap because it strips away the natural oils that protect the skin from drying and cracking, and can make a sore or cracked nipple worse. Always treat your breasts gently—don't rub them dry but carefully pat them dry instead.

There's no need to wash your nipples before or after each feeding, but before you fasten or put on your bra after feeding, let your nipples dry in the air. Always wash your hands before handling your breasts to prevent infection.

Engorgement Three or four days after you've given birth, your breasts will fill with milk. They'll become larger and heavier, and feel tender and warm when you touch them. They can get too full—this is called engorgement. Engorgement usually only lasts a day or two, but it can be uncomfortable and may happen again.

To ease engorged breasts, express some milk with your hands or by feeding your baby—you'll probably have to express a small amount of milk first so that he can latch on (see also pp.328 & 330). It also helps to bathe your breasts with warm water or cover them with warm towels, and to stroke them gently but firmly toward the nipple.

Engorgement can come back at any time during breastfeeding, particularly if your breasts are never thoroughly emptied or if your baby misses a feed.

Blocked ducts In the early weeks of breastfeeding you can get a blocked milk duct. This can be caused by engorgement, from a bra that is too tight, or from dried secretions on the nipple tip blocking a nipple opening. If you get a blockage, your breast will feel tender and lumpy and your skin may redden.

To clear a blocked duct, start feedings with your affected breast and gently massage it just above the sore area while feeding to ease the milk gently toward the nipple. If the blockage doesn't clear, don't offer the breast to your baby; check with your doctor immediately. Your breast could become infected and cause a breast abscess, which is painful, although not disastrous.

Sore nipples When you begin breastfeeding, your nipples may feel slightly tender for the first minute or so of suckling. This tenderness is quite normal, and it usually disappears after a few days. Sore nipples, though, are a common problem in the early weeks and can turn what should be a pleasure into something of an ordeal. The main causes of sore and cracked nipples are your baby not latching on properly and not being careful enough when taking your baby off your breast (see p.328). Taking care to start and finish feeding properly can prevent these problems, and is essential if nipples are to heal after they have become sore or cracked.

Sore nipples heal quickly when they are exposed to the air so, if possible, go topless or braless occasionally, especially when resting, in order to let the air circulate over them.

Cracked nipples If a sore nipple becomes cracked, you may need to keep your baby off that breast for up to 72 hours and express milk from the breast to prevent it from getting engorged. Cracked nipples can be very painful, and they can lead to breast infection. To help avoid cracked nipples, apply a drop of baby lotion to your breast pad.

Mastitis The first signs of mastitis (breast infection) are swelling, tenderness, and reddening of the affected area. You'll also have flulike symptoms, including a high temperature, chills, aches, headaches, and perhaps nausea and vomiting. If you think you've developed an infection, call your doctor. If it's treated promptly with antibiotics, mastitis usually improves within a day or so. The infection only affects your breast tissue, not your milk, so you can't pass it on to your baby.

PROTECTING SORE NIPPLES

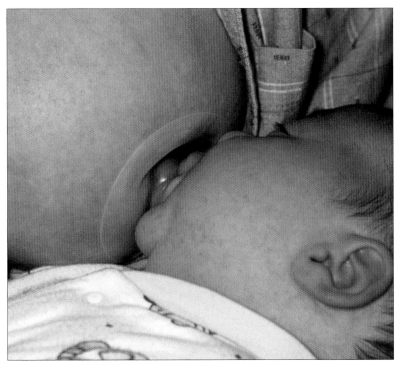

CONSTIPATION

Constipation is quite common after giving birth, but eating sensibly and drinking lots of fluids helps you deal with it.

After delivery, the passage of feces through your bowels tends to slow down, and this can lead to constipation. The slowing down happens mainly because your abdominal muscles are relaxed and stretched and so the pressure within your abdomen is lower than normal. Your bowel muscles might also be relaxed because of the high levels of progesterone during pregnancy. And if you've had an episiotomy you might, consciously or unconsciously, hold back from passing stools for fear of pain.

Medication, such as laxatives, stool softeners, or suppositories, can help get things moving again, but if you're breastfeeding, it is best to avoid taking any such drug by mouth. It can be passed on to your baby via your milk, and can cause stomach cramps and watery stools.

The best remedy for constipation (and a good way to prevent it) is to eat dried prunes or figs. It also helps to drink plenty of fluids; eat plenty of fiber-rich foods; and keep active. After your lochia discharge has stopped, do some exercises to tone up your abdominal muscles (see p.358) and do pelvic floor muscles exercises to return tone to your anal muscle and the anal sphincter.

Using a breast shield
If your nipples get sore, use breast shields to protect them during feeding. The shield fits over your nipple and the baby sucks through it. To ease your nipple into the shield, slip your hand between breast and rib cage and push gently upward. Your baby will soon get used to the feel and taste of the shield.

Postnatal exercises

FIRST DAYS

It's fine to do a few gentle exercises just days after giving birth. When you're lying down, or sitting in a chair, try to get into the habit of doing something to tone your muscles.

Start doing your pelvic floor exercises again (see p.148). Strengthening these will help to prevent incontinence.

To tone up your stomach muscles, pull them in as you breathe out, hold for a few seconds, then relax. Repeat whenever you can.

To prevent or reduce swelling in your ankles and feet, simply move your feet up and down as though you were pedaling a bicycle.

TAKE CARE

If you've had a cesarean, wait for 4–6 weeks before starting to exercise, and check with your doctor first. If you've had a tear or an episiotomy, don't practice stretching exercises until you've healed.

A few weeks after giving birth, try to get into the habit of doing some exercise every day. This may seem like an impossible task when you're faced with all the demands of being a new mother, but exercise will tone muscles that were stretched during pregnancy and delivery and help to give you more energy. You'll feel better about yourself, too.

You don't have to exercise for long—several short sessions are just as good, and easier to fit around the demands of caring for a new baby. Even 10 minutes here and there during the day will help. Take it carefully at first and don't exercise if you feel exhausted or unwell.

Side bends
Stand with your feet about 3 ft (1 m) apart. With your left hand on your thigh, slowly bend over to the left. Run your left hand down your leg as far as you can without straining, raise your right hand over your head, and breathe deeply. Hold your breath for a moment, then straighten up as you breathe out. Repeat the exercise, bending over to the right.

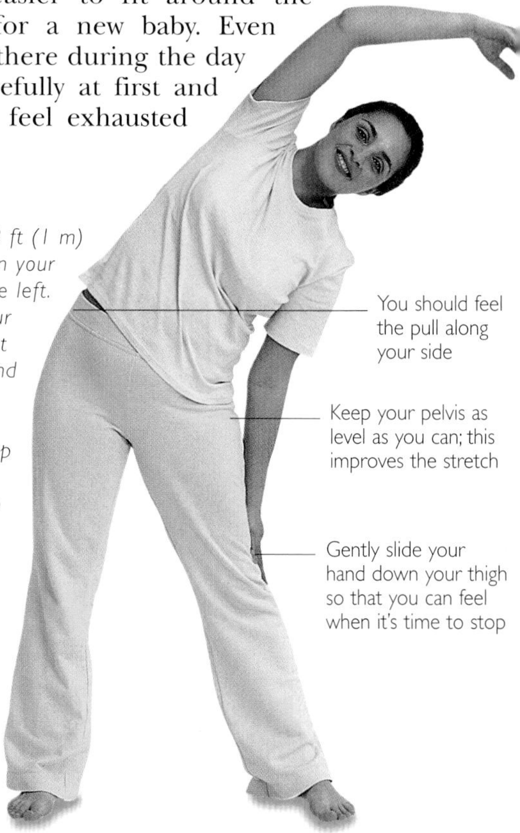

You should feel the pull along your side

Keep your pelvis as level as you can; this improves the stretch

Gently slide your hand down your thigh so that you can feel when it's time to stop

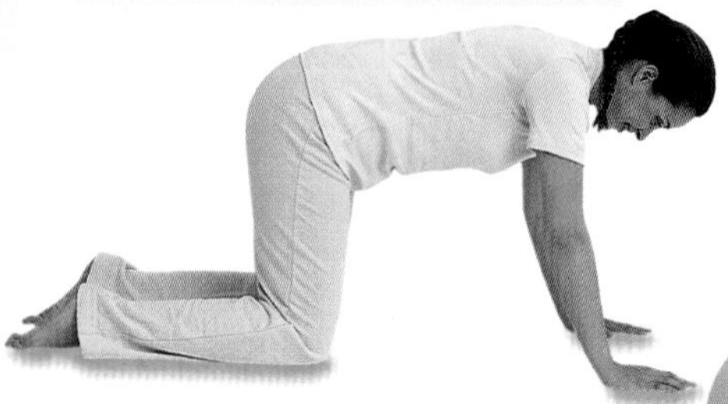

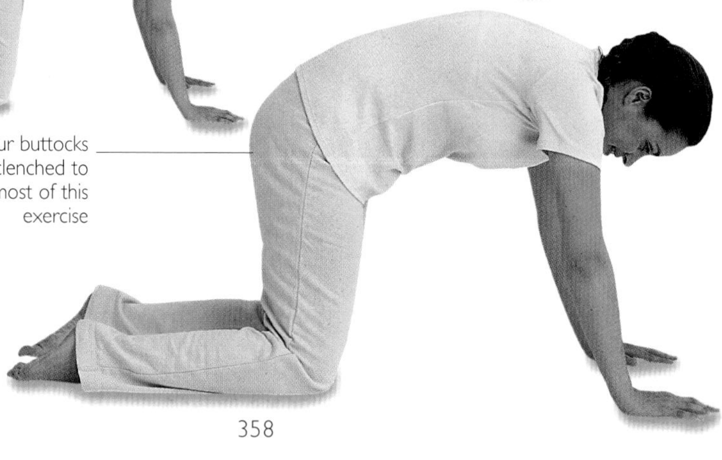

Keep your buttocks tightly clenched to make the most of this exercise

Pelvic tuck-in
You may have practiced this exercise before giving birth as it helps to correct the tilt of your pelvis. Kneel down on all fours with your knees about 12 in (30 cm) apart. Tighten your buttock muscles, tucking in your pelvis and arching your back upward into a hump. Hold for a few seconds, then release. Don't let your back sink downward. Repeat a few more times.

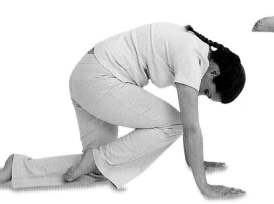

Stretch your neck and push your chin forward

Your thigh muscles contract and stretch in a steady rhythm

Cat arching
Kneel on all fours with your back straight. Breathing in, bend a leg up and lower your forehead toward your knee. Hold for a second. Breathing out, stretch, raising the leg behind you and lifting up your head. Hold for a few seconds, then change legs.

Keep knees bent and feet flat on the floor

Breathe out as you tense your stomach muscles

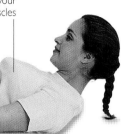

Abdominal toner
Lie on your back on the floor with your knees bent and your arms by your sides. Breathe deeply. As you breathe out, raise your head and arms, palms down. Hold for a couple of seconds, then relax. Repeat 10 times. You'll be able to lift your head higher with regular practice.

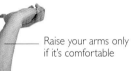

Raise your arms only if it's comfortable

Keep your back as straight as you can; this will make the exercise far more effective

Forward bend
Place your feet 12 in (30 cm) apart, keeping them parallel, and loosely clasp your hands behind your back. Keeping your back straight, bend slowly forward from your hips. Then raise your hands until they are as far above your head as you can possibly reach. Breathe deeply for a few breaths, then rise slowly and repeat.

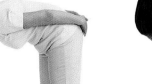

POSTNATAL CHANGES

After childbirth there's a sudden dramatic drop in your hormone levels. This is probably the main cause of the feelings known as baby blues and of postpartum depression.

Soon after you conceive, the levels of certain hormones in your body, especially progesterone and estrogen, rise steeply and stay high throughout your pregnancy. Then, during the first 72 hours after giving birth, the levels of these hormones crash.

The amount of progesterone in your blood falls from about 150 nanograms (thousand millionths of a gram) per milliliter to less than 7 ng/ml. The amount of estrogen falls from around 2,000 ng/ml to 20 ng/ml. After that, the amount of progesterone dwindles to zero and the estrogen settles down at about 10 ng/ml.

When the levels of estrogen and progesterone drop, your body finds it very difficult to adjust. This can affect your emotions and mental well-being, and, along with other factors, such as personal or relationship problems, can lead to baby blues or even postpartum depression. Eight in ten women experience baby blues, so don't be afraid to ask for help from family or friends, and tell your doctor.

Severe exhaustion, another possible postnatal problem, may be worse if you lack potassium. You can easily correct your potassium levels by eating plenty of potassium-rich foods such as bananas or tomatoes.

Your changing emotions

During the first days and weeks after the birth, you're likely to be very volatile emotionally because of the abrupt drop in your hormone levels (see column, left). And, because giving birth is such a major event in your life, it's likely to accentuate any underlying personal or emotional problems you may have, and to bring any unresolved issues to the surface. It's difficult to predict just how you will feel about the birth of your baby—sometimes an elated, trouble-free pregnancy can be followed by a low-key postnatal period.

The nature and severity of postnatal emotional problems and the length of time they last varies greatly from one woman to another, and from one pregnancy to another. A woman can be fine after the birth of one child, then have a rough time following the birth of the next one.

THE "BABY BLUES"

Because the most important single cause of emotional problems after a birth is the abrupt and unavoidable drop in hormone levels, don't be surprised if you suffer from the baby blues to some extent. As many as 80 percent of mothers do, so it's really the norm rather than the exception. Women who escape these feelings entirely are a very lucky minority. For the nine months of pregnancy, you've had very high levels of hormones, and suddenly they're plunged back to the comparatively low normal levels. This drastic swing makes most women weepy, susceptible to sudden mood swings, irritable, indecisive, and anxious.

The baby blues usually start about three to five days after the birth and last for about a week to 10 days. The onset often coincides with your milk coming in (which itself is governed by your changing hormones), and for this reason the baby blues used to be known as "milk fever."

Becoming a mother If you get the baby blues, you'll probably find that the reality of motherhood seems difficult to cope with once the initial euphoria of the birth wears off. As well as the symptoms mentioned above, you might feel confused, anxious about your ability to care for your baby, and frustrated because it seems to be taking you so long to learn to be a good mother. Be easy on yourself; no woman has the expertise for instant motherhood—it's something that only happens with time.

Relationship changes You might also find that you feel differently about your partner. This doesn't mean that you are feeling less for him, you're just feeling different. This isn't a sign that your relationship is deteriorating—it's more likely that eventually it will mature and become richer. One of the best ways to keep the stresses and strains of motherhood in perspective, and prevent them from turning into a serious emotional disturbance, is to talk things through openly with your partner and share your worries.

It's also important not to overdo things. Of course you'll be tired in the early days, but don't ignore your feelings. If you're tired, stop whatever you are doing if it's not essential, and lie down with your feet raised slightly above your head. You don't have to go to sleep to conserve your strength; a good rest may be all you need.

POSTPARTUM DEPRESSION

About 10 percent of all mothers develop postpartum depression. In many ways this is different and separate from the baby blues. Postpartum depression is longer-lasting, more serious, and needs rapid medical attention. It's a psychiatric disorder that can get out of hand if left untreated, and it's vital to get medical help early. With treatment, your depression should improve in a few weeks; the longer it is untreated, the longer it will take to resolve.

Symptoms   Postpartum depression has many symptoms, and different women experience these in varying combinations. As well as depressive symptoms, such as hopelessness and despondency, sufferers can experience lethargy, anxiety, tension, panic, sleep difficulties, loss of interest in sex, obsessional thoughts, feelings of guilt, and lack of self-esteem and concentration.

Treatment   Drugs will help you recover from postpartum depression, but you'll need lots of support from family and friends, too. There are also things you can do for yourself (see column, right). Your doctor will normally prescribe antidepressant drugs, taking breastfeeding into account. Over a period of time, these will bring about a gentle and gradual improvement, so it's important to keep taking your medication even after you start feeling better. Some drugs may have side effects such as a dry mouth, drowsiness, and confused thoughts. If you find that any of these side effects interfere with your daily life or upset you, ask your doctor about changing your medication.

If you find that your feelings of depression get worse before your period, tell your doctors. They may be able to prescribe further medication, such as progesterone suppositories or injections, to prevent this severe form of premenstrual syndrome.

PUERPERAL PSYCHOSIS

This rare psychotic form of postpartum depression affects about one in 1,000 mothers. The sufferer loses contact with reality, may experience delusions or hallucinations, and always has to spend some time in the hospital. Treatment may include drugs, psychotherapy, and/or electroconvulsive therapy.

SELF-HELP FOR DEPRESSION

If you're feeling low, there are things you can do to help yourself. The most important thing is to tell yourself that you will get better, no matter how long it takes.

Rest as much as you can. Being tired definitely makes depression worse and harder to cope with. Catnap during the day and, if possible, get someone to help with night feedings.

Eat well Have plenty of fruit and raw vegetables; don't snack or binge on chocolate and cookies. Eat little and often. Don't go on a strict diet.

Take gentle exercise Give yourself a rest from being indoors or taking care of the baby. Get out of the house, even for a short walk, either with or without the baby. The fresh air will make you feel better.

Avoid major upheavals Don't move house or redecorate.

Try not to worry unduly Aches and pains are common after childbirth, and more so if you're depressed. Try to take them in stride; they'll almost certainly fade away as soon as you can relax.

Be kind to yourself Don't force yourself to do things you don't want to do or that might upset you. Don't fret about housework—you don't have to keep things spotless at this time. Take on small, undemanding tasks, one at a time, and reward yourself when you finish them.

Talk about your feelings Don't bottle up your worries; this will only make matters worse. Talk to others, particularly your partner, about what you're going through.

The depressed mother

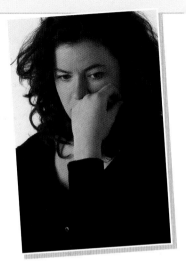

Case study

Name Christine Rance
Age 33 years
Past medical history Nothing abnormal
Obstetric history Three children, a boy aged four,
a girl aged two and a half, and a boy of four
months. All pregnancies and deliveries normal

Christine sailed through all her pregnancies, although afterwards she came
down with a crash. After the birth of her first baby, she went through
a short spell of "baby blues," although she recovered in a few days. After her
second baby was born, she felt tired and dejected for about two weeks. She
also put on a lot of weight, which she hasn't been able to lose. Three weeks
after the birth of this third baby, Christine's depressed and unable to cope.
Her doctor says she has postpartum depression.

Mild feelings of depression are not uncommon for a few days after a birth, but depressive feelings that deepen and last longer than about two weeks may be a sign of something more serious that needs medical treatment. Women with postpartum depression become increasingly withdrawn and lose touch with reality and their baby.

EARLY WARNING SIGNS

Christine's never been very good at handling changes in her life; she likes things to stay the same. She's always felt a little inferior and unsure of herself, doesn't have a particularly clear sense of her own identity, and lacks self-respect. Her weight has become a problem for her, particularly since she tends to overeat when she's depressed. She's put on weight with each pregnancy, which she's found increasingly difficult to lose. After her first pregnancy, she was almost 15 pounds overweight and it took a year to slim down. She then got pregnant with her second child, Laura, and the weight piled on again. After Laura's birth, she found it impossible to lose weight and in fact put on more in the first months of Laura's life than she had when she was pregnant.

Christine's husband, Stephen, often complains that she no longer looks like the woman he married, and Christine has been on countless diets to try to get herself back into shape, without success. She feels extremely self-conscious about her size, and tries to hide her figure in shapeless clothes. Sometimes she thinks that she hasn't been a very good mother, and she often worries about her maternal instincts.

FEELING HELPLESS

Christine is used to the feeling of baby blues and was expecting to feel sad after her third child. When depression set in it was almost a self-fulfilling prophecy. By the third day after the birth she was extremely weepy. The smallest problem was too much for her, and molehills became mountains. She started behaving in a helpless way, and refused to get out of bed.

Stephen's mother came to live with the family to take care of Thomas and Laura and to help with running the house. She tried to be helpful, but Christine did nothing but criticize her efforts. The atmosphere became tense, and Christine's mother-in-law tended to leave her alone rather than risk upsetting her.

Christine and Stephen then began to have arguments. Christine felt that Stephen didn't really understand her situation. She wanted him to take time off from work so he could support and comfort her. Stephen didn't really know what was going on and started to become depressed himself, so his work suffered.

Christine was so submerged in her own misery—at feeling so exhausted, hopeless, and guilty, at having three children to look after (especially as the two eldest had started to be difficult and misbehave), having to coordinate the household, and the tense relationships between herself and Stephen, and with her mother-in-law—that she could think of nothing else. She stopped communicating with her family and talked only to her baby. After a week of this, she found herself unable to even relate to baby Oliver, and began thinking of the awful things she could do to keep him from crying. She didn't care about feeding him anymore, and started to let him scream, instead of picking him up.

HELP IS OFFERED

After about two weeks of Christine's increasing depression, during which her midwife reassured her that everything would get better soon, she finally realized that Christine's reactions were far from normal and that she needed help. She contacted Christine's doctor and made an appointment for Christine to visit him three weeks after the delivery. He diagnosed early postpartum depression and referred her to a therapist specializing in new mothers suffering from depression.

About two weeks after her first visit to the therapist, Christine started to improve, mainly because of the advice that he gave her. First, he suggested she forget what was happening in the rest of the house. She should think only about her baby and herself and let everything else take care of itself. Second, he advised her to let someone else take care of her baby overnight so she could get a full night's sleep. Third, he suggested that she should attend group therapy sessions twice a week, where she could talk to other women who were going through a similar experience. He also advised her to contact DAD (Depression After Delivery – see Addresses, p.370), for additional advice and support.

Christine's doctor prescribed an antidepressant and a mild sleeping pill to tide her over the first few difficult weeks. He said that he'd continue to give her antidepressants after this, and they agreed that he'd reduce the dosage gradually as soon as Christine felt able to take charge of herself and her life.

YOUR PARTNER'S ROLE

There's quite a lot of research that shows that a crucial factor in determining whether a woman succumbs to postpartum depression is having a supportive and helpful partner; second is an understanding family. So I suggested to Christine that she and Stephen might think of ways that he could take the pressure off her. There are many ways in which he could really help, such as:
• hold Christine close and tell her that he's proud of her
• stay with Christine and Oliver whenever possible, hold them both, or feed Oliver for Christine
• get used to carrying Oliver around the house in a baby sling whenever he's at home
• do the shopping, run errands, and cook whenever he can
• take Oliver with him whenever he goes out to give Christine a real break
• take the children out as much as possible so that Christine can have plenty of time to be by herself.

FUTURE LOOKS BRIGHT

After six weeks, Christine was sleeping so much better that she asked her doctor to go off the sleeping pills. She's continuing to take the antidepressant medication and is determined to cut down the dose over the next four weeks and be free of it in another six. Stephen feels much happier now that she is almost back to normal, and the children, too, are more relaxed.

Christine's children

No permanent harm will have been done to Christine's ability to bond with her baby, and once she started to feel better, she was able to rebuild her relationships with her older children.

• However, while she was feeling depressed and was unable to give them much attention, her children became anxious and constantly acted out their frustrations. They rebelled against their grandmother's care, and made more demands on their parents' attention and affection.

• In cases of postpartum depression, children can get support, either before or after their mother has improved, from therapists and child psychologists. Friends who have gone through similar experiences may also be able to help.

BIRTH CONTROL

When you want to start making love again after the birth you'll need to decide on what form of contraception to use. Ovulation could start at any time.

If you start making love before your periods have come back, don't assume that you won't get pregnant because you're not menstruating. You'll ovulate two weeks before your first period, so if you put off using contraception until after that, you may have waited too long. Even when you're breastfeeding your baby, and your periods won't start until you wean her, you may still ovulate, so you could get pregnant if you don't use any contraception.

Contraception If you're breastfeeding, you won't be given pills containing estrogen—estrogen reduces milk production. You may be prescribed progestogen-only "mini-pills" instead. These don't affect milk production, but their long-term effects on babies aren't yet known. Some experts think they may also make any postpartum depression worse because they inhibit the natural production of progesterone.

If you're breastfeeding, you might prefer to avoid the pill and use a different kind of contraception, such as condoms with contraceptive gel or cream. If you want to use a diaphragm or an IUD (coil), you'll have to wait until your six-week checkup before you can get one. If you used a diaphragm before your pregnancy, you'll need to be fitted for a new one because your cervix may have enlarged and your old diaphragm may no longer fit. Use condoms and spermicidal cream until you can get your new diaphragm or IUD.

Making love again

You probably won't feel like making love in the first days, or even weeks, after giving birth. The sheer physical exhaustion of labor and the drastic changes in your hormone levels after delivery combine to lessen sexual desire. A lack of interest in sex at first is both natural and desirable, because your body needs time to recover from the changes and stresses of pregnancy and childbirth, and you need time to adjust to your new baby. Talk to your partner—you'll probably find that he's totally sympathetic and understanding.

YOUR PARTNER

Your partner's libido may also be affected by the arrival of your baby; it's not uncommon for a new father to feel a lack of desire and even to lose his ability to maintain an erection. He might also find it difficult to adjust to his and your dual, sometimes contradictory, roles as parents and lovers.

It'll help if you're both aware that there may be such problems and you don't take them personally. The best solution is to be philosophical and open about these things, and discuss them lovingly and sympathetically. This will stop them from developing into long-term difficulties.

WHEN TO START AGAIN

Couples differ greatly as to when they feel like starting to make love again after the birth of a child. Your feelings may even differ from one pregnancy to another. A woman might have been eager to have sex three weeks after one pregnancy, but have no interest in it for three months or more after the next one.

Many couples also worry about when it's physically safe for intercourse to take place. At one time, couples were advised to give up sex six weeks before the expected date of delivery and not to start again until six weeks afterward (until after the six-week checkup). The general opinion today is that the old advice was overcautious and you can go on having penetrative sex as long as you want—provided there are no medical reasons to avoid it (see p.234)—and you can begin again as soon as you like. You can also have nonpenetrative sex as soon as you like after giving birth. If you or your partner are at all unsure about whether it's safe to make love again, talk to your doctor or obstetrician.

If you're both happy about it, and there's no medical objection, you can start making love again as soon as you feel the desire to. This can be a good idea for a number of reasons. For one thing, lovemaking reaffirms your affection and desire for one another and so helps strengthen your relationship at what can be a difficult time. Also, the hormones that are released during sexual activity cause contractions of your uterus, which help it to return to its prepregnant state.

LACK OF DESIRE

Don't worry about loss of libido—it's natural after childbirth. But there are some things that can affect both your desire for and your enjoyment of postnatal sex. Apart from any lingering discomfort you might feel, it's quite common to feel unattractive at first, and this can make you shy away from sex or think negatively. If your still-bulging tummy is making you feel unsexy, try to start doing some exercises to get back into shape (see p.358). Exercise will help your self-esteem, and pelvic floor exercises will help to reduce the slackness of your vagina.

You may also have anxieties and distractions that lessen your sexual desire or enjoyment. Perhaps you're afraid of getting pregnant again or worried about coping with birth control again. Even your baby can affect your enjoyment of lovemaking—it can be hard to adjust to this new presence in the house. You may not feel as free as before or as able to abandon yourself, and it may be harder to relax and enjoy lovemaking because you half expect your baby to cry for attention at any time. You can also find that you get so absorbed with your baby that you have little need for other emotional ties or physical contact—even with your partner. Even your sexual responses may become focused on your baby because oxytocin, the hormone that's produced during breastfeeding, is sexually stimulating. During a feeding a woman can be stimulated up to and even including orgasm.

ENJOYING SEX AGAIN

It can take a while for you both to get back to your previous level of sexual interest. You may need to spend more time on fondling, kissing, and other foreplay before you become sexually aroused. For the first few times you make love, it's best to avoid penile penetration and stick to gentle oral or manual sex. And because an episiotomy site can be surprisingly painful during intercourse and may take months to become totally pain-free, please be honest with your partner and tell him if sex causes you discomfort or pain. Getting him to touch your scar will help him to understand how you feel and be sympathetic. Taking a warm bath before lovemaking and using a water-soluble vaginal lubricant or saliva can be a great help.

Whether or not you've had an episiotomy, you'll probably need extra lubrication. Until your hormone levels are back to normal, your vagina won't lubricate itself as quickly as in prebirth days, no matter how much foreplay you have. Avoid non-water-soluble lubricants such as petroleum jelly because they can prevent air from reaching the lining of your vagina and encourage the growth of harmful bacteria.

When you start making love again, you may well find that man-on-top positions are uncomfortable. Experiment with other positions (see p.234)—side-by-side positions are especially good to try if you're suffering from a sore episiotomy site. Whichever positions you use, be patient, don't do too much at first, and build up your sexual activity again gradually.

POSTNATAL CHECKUPS

Your last visit to your obstetrician will be about six weeks after delivery, when you'll be thoroughly checked.

Your checkup At your visit, you'll be weighed and your blood pressure will be checked. Your breasts may be examined for lumps, although this isn't always done if you're breastfeeding, because lumps aren't easy to distinguish from milk glands. You'll have a pelvic examination to check that, among other things, an episiotomy has healed well, your cervix is closed, and your uterus is back to normal. The doctor will usually ask you how you're feeling emotionally and how you're coping. It's also a good time to talk about future methods of contraception and get a diaphragm or an IUCD if you want one.

Your baby's first checkup This will usually be a separate visit. The doctor will check your baby's ears, eyes, limbs, and muscle tone, listen to his heartbeat, check his control over his head movements, and check for hip displacements. His head circumference will be measured and he'll be weighed. His weight will be recorded on his chart every time he goes to the clinic after this, and the chart will be an important record of how he's developing.

MAKE TIME FOR YOURSELVES

It's important to find some time in your daily routine when you and your partner can be alone together. This will help keep your relationship alive and well.

At home Keep up the small rituals of your daily life together. If you've always made the time to catch up with each other's news at the end of the work day, shared a bath or the crossword puzzle in the evenings, or simply spent time watching TV, continue to do so. Not only are these ways of spending precious time together as a couple, they'll also help you keep some normality in your everyday lives.

Going out Your new baby's surprisingly easy to take along in the first few months of her life, but you'll also need time together without your baby. Ask someone you really trust to babysit. If you're breastfeeding, express your milk so that your baby can be fed while you're out. It may seem difficult or too much hassle to organize but persevere. It's important for you and your partner to have time together away from your baby.

As a couple If you want to learn a new sport or skill, or take up an old one again, why not plan to do it together now? Setting aside two or three hours every week to do something as a couple will make sure that you have time together as individuals rather than always as parents.

Changes to your lifestyle

Many people underestimate just what's involved in caring for a new baby. It's a demanding and exhausting job that can turn your lives upside down. You'll probably find yourself wondering whether you and your partner will ever be able to spend time together again. Fitting in all the demands on your time and energy can be difficult, but if you approach the situation sensibly and make plans together before the birth, you should be able to cope with the disruption and manage to spend some time alone. It takes planning, but it's possible.

KEEPING ON TOP OF IT ALL

Taking care of your newborn baby will probably be much harder than you ever expected. For one thing, labor and birth are physically and emotionally draining; for another, you'll find that in the first days, there always seems to be one job after another, almost without a break.

Getting enough rest is vital. It's rare for a new baby to allow you more than four hours' sleep at a time at night, so it helps if you can catnap during the day. You need to eat well, too, especially if you're breastfeeding. Keep eating as well as you did throughout your pregnancy, and drink plenty of fluid.

Taking shortcuts, such as occasionally buying convenience foods, at least for the first few months, will help you manage, as will getting your priorities right—getting enough rest, for example, is far more important than cleaning the house.

Avoid guilt Feeling guilty seems to be a burden carried by most new parents and quite a few well-established parents. Remember that you can only do your best, and that it's important to put yourself and your own health high on your list of priorities. Bear in mind, too, that it takes about a year for your body to get back to its prepregnancy state. Don't expect too much of yourself at first, because just after delivery you'll find that you have very little stamina and you'll get exhausted easily.

Find a routine This doesn't mean training your baby to eat, sleep, and play according to your timetable but following his lead and fitting your life around his daily routine. You won't necessarily have to rearrange your entire lives to accommodate him; much of your routine and lifestyle can continue as before.

APPRECIATE YOUR NEW ROLES

At first, it may be more difficult than you'd thought to settle into your new roles as parents. If you're on maternity leave and at home for while while your partner's gone back to work, you may find yourself resenting his relatively free and independent lifestyle. Your partner, on the other hand, may feel shut out from your intimate relationship with your baby. He may also feel envious of your being at home, especially if he doesn't appreciate how demanding a baby can be.

These different experiences can leave you wondering where the closeness and intimacy of pregnancy went, and also whether you will ever get back to the easy understanding you had before you became pregnant. You will, but you need to keep talking to each other. Explain your thoughts and feelings, and try not to let little misunderstandings alienate you from each other. When your partner is at home, don't cut him off from your baby. Let him take over some of the care and give you a break.

MAKING TIME FOR YOURSELVES

One of the most difficult changes to manage is lack of time. Most of your waking and sleeping hours will be devoted to the care of your new baby at first. This can be frustrating and might make you feel resentful. If you can keep up some of your contacts with friends, continue with as much of your usual lifestyle as you can, and keep the lines of communication open between you and your partner, it'll go a long way toward helping you cope with the various conflicting demands on your time and energy.

Sharing Doing things together is especially important once you have a baby. Your infant is easy to take with you, so don't hesitate to include him in your plans. He can come along when you visit friends, and you may be surprised at how easy it is to keep up your social life in the first few months of his life.

You also need time together alone and, although it may seem odd having to make a formal appointment to spend time with your partner, it really can help you to keep up a healthy relationship. One of the problems you'll have following the birth of your first child is that the spontaneity you had as a free and easy couple tends to get lost, so planning to spend time together becomes even more important. It needn't be elaborate—it could be something as simple as always having a cup of decaf and a chat together at the end of the day, or planning to go swimming, jogging, or walking together for an hour or two every Sunday while a friend or relative cares for your baby.

Time alone We all need time and space to recharge our batteries. When you have a baby it's very easy to get so caught up in the never-ending round of babycare that you lose sight of this need.

It's important to have at least a few hours every week when you can just please yourself—whether on a special outing, seeing a friend, or doing something you enjoy. Make an arrangement with someone you trust to babysit for you—your partner, a close friend, or a relative. You'll be all the better for it, and your baby will also benefit from social contact with other people.

SHARING YOUR BABY'S CARE

You'll get lots of offers from friends and relatives to babysit. Take advantage of these and let others help you take care of the baby.

Father As far as your baby's concerned, her father is the second most important person in her life after you. Daddy can do anything that Mommy can—he can even give breast milk in a bottle—so encourage your partner to take equal responsibility for the care of your baby.

Grandparents They're usually itching to help and thoroughly experienced in childrearing, so can be the ideal people to help with babysitting and general babycare. Both grandparents and your baby will relish the contact, and this will help them to form strong bonds of affection from the very beginning.

Relatives and friends Your relatives will probably enjoy helping you care for the new addition to the family. Friends may also be enthusiastic about babycare—and the ones who've already had children can be invaluable support. Always make sure that non-parents or young assistants know how to handle a baby properly, but try not to watch so closely or anxiously that you make them feel uncomfortable—young babies are more resilient than they look.

The new father

Case study

Names James and Sarah Blake
Age 34 and 30 respectively
Past medical history Nothing abnormal
Obstetric history Sarah recently gave birth to a
baby girl, Emma

Emma is James and Sarah's first baby. She was a born in the hospital one day
before Sarah's due date. The medical staff had undertaken routine
examinations and decided that the baby was "small for dates." They advised
James and Sarah that it was better to induce the birth rather than wait for
nature to take its course. James had been to prenatal classes for dads and was
at Sarah's side throughout the birth.

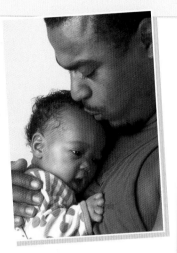

*During Sarah's pregnancy, James wanted to find
out all he could about pregnancy, childbirth,
and parenthood. He and Sarah read books,
attended prenatal classes, and got hands-on
experience with friends' children. But they
discovered that nothing totally prepares you
for parenthood and that you need to be
adaptable and flexible.*

LABOR AND BIRTH

To induce the birth Sarah was given a prostaglandin
suppository. About three hours later, she was feeling
waves of substantial pain and couldn't sit down. In
another two hours, she was in tremendous and constant
pain, which James found very upsetting. There was very
little he could do to help—nothing he'd learned in
class about breathing or massage seemed appropriate,
especially since Sarah's pain was constant, and she felt
compelled to keep moving around.

Sarah was admitted to a delivery room just before
seven in the evening. Fortunately, the constant pain
began to resolve itself into definite, spaced contractions,
so James was able to anticipate them and comfort her.
It still makes him wince to think about how the midwife
broke Sarah's water with a big blue plastic hook.

The next part of the labor was a bit of a blur for both
of them, with just 40 seconds between contractions that
each lasted about a minute. At 8:30 p.m. Sarah was
asked whether she wanted more pain relief, and she was
given an injection of Demerol. However, the remaining
dilation was quick and the baby's head began to crown
before the pain medication took effect.

At around 9 p.m. the midwife decided that Sarah
needed an episiotomy to avoid possible distress to the
baby. James will never forget the sound of the snipping.
And suddenly, at 9:13, they had a new baby girl. She was
given straight to Dad, who held her for a few seconds
before giving her to Mom, where she started to suckle
immediately. James can't remember whether he cut the
cord—he thinks the midwife did it. The baby weighed a
healthy 6 lb 8 oz (2.9 kg). Not being squeamish, James
watched the placenta being delivered and the
episiotomy being stitched up again. There was quite a
lot of blood, but Sarah didn't seem to mind.
Thinking back, Sarah thinks that physically, she got off
fairly lightly—labor and birth were relatively short and
free of complications. Emotionally, though, both
parents were shattered—a state of elation and mild
shock that lasted for about two weeks.

IN THE HOSPITAL

James had to go home by about midnight, leaving Sarah
and Emma in the maternity ward. He was back the next
morning to see how Mom and daughter were coming
along. Sarah stayed a second night in the hospital
because she'd chosen to breastfeed and needed help
getting it started. The staff gave lots of advice and help,
and Sarah and Emma were discharged from the hospital
after a successful feeding around noon on day two.

BACK HOME

Taking Emma home was a scary moment for James and Sarah, since she seemed so tiny and fragile, but everything went smoothly. Sarah's stitches took time to heal, and she had to rest as much as she could. James took two weeks off work, which was great because there was so much for them both to get used to.

They had lots of visitors in the first two weeks, which, looking back, they decided was overdoing it. I usually recommend limiting visitors if at all possible—people are very understanding.

SLEEPING

At first, Emma woke about every three hours and was breastfed on demand, so Sarah in particular didn't get very much sleep. Emma wasn't a bad sleeper, though, and after about three months her sleeping patterns began to settle down so she generally woke just once in the night. Because she was breastfeeding, Sarah was usually the one who got up to see to Emma in the night, though James was nearly always woken up, too.

Throughout the night Emma would make lots of coughing noises and grunts in her sleep. After a few days of this, James couldn't sleep in the same room, so he slept on the couch for several weeks until Emma was ready to sleep in her own room. He felt bad about it, but fortunately Sarah was understanding. Emma only began sleeping through the night after eight months.

WHO DOES WHAT?

James helps however he can. Sarah concentrates on the feeding and cooking, and James generally does the laundry and bathing, cleans up messes, and deals with the nastiest diapers. Sieving poop out of the bathtub is the latest in a long series of new experiences for him.

From early on, they came to an agreement that James shouldn't expect any thanks from Sarah for doing things that just need doing—they're in this together. This is a very sound thing to have decided. Good communication is essential between new parents, and roles and responsibilities often need to be talked through carefully.

Sarah didn't have a job to go back to, so she has been at home since the birth. James is lucky to have an employer who allows him to be relatively flexible in his working hours. He's also been able to take time off to care for Sarah when she's been ill (she had mastitis twice) and to help take the baby for her vaccinations.

BEING PARENTS

James feels that when he watches his baby making her mark in the world, he doesn't miss their past life. Neither of them goes out as much in the evenings now, if at all. Because caring for Emma is such hard work, they're usually too tired anyway.

Overall, being parents has been an amazing experience for James and Sarah—as well as giving them lifetime membership of a wonderful new club. Everyone else who's had children understands what it's like and—more than likely—offers advice and help. Support often comes from surprising directions—not least from other new parents—and they both say that despite the hard work, every smile from their baby and every grin from a granny in the supermarket make it all worthwhile.

James and Sarah's baby

James decided that he wanted to be as involved as possible in his baby's life right from the start. She's pretty much a full-time occupation when he's not at work, but he wouldn't have it any other way. There are lots of things he can do.

• Now that Emma is being weaned on cow's milk instead of breast milk, James is getting up earlier to give her breakfast before he goes to work.

• James is able to get home in time to give Emma a bath and cuddle her at bedtime. Then he and Sarah have some much-needed time to themselves.

• Emma loves being with her father on weekends, and James is good at organizing baby-friendly activities—walks in the country, a trip to the beach, or just sitting in the backyard playing games.

• Sarah is at home during the day with Emma, and James understands that she needs an evening off once in a while to see friends.

Useful addresses

American Academy of Husband-Coached Childbirth (Bradley)
P.O. Box 5224
Sherman Oaks, CA 91413
(800) 422-4784
www.bradleybirth.com
Coaching information for parents

American College of Nurse Midwives
8403 Colesville Road, Suite 1550
Silver Spring, MD 20910
(240) 485-1800
www.midwife.org
Nurse midwives organization; will provide directory of practices

American College of Obstetricians and Gynecologists
P.O. Box 96920
Washington, DC 20090-6920
(202) 638-5577
www.acog.org
Obstetricians' and gynecologists' organization; has informational pamphlets for the general public

American Diabetes Association
1701 North Beauregard Street
Alexandria, VA 22311
(703) 549-1500
www.diabetes.org
Publications and an informational hotline for diabetic pregnant women

American Foundation for Maternal and Child Health
(212) 759-5510

American Society for Reproductive Medicine
1209 Montgomery Highway
Birmingham, AL 35216-2809
(205) 978-5000
www.asrm.org
Conducts research into various aspects of infertility; informational booklets available

Cascade HealthCare Products
1826 NW 18th Avenue
Portland, OR 97209
(800) 443-9942
www.1cascade.com
Catalogs on birthing supplies, baby products, baby clothes, and more

Cesareans/Support Education and Concern (C/SEC)
22 Forest Road
Framingham, MA 01701
(508) 877-8266
Cesarean birth information

Depression After Delivery (DAD)
P.O. Box 278
Belle Mead, NJ 08502-0278
(800) 944-4733
www.depressionafterdelivery.com
Information and support for PPD

First Candle/SIDS Alliance
1314 Bedford Avenue, Suite 210
Baltimore, MD 21208
(800) 221-7437
www.sidsalliance.org
Research group provides information, support services, and counseling

InterNational Association of Parents & Professionals for Safe Alternatives in Childbirth
Route 4, Box 646
Marble Hill, MO 63764
(573) 238-2010
www.napsac.org
Alternative childbirth information

La Leche League International
1400 N. Meacham Road
Schaumburg, IL 60173-4808
(847) 519-7730
www.lalecheleague.org
Breastfeeding help and information

Lamaze International
2025 M Street NW, Suite 800
Washington, DC 20036
(800) 368-4404
www.lamaze.org
For parents and doctors interested in Lamaze method of childbirth

March of Dimes Birth Defects Foundation
1275 Mamaroneck Avenue
White Plains, NY 10605
(914) 428-7100
www.modimes.org
Fights various birth defects

Maternity Center Association
281 Park Avenue South, 5th Floor
New York, NY 10010
(212) 777-5000
www.maternitywise.org
Birthing center

Midwives Alliance of North America
375 Rockbridge Road, Suite 172-313
Lilburn, GA 30047
(888) 923-MANA
www.mana.org
Midwives organization; will provide directory of midwives

National Association of Childbearing Centers
3123 Gottschall Road
Perkiomenville, PA 18074
(215) 234-8068
www.birthcenters.org
Information on birthing centers in parents' area and how to select one

National Healthy Start Association, Inc.
P.O. Box 25227
Baltimore, MD 21229-0327
(410) 525-1600
www.healthystartassoc.org
Promotes community-based maternal and child health programs

National Women's Health Network
514 10th Street NW, Suite 400
Washington, DC 20004
(202) 347-1140
www.womenshealthnetwork.org
Advocacy group for women's health and rights issues

North American Vegetarian Society
P.O. Box 72
Dolgeville, NY 13329
(518) 568-7970
www.navs-online.org
Articles on healthy vegetarian eating, lists of events, and helpful links

Parents of Premature Babies Inc. (Preemie-L)
www.preemie-l.org
Provides support to families and caregivers of premature babies

Peaceful Beginnings
29 School Street
Limerick, ME 04048
(800) 370-1683
www.midwifesupplies.com
Provides products for midwives, mothers, and babies

SIDS Alliance
See entry for First Candle/SIDS Alliance, above

Slowlane.com
1216 East Lee Street
Pensacola, FL 32503
(850) 434-2626
www.slowlane.com
Online resource dealing with issues of fathering, family and being a stay-at-home dad

Index

A

Abnormalities in babies: fetal problems 196–203
  genetic 24–5
  tests for 184–9
Abortion 189
  spontaneous see Miscarriage
Acrosome test 41
Acupuncture 283
AFP (alphafetoprotein) test 184–5, 189
Afterpains 354
Age of mother 17, 34, 185
AIDS 17, 19
Air travel 171
Alcohol 16–17
Amenorrhea 60
Amniocentesis 185–6, 189
Amniotic fluid 77, 87, 89, 192, 267, 273
Amniotic sac 72, 87, 231
Amniotomy 109, 301
Anemia, in fetus 187, 200
Anesthesia: cesarean delivery 99
  epidural 274, 281–2, 303, 308, 309
Animals, safety 169
Antibodies: in colostrum 246
  fetal blood transfusions 201
  fetus 89
  infertility 39, 43
  Rhesus incompatibility 202–3
Anus, imperforate 196
Apgar score 292
Areola 66, 74, 158
ART (assisted reproduction technology) 48–57
Asthma 18
Au pairs 255

B

Babies: bathing 99, 340–1
  bonding with 92, 94, 99
  death 312–13
  delivery 284–7
  diapers 336–9
  feeding 246–7, 326–35
  first hours 292–3
  first weeks 352–3
  health 342–3
  holding and handling 324–5
  newborn baby 316–21
  premature babies 299
  preparing for 240–61
  registering birth 323
  sleep 102
  special care babies 344–9
Baby blues 100, 360–1, 362
Baby carriers 242
Baby chairs 243
Backache 206–7
  avoiding 69, 85, 160, 163, 207
  causes 69, 85
  in labor 272, 279, 282, 283, 296
Backpacking 145
Baths: bathing baby 99, 340–1
  in pregnancy 169

Bearing down 284–5, 286, 290, 304
Bilirubin 187, 203, 342
Birth see Childbirth
Birth plans 67, 95, 122–3, 274
Birthing centers 114–115, 264–265
Birthing pools 107, 282
Birthing rooms 119
Birthing stools 285
Birthmarks 318
Blastocysts 32, 33, 72, 224
Bleeding: after delivery 291
  clots 322
  placenta 222
  vaginal 218, 219, 237
Blood cells, fetal 77
Blood pressure 70, 178, 208–9, 224, 226
Blood tests 61, 71, 177–8, 322
Blood transfusions, intrauterine 200, 201
Body care 158–61
Bonding 293, 352
  fathers 92, 94, 99, 293
  premature babies 347, 349
Bottlefeeding 246, 247, 332–5
  and bowel movements 337
  equipment 332
  measuring and mixing formula 333
  and newborn health 342, 343
  sterilizing equipment 333
Bowel movements: after delivery 354–5, 357
  baby 337
  fetus 89
  in pregnancy 68
Bradley method 112
Brain, fetal problems 197–8
Bras: maternity 67, 330, 356
  in pregnancy 163
Braxton-Hicks contractions 71, 87, 270–1, 354
Breast pads 330, 356
Breast shields 357
Breastfeeding 246–7, 323, 326–30
  and bowel movements 337
  breast care 330
  and contraception 364
  on demand 326
  expressing milk 257
  latching on 327, 329
  maintaining milk supply 326–7
  and newborn health 342, 343
  refusal 327
  switching to bottlefeeding 334
Breasts: blocked ducts 356
  bras 67, 163, 330, 356
  care of 330, 356
  colostrum 85
  engorgement 327, 356
  mastitis 357
  newborn baby 318
  painful 212–13, 237
  in pregnancy 61, 66, 72, 74, 176, 230
Breathing: fetus 83, 85
  in labor 107, 277, 282, 284, 289
  newborn baby 293, 305, 321
  in pregnancy 66, 70, 81
  premature babies 299, 347, 349
Breech birth 110, 307
Breech position 87, 259
Burping baby 335

C

Calcium 133, 134, 135, 136, 137
Calories 128, 132, 137, 246
Candida albicans 212–13
Car seats 242
Car travel 171, 267
Carbohydrates 132, 134
Carpal tunnel syndrome 206–7
Caudal anesthesia 281
Cerebral palsy 198
Cervix: after delivery 355
  dilatation 109, 272–3, 274, 297
  incompetent 219, 223
  mucus plug 72, 231, 237, 267, 271
  sutures 223
Cesarean section 308–11
  anesthesia 282, 309
  emergency 309, 310–11
  fathers and 98–9
  stitches 309, 311, 322–3
  wound 322, 355
Chemicals, safety 169, 170
Chickenpox 170
Childbirth/labor:
  birth plans 67, 95, 122–3, 274
  birthing centers 114–115, 264–265
  cesarean section 308–11
  choices in 106–25
  classes 124–5
  comfort aids 268–9
  contentious issues 108–10
  expected arrival date 62–3
  fathers at 95, 96–9
  fears 155
  first stage 272–9
  home birth 304–305
  hospital birth 116–19, 265, 266–7, 274–5
  induction of labor 109, 300–3, 368
  length of labor 110, 125, 273
  managed birth 107
  natural birth 106–7
  pain relief 280–3
  partner's role 276–7, 288–9
  philosophies 112–13
  positions 278–9, 282
  prelabor 270–1
  second stage 284–9
  "special deliveries" 306–13
  special types of labor 296–9
  sudden birth 99, 267, 304–5
  third stage 290–1
  twins 182
  in water 107
  see also Delivery
Childcare 254–5, 256
Children (siblings): and new baby 353
  preparing for new baby 252–3
Chlamydia 37, 43, 44
Chloasma 158–9
Chorion 72, 77
Chorionic villus sampling (CVS) 186–7, 189
Chromosomes 22–3
  chorionic villus sampling 186
  disorders 24, 25, 198
  fertilization 32

Chromosomes *(continued)*
  infertility 38
  sex chromosomes 31, 33
Circulation: fetus 76
  in pregnancy 74, 77
Cleft lip and palate 197
Clomiphene 42, 46, 50
Clothes: baby 71, 244–5, 266
  in pregnancy 67, 162–3
Club foot (talipes) 199
Cognitive control, pain relief 125
Colic 343
Colostrum 321
  antibodies 246, 326
  breastfeeding 330
  nutritional value 326
  in pregnancy 68, 85
  premature babies 344, 349
Conception 28–35
  problems 34–57
Constipation 68, 71, 206–7, 343, 354, 357
Contraception: after delivery 355, 364
  and breastfeeding 327
  stopping 17
Contractions: afterpains 354
  Braxton-Hicks 71, 87, 270–1, 354
  delivery 284, 285
  false labor 272
  first stage 272
  induction of labor 301, 303
  pain 280
  prelabor 265, 266, 267
  premature labor 299
Cordocentesis 187, 189, 203
Corpus luteum 28, 29, 72, 230
Cortisone 89
Counseling: genetic 24, 26–7
  infertility 35, 37, 48, 54, 57
Cramps 206–7
Cribs 243
Cravings 60–1
Crowning 97, 285, 286, 289, 291, 305
Crying, newborn baby 321
Cryopreservation, infertility treatments 49, 53, 55
Cystic fibrosis 24–5, 26

D

Dancing 145
Death, of baby 312–13
Dehydration 342
Delivery 284–7
  breech birth 307
  cesarean section 308–11
  placenta 290–1, 305
  positions 97
  "special deliveries" 306–13
  sudden birth 304–5
  see also Childbirth/labor
Demerol 280, 281, 282, 299
Depression, postpartum 361, 362–3, 364
Desensitization, pain relief 125
Diabetes 18, 140–1, 177, 198
Diaper rash 336, 338
Diapers 336–9
Diaphragm, contraceptive 364
Diaries 67, 156
Diarrhea 208–9, 342
Dick-Read, Dr. Grantley 112
Diet *see* **Food**

Digestive problems 68
Dilation and curettage (D and C) 219
Discharges, lochia 291, 322, 354
Disproportion, pelvic 260, 261, 298
DNA 22–3, 26
Doctors 120
  when to call 342
Donors, infertility treatments 49, 54–5
Doppler scans 178, 185, 187, 203, 265
Down syndrome 17, 24, 184, 185, 186, 188–9, 198
Dreams 155–6
Drinks 139
Drugs: and infertility 37
  infertility treatment 46–7
  pain relief 280, 281–2
  preconception 17
  in pregnancy 168
  premature labor 299
Duchenne muscular dystrophy 25
Dysentery 139

E

Ear infections 343
Echocardiography 196
Eclampsia 224–5
Ectopic pregnancy 224, 225
Egg *see* **Ovum**
Egg penetration test 41
Ejaculation 30, 31, 38
Electronic fetal monitoring 109, 178, 260, 275
Embryo: development of 33, 72–5
  infertility treatments 51, 53, 55
  see also Fetus
Emergencies 218–27
Emotions: father's 94, 97
  postnatal period 360–3
  prelabor 270
  in pregnancy 154–7
  stillbirth 313
  and unborn child 193
Endometriosis 43, 47
Endometrium 29, 33, 44, 55
Engagement of head 85, 89, 261, 270, 271
Engorgement, breasts 327, 356
Entonox 282
Epidural anesthesia 274, 281–2, 303, 308, 309
Epilepsy 18
Episiotomy 108, 109–10, 285
  breech birth 307
  pain 110, 354, 355, 365
  premature labor 299
  stitches 110, 293, 355
  wound 110, 355
Epispadias 199
Equipment: for baby 242–3
  bottlefeeding 332
  diapers 336–7
Essential oils, massage 153
Estrogen: and contraception 364
  ovarian cycle 28, 29
  postnatal emotions 360
  in pregnancy 87, 230
Ethics, infertility treatments 48–9
Exercise: classes 124
  postnatal 358–9
  preconception 17
  in pregnancy 144–51

Expected date of delivery(EDD) 62–3, 260
Expressing milk 257, 327
Eyes, newborn baby 317–18

F

Faintness 208–9
Fallopian tubes 28
  ectopic pregnancy 224, 225
  fertilization of ovum 32
  and infertility 43, 44–5
  infertility treatment 46, 47
False labor 272
Familial hypercholesterolemia 24
Fathers/partners 92–103
  after the birth 110
  at birth 95, 96–9
  bonding with baby 92, 94, 99, 293
  childcare 254
  communication with 157
  death of baby 312
  lifestyle changes 366–9
  and postpartum depression 363
  prenatal classes 125
  relationship with 231, 360–1
  resuming sex 364
  role at birth 276–7, 288–9
  and unborn child 193
  and working mothers 165
Fatigue *see* **Tiredness**
Fears 155
Feeding: premature babies 347
  see also Bottlefeeding;
  Breastfeeding
Feet: club foot 199
  newborn baby 317
Fertility 29
  see also Infertility
Fertilization 32–3
  infertility treatments 51, 53
Fetal alcohol syndrome 17
Fetus: abnormalities 196–203
  communication with 192–3
  development 76–89
  distress 275, 301, 310
  engagement 85, 89
  heartbeat 178
  monitoring in labor 109, 178, 274, 275
  movements 77, 78–9, 81, 85, 87, 89, 193, 194–5, 260, 271
  overdue babies 260–1
  position in uterus 175, 259, 296
  problems 196–203
  surgery 200–1
  see also Baby; Embryo
Fevers 170, 343
Fibroids 43
Fimbrioplasty 46, 47
Fluid consumption 133
Folic acid 17, 18, 20–1, 133, 137
Follicle-stimulating hormone (FSH) 28, 30, 34, 42, 43, 46
Fontanelles 316, 317, 342
Food: and breastfeeding 327
  cravings 60–1
  folic acid in 21
  hazards 139
  in labor 108
  nutrition 132–9

Food (*continued*)
  preconception 17
  in pregnancy 128–39
  vegetarianism 131, 136–7
Forceps delivery 109, 306
  premature labor 299
Fruit 134

G

Gas (anesthetic) 280, 282
Gas (gastrointestinal condition) 335
Gender-linked diseases 25, 185
Genes 22–7
Genetic counseling 24, 26–7
Genetic disorders 24–5, 186
German measles (rubella) 19, 26, 170, 178, 322
GIFT (gamete intrafallopian transfer) 49
Girdles 163
Gonadotrophin releasing factor (GnRH) 46, 47
Grandparents 156, 157, 254–5, 367
Grasp reflex 253, 320
Gum problems 68, 81, 159

H

Hair: lanugo 81, 83, 85, 88, 317
  in pregnancy 159
Hands: newborn baby 317
  swelling 176
Harelip 197
Hawthorne effect, pain relief 125
Head, newborn baby 316
Health: newborn baby 342–3
  preconception 18–19
  in pregnancy 206–13
Hearing: newborn baby 320
  in unborn child 83, 94, 192, 193, 253
Heart: congenital disease 196–7
  disease in pregnancy 19
  fetal heartbeat 178
  maternal heartbeat 192
  in pregnancy 66, 79
Heartburn 68, 81, 83, 208–9
Height of mother 176
Hemolytic disease of the newborn 202, 342
Hemophilia 25, 27, 185
Hemorrhage: emergencies 222–3
  postpartum 291
Hemorrhoids 355
Hepatitis B 177
Hereditary disorders *see* **Genetic disorders**
Hernia, umbilical 196, 318
Herpes 19
Hiccups, newborn baby 321
High blood pressure (hypertension) 208–9
Hips, congenital dislocation 197
HIV 17, 19, 177
Holding baby 324–5
Home birth 265 304–305
Hormones: after delivery 355
  breastfeeding 326–7
  and emotional changes 154
  and infertility 34, 42–3, 44
  male 30
  and miscarriage 221
  ovarian cycle 28)

Hormones (*continued*)
  placental 73, 79, 87, 89
  postpartum depression 360
  prelabor 270, 271
  in pregnancy 69, 77
  and sexuality 230, 231, 236
  and unborn child 193, 194–5
Hospitals: birth 107, 108–9, 116–19, 265, 266–7, 274–5, 322–3
  intensive care babies 344–7
Housing 157
Human chorionic gonadotrophin (hCG) 42, 60, 61, 62, 73
Human menopausal gonadotrophin (hMG) 42, 50, 62
Hydrocele 38
Hydrocephalus 20, 197–8, 200
Hydronephrosis 201
Hyperemesis gravidarum 177
Hyperprolactinemia 42–3
Hypertension 70
Hypnosis, pain relief 283
Hypospadias 199
Hysterosalpingogram 45

I

ICSI (intracytoplasmic sperm injection) 49, 52–3, 57
Identical twins 33, 183
Identification, baby 293
Immune system 72, 221
  infertility 39
Immunizations, in pregnancy 169, 171
Implantation 33, 72
  ectopic pregnancy 224, 225
  infertility treatments 53
Incubators 344, 345, 346–7, 348–9
Indigestion 83
Induction of labor 109, 300–3, 368
Infections: postnatal 225
  in pregnancy 170
Infertility 34–57
  female 42–7
  male 38–41, 56–7
  treatments 35, 36, 46–57
Insemination, artificial 54–5
Insomnia 210–11, 258
Intensive care units 346–347
Internal examinations 61
Intrauterine devices (IUDs) 17, 364
Iron 131, 133, 135, 136–7, 327
Isolation, social 157
Itching 161
IVF (in vitro fertilization) 48, 49, 50–1, 53, 57

JKL

Jaundice of the newborn 342, 345
Jogging 145
Ketones 177
Kick charts 195
Kidneys: disease in pregnancy 19
  fetal problems 201
Kitzinger, Sheila 113
Klinefelter syndrome 38
Labor *see* **Childbirth**
Lamaze method 113

Lanugo 81, 83, 85, 88, 317
Laparoscopy 45, 47, 51
Latching on, breastfeeding 327, 329
Leboyer, Frederick 112–13
Legs, swelling 176
Letdown reflex 354
Libido, loss of 236, 364, 365
Lifestyle changes 366–7
Lifting, safety 160, 206
Lightening 270
Linea nigra 69, 79, 87, 158
Lip, cleft 197
Listeriosis 139, 219
Lochia 291, 322, 354
Lovemaking *see* **Sexual intercourse**
Luteinizing hormone (LH) 28, 30, 34, 42, 43, 46, 221

M

Malnutrition 138–9
Massage: in labor 268, 282, 283
  in pregnancy 152–3
  sensual 232–3
Mastitis 357
Masturbation 237
Maternity care units 119
Maternity leave 64, 256
Maternity nurses 255
Meconium 89, 109, 301, 337
Membrane rupture: artificial 109, 110, 297, 301
  natural 267, 273, 298, 302
Meningitis 343
Menstruation: after delivery 355
  missed periods 60
  ovarian cycle 29
MESA (microepididymal sperm aspiration) 49, 52
Metabolism, in pregnancy 66, 74, 81
Micromanipulation, infertility treatments 52–3
Midwives 121
  birthing centers 114–115, 264–265
  prenatal care 174
  delivery of baby 97
  hospital birth 107, 116, 121, 274
Milia 318
Milk: bottlefeeding 247, 332
  breastfeeding 246, 326–7
  expressing 257, 327
Minerals 133, 135
Miscarriage 218–21
  incompetent cervix 223
  prenatal tests and 186, 187, 189
MIST (microinsemination sperm transfer) 49
Mongolian spots 318
Monitoring, fetal 109, 178, 260, 275
Montgomery's tubercles 66
Mood swings 210–11, 236
Morning sickness 61, 74, 210–11, 236
Moro reflex 321
Multiple pregnancy 182–3
  death 313
  delivery 306
  fertilization 33
Multiple sclerosis (MS) 214–15
Mumps 38, 56, 170
Muscular dystrophy 25
Mutant genes 23

N

Nails: newborn baby 317
  in pregnancy 161
Names, choosing 248–50
Nannies 167, 255
Narcotics 282
Navel 318, 341
Neonatal death 313
Neonatal intensive care units (NICU) 346–347
Nesting instinct 89, 114, 271
Nipples: bottlefeeding 332, 333, 334
  breastfeeding 323, 328, 329, 330
  care after delivery 356
  cracked 330, 357
  pigmentation 231
  in pregnancy 61, 66, 68, 79
  sore 330, 356–7
NSU (nonspecific urethritis) 56
Nuchal scans 184, 185, 189
Nurseries 240–1
Nutrition see Food

O

Obstetricians 120, 365
Obstructed labor 297, 298
Odent, Dr. Michel 108, 113
Oral sex 237
Orgasm 230–1, 237, 365
Otitis media 343
Ovaries 45
  infertility 42, 43
  infertility treatments 46, 50
  ovarian cycle 28, 29
Overdue babies 260–1, 300
Ovulation 72
  after delivery 355, 364
  infertility treatments 46–7, 51
  ovarian cycle 29
  problems 34, 42, 44
  sex of baby 31
Ovum (egg): development of 28–9
  donor eggs 49, 54–5
  fertilization 32–3
  genes 22, 23
  infertility 34, 42
  infertility treatments 49, 50–3
  ovarian cycle 28, 29
  twins 33
Oxytocin: afterpains and 354
  breastfeeding and 246, 326–7
  effects on uterus 246, 291, 305
  inducing labor 300, 301, 302
  resuming sex 365
  speeding up labor with 110

P

Pacifiers 332
Pain: backache labor 296
  contractions 272
  episiotomy 110, 354, 355, 365
  in labor 96, 107, 272, 273, 277
  in pregnancy 83
Pain relief: in labor 274, 280–3
  prenatal classes 125
  without drugs 282–3

Palate, cleft 197
Pantyhose 163
Parents: grandparents 156, 157, 254–5, 367
  parenting classes 124
  see also Fathers/partners
Partogram 297
Pelvic floor exercises 148, 355, 357, 358, 365
Pelvic inflammatory disease (PID) 44, 225
Pelvis: disproportion 260, 261, 298
  engagement of head 85, 89, 261, 270, 271
  size 176
Penis 31
  fetal problems 199
Perineum, tears 110, 285, 291
Periods *see* **Menstruation**
Demerol 280, 281, 282, 299
Pets, safety 169
Phenylketonuria (PKU) 318
Photographs 288, 313
Pigmentation 68, 69, 79, 158–9, 161, 231
Pill, contraceptive 17, 364
Pimples 159
Pinnard stethoscope 178, 265
Pitocin 291, 297–8, 302
Pituitary gland 28, 30, 42, 43, 46, 326–7
Placenta: delivery of 290–1, 305
  development of 33, 72, 73, 77, 79, 89
  emergencies 222–3
  hormones 79, 87, 89
  insufficiency 223, 261, 300
  overdue baby 261
  preeclampsia 226–7
  stillbirth 312
Polycystic ovary syndrome 21, 42, 46
Port wine stains 318
Positions: delivery 285, 288–9
  in labor 106, 278–9, 282
  lovemaking 231, 234, 237, 365
Postmaturity 260, 261
Postnatal period: checkups 365
  emotions 360–3
  exercises 358–9
  health 354–7
  infections 225
Postpartum depression 361, 362–4
Postpartum hemorrhage 223, 291
Posture, in pregnancy 69, 89, 160
Preeclampsia 70, 177, 224, 226–7
Pregnancy: body care 158–61
  complaints 206–13
  emergencies 218–27
  exercise 144–51
  food 128–39
  late stages 258–9
  prenatal care 174–89
  preparation for 16–27
  signs of 60–1, 72
  tests 61–2
  trimesters 66–89
Prelabor 270–1
Premature babies 80, 84, 348–9
  breathing problems 299, 347, 349
  intensive care units 344, 345, 346–7
Premature labor 298–9
Prenatal care 67, 69, 71, 174–89
  classes 95, 124–5
  clinics 174–5
  multiple pregnancy 182
  preeclampsia 227
  tests 176–81, 184–9
  ultrasound scan 178, 180–1

Preserved food 139
Processed foods 138–9
Progesterone: and contraception 364
  and infertility 42, 44
  ovarian cycle 28, 29
  postnatal emotions 360
  in pregnancy 60, 72
  sensual pregnancy 230
Projectile vomiting 199
Prolactin 43, 47, 326, 327
Prolonged labor 296–7
Prostaglandins, induction of labor 300, 302, 303, 368
Proteins 131, 132, 134, 136, 137
Pudendal block 281
Puerpural psychosis 361
Pumps, expressing milk 327
Pushing, in labor 284–5, 286, 289
Pyloric stenosis 199

QR

Quickening 79, 194
Rashes: diaper rash 336, 338
  in pregnancy 161
Red blood cells, Doppler scans 187
Reflex actions, newborn baby 320–1
Registering birth 323
Relaxation: in labor 289
  massage 152–3
  pain relief 125
  in pregnancy 151, 258–9
Reproductive tract: female 28
  male 31
Respiratory distress syndrome (RDS) 198–9, 345
Rhesus incompatibility 54, 177, 185, 187, 200–1, 202–3, 342
Rib pain 212–13
Rooting reflex 321, 328
Rubella *see* **German measles**

S

Safety: babies 243
  food hazards 139
  nurseries 241
  in pregnancy 17, 168–71
  working mothers 164, 165, 169–70
Salmonella 139
Screening tests 184–5, 188–9
Scrotum 38
Seminal fluid (semen) 30
  donor insemination 55
  ejaculation 31
  infertility tests 39, 40–1
Sensual pregnancy 230–7
Serum screening 184
Sex, of baby 31, 33, 81
Sex chromosomes 31, 33
  abnormalities 25
Sexual intercourse: after childbirth 100
  after delivery 364–5
  in pregnancy 69, 230–1, 234–7
Sexually transmitted diseases 19
Shivering 291
Shoes 162–3
Show 237, 267, 271
Shunts, urinary tract problems 201
Siblings *see* **Children**

Sickle-cell anemia 25, 26, 178, 186
Sight: newborn baby 320
  in unborn child 192, 193
Single parenthood 166–7
Sit-ups 145
Skin: birthmarks 318
  care of 158
  newborn baby 316–17, 318
  pigmentation 68, 69, 79, 158–9, 161, 231
  in pregnancy 158–9
  problems 161
  spider veins 81, 159
  stretch marks 81, 159
Sleep: after delivery 356
  baby 102
  in pregnancy 70–1, 85, 89, 210–11, 258
Small-for-dates babies 344
Smell, sense of 61
Smoking 16
Sneezing, newborn baby 321
Socks 163
Special care/Intensive care babies 346–347
Sperm: donor insemination 49, 54, 55
  ejaculation 30, 31
  fertilization 32–3
  genes 22, 23
  infertility 34, 38–41
  infertility treatments 49, 52
  production of 30
  and sex of baby 31
Spider veins 81, 159
Spina bifida 17, 20–1, 197, 293
Sports 144–5
Squatting 151
Squint 318
Step reflex 320
Sterilization: bottlefeeding equipment 332, 333
  reversal of 47
"Sticky eye" 317–18
Stillbirth 261, 312
Stitches: cesarean section 309, 311, 322–3
  episiotomy 110, 293, 355
Stockings 163
Stork bites 318
Strawberry birthmarks 318
Stretch marks 81, 159
Stretching exercises 146–7
Strollers 242
Sucking reflex 321
Superstitions 156
Surgery: cesarean section 308–11
  fetal 200–1
  infertility treatment 46, 47
Surrogate mothers 54, 55
SUZI (subzonal insemination) 49
Swimming 145, 182

T

Tailor sitting 150
Tay-Sachs disease 25, 26
Tears, perineum 110, 285, 291
Teeth, in pregnancy 159
Teething rings 332
Telemetry, fetal monitoring 275
Television, safety 169
Temperature: after delivery 291
  baby's 343

TENS 283
Tense and relax technique 258–9
Termination of pregnancy 189
TESE (testicular sperm extraction) 49, 52
Testes (testicles) 30, 38, 39
Testosterone 30
Thalassemia 25, 178, 186
Thrush 18, 212–13
Tiredness: after delivery 356, 361
  in labor 98, 277
  loss of libido 236
  in pregnancy 60, 70–1, 164
"Topping and tailing" 340
Toxoplasmosis 139, 169, 178
Toys 241
Trains 171
Transition stage 273, 279
Travel: in pregnancy 171
  to hospital 267
  with baby 242–3
Trial of labor 298, 308
Trimesters 66–89
  first 66–7, 72–5
  second 68–9, 76–85
  third 70–1, 86–9
Triple serum screen 184, 189
Trisomies 25, 198
Tuboplasty 47
Twins 182–3
  death of 313
  delivery 306
  fertilization 33
  naming 250

U

Ultrasound scans: embryo/fetus 61, 75, 77, 79, 83, 85, 87, 89
  fetal surgery 200–1
  infertility treatments 44, 50, 51
  overdue babies 260
  in pregnancy 69
  prenatal care 178, 180–1
  twins 183
Umbilical cord 77, 87, 137
  around baby's neck 285
  childbirth 99
  cleaning stump 341
  cutting 97, 292–3, 318
  delivery of placenta 290, 291
  Doppler scans 187
  prolapse 304, 310
  sudden birth 305
  umbilical vein sampling 187, 189
Umbilical hernia 196, 318
Umbilicus 318
Underwear 163
Urinary problems, baby 201, 343
Urination: after delivery 355
  in pregnancy 60, 66, 85
Urine tests 18, 61, 62, 71, 176–7
Uterus: after delivery 354
  baby's position 175, 259, 296
  Braxton-Hicks contractions 270–1, 354
  contractions 272
  delivery of placenta 290, 291
  fetal surgery 201
  fibroids 43
  fundal height 77, 175
  implantation 33, 53, 72
  in pregnancy 66, 69
  septum 219

V

Vacuum extraction 109, 306, 307
Vagina: after delivery 355
  bleeding 218, 219, 237
  in pregnancy 74
  sexual intercourse 230–1, 365
Varicocele 38, 39
Varicose veins 212–13
Vas deferens 31, 38
Vegan diet 136
Vegetables 134
Vegetarianism 131, 136–7
Vernix caseosa 81, 86, 87, 88, 316–17
Visualization, pain relief 283
Vitamins 131, 132–3, 134–5
Vitamin B12 136, 137
Vitamin D 133, 135
Vomiting: babies 199, 342
  morning sickness 61, 74, 210–11, 236

WYZ

Walking 145
"Walking" epidural 303
Washing diapers 337
Water, drinking 133
Water birth 107, 283
Water retention 212–13
Waters, breaking 267, 273, 302
Weight: low birthweight babies 344
  in pregnancy 66, 68, 69, 70, 83, 128, 129, 154, 176
Womb see Uterus
Working mothers 164–5
  childcare 256–7
  clothes 162
  rights 64–5, 164
  safety 164, 165, 169–70
  single mothers 167
Wounds: cesarean section 355
  episiotomy 355
Yeast infections 212–13
Yoga 125, 145
Yolk sac 72, 73, 77
ZIFT (zygote intrafallopian transfer) 49
Zinc 135
Zygotes 32

Acknowledgments

PHOTOGRAPHY for new edition
Ian Hooton
ART DIRECTION FOR PHOTOGRAPHY
Sally Smallwood
ILLUSTRATIONS Annabel Milne: 23, 28, 29, 31, 33, 45, 109, 183, 186, 203, 219–221, 224, 271, 273, 275, 281, 298, 301, 329 Howard Pemberton: 45, 73, 75, 77, 79, 81, 83, 85, 87, 89, 286, 287, 309
MEDICAL CONSULTANTS FOR THIS EDITION
Dr. Sarah Reynolds;
Dr. Courtney D. Stephenson
ADDITIONAL PHOTOGRAPHY Ranald Mackechnie; Dave King; David Murray; Ray Moller; Stephen Oliver; Susanna Price; Jules Selmes
INDEX Hilary Bird

PICTURE CREDITS
Picture research: Franziska Marking, Anna Bedewell.
Picture library: Romaine Werblow.

The publisher would like to thank the following for their kind permission to reproduce their photographs/ (Abbreviations key: t=top, b=bottom, r=right, l=left)

1: Powerstock/Super Stock; 2-3: Getty Images/Britt Erlanson; 6: Corbis/LWA-Dann Tardif (tl); 9: Mother & Baby Picture Library (cr); 14-15: photolibrary.com; 28: Retna Pictures Ltd/Philip Reeson (cl); 29: Science Photo Library; 30: Science Photo Library (cl), James Stevenson (b); 32: Science Photo Library (tl), (cl), (bl), (br); 33: Getty Images (b), Science Photo Library (c); 37: Mother & Baby Picture Library/Ian Hooton (b); 39: Science Photo Library (tr), Science Photo Library (cr), University of Nottingham (b); 40: Science Photo Library/John Walsh (bl), Stevie Grand (bl); 41: Parthenon Publishing Group/Dr John Yovich (t); 42: Science Photo Library/David Leah (cl), P M Motta & S Makabe (bl); 45: Science Photo Library (tr), (c), Science Photo Library/Antonia Reeve (b); 48: Science Photo Library/Hank Morgan (bl); 50: Science Photo Library/Hank Morgan (b), Petit Format/CSI (cr); 52: CARE/Centres for Assisted Reproduction, Nottingham (cr), The Wellcome Institute Library, London (tl); 66: Bubbles/Frans Rombout (bl); 68: Bubbles/Frans Rombout (bl); 70: Bubbles/Frans Rombout (bl); 72: Science Photo Library (br); 73: Science Photo Library (br); 74: The John Hillelson Agency/Howard Sochurek; 75: Science Photo Library (b); 76: Bubbles/Frans Rombout (l); 77: The John Hillelson Agency/Howard Sochurek (cb), Science Photo Library (bl); 78: Bubbles/Frans Rombout (l); 79: Science Photo Library (c), (b); 80: Bubbles/Frans Rombout (l); 81: Genesis Space photo library (cl), (cr). 82: Bubbles/Frans Rombout (l); 83: Genesis Space photo library; 84: Bubbles/Frans Rombout (l); 85: The John Hillelson Agency/Howard Sochurek (crb), Science Photo Library (clb); 86: Bubbles/Frans Rombout (l); 87: The John Hillelson Agency/Howard Sochurek (cbl), (br); 88: Bubbles/Frans Rombout (l); 89: The John Hillelson Agency/Howard Sochurek (bl), Science Photo Library/Stevie Grand (r); 106: Mother & Baby Picture Library/Moose Azim (b); 111: Telegraph Colour Library/Getty Images/Antonio Mo; 115: Mother & Baby Picture Library/Moose Azim (b); 117: Sally & Richard Greenhill (bl); 121: Sally & Richard Greenhill (bl); 128: Bubbles/Frans Rombout (bl), (bc), (br); 136: Bubbles/Lucy Tizard (tr); 137: Science Photo Library (b); 139: Science Photo Library/Hank Morgan (br); 155: Bubbles/Daniel Pangbourne; 166: Bubbles/Chris Rout (tr); 179: Getty Images/Chris Harvey; 181: The John Hillelson Agency/Howard Sochurek (b); 183: Zefa Visual Media/Howard Sochurek (cr); 188: Mother & Baby Picture Library/Ian Hooton (t); 193: Science Photo Library (bl); 196: Dr I D Sullivan (cl); 199: Science Photo Library/Secchi (bl); 202: Bubbles (tr); 214: Zefa Visual Media/M. Moellenberg (tr); 226: Bubbles/Peter Sylent (tr); 235: Telegraph Colour Library/Getty Images/Antonio Mo; 244: Mother & Baby Picture Library/Ruth Jenkinson (bl); 251: Getty Images/Steve Smith; 252: Telegraph Colour Library/Getty Images (b); 256: Bubbles/Frans Rombout (tr); 262-263: Mother & Baby Picture Library/Ian Hooton; 275: Mother & Baby Picture Library/Ruth Jenkinson (tr); 281: Mother & Baby Picture Library/Moose Azim (b); 284: Mother & Baby Picture Library/Moose Azim (br); 286: Sally & Richard Greenhill (b); 287: Sally & Richard Greenhill (t), (c), (b); 292: Mother & Baby Picture Library/Mampta Kapoor (b); 293: Hutchison Library (br); 302: Bubbles/Chris Rout; 307: Collections/Anthea Sieveking; 309: Science Photo Library/Moredun Animal Helth Ltd (l), The Wellcome Institute Library, London (br); 310: Bubbles/John Powell; 316: Hutchison Library (bl); 318: Sally & Richard Greenhill (bl), (bc), (br); 319: Telegraph Colour Library/Getty Images/Ian McKinnell; 331: Mother & Baby Picture Library/Ian Hooton; 338: Science Photo Library (cra), Science Photo Library/Andy Walker (tl); 345: Science Photo Library/Manfred Kage (bl); 346-347: Science Photo Library/Bsip Bajande, Science Photo Library/Stevie Grand (cl); 347: Sally & Richard Greenhill (br), Science Photo Library/Jim Stevenson (cb), Science Photo Library/John Greim (ca), Getty Images/David Joel (cl); 348: Bubbles/Loisjoy Thurston; 353: Getty Images/Tim Brown (b); 357: Science Photo Library/Dr P. Marazzi (b); 368: Bubbles/Loisjoy Thurstun (tr).

All other images © Dorling Kindersley. For further information see www.dkimages.com